AMERICAN RED CROSS

Home Nursing

TEXTBOOK

SEVENTH EDITION
1963

PREPARED BY
Nursing Services, American Red Cross

DOUBLEDAY & COMPANY, INC.
NEW YORK

THE MISSION OF THE RED CROSS

The American Red Cross is the instrument chosen by the Congress to help carry out the obligations assumed by the United States under certain international treaties known as the Geneva or Red Cross Conventions. Specifically, its Congressional charter imposes on the American Red Cross the duties to act as the medium of voluntary relief and communication between the American people and their armed forces, and to carry on a system of national and international relief to prevent and mitigate suffering caused by disasters.

All the activities of the American Red Cross and its chapters support these duties.

Nationally and locally the American Red Cross is governed by volunteers, most of its duties are performed by volunteers and it is financed by voluntary contributions.

The Home Nursing program of the American National Red Cross, for which this book is a teaching text, stems from the Congressional charter provision that the organization shall devise and carry on measures for relieving and preventing suffering.

6th PRINTING
DECEMBER, 1965

Printed in the United States of America
8

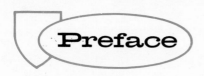

Preface

The first edition of the Red Cross home nursing textbook, published in 1913, was designed as a guide to prepare families to care for those ill at home. The seventh edition has the same purpose but takes cognizance of the changing patterns for the care of the sick at home and the scientific advances that influence these patterns.

The present revision of the text incorporates the new concepts concerning the care of the sick and the aged at home and explains the procedures and attitudes necessary to assist in the rehabilitation of such patients. Increased longevity in the United States has also necessitated the inclusion of material on the maintenance of health in the later years. Because the problem of survival is primarily an individual and family responsibility, information on survival and on the care of disaster victims has also been added.

It is our belief that this text will be a helpful reference for those who enroll in classes sponsored by the Red Cross Nursing Services and a valuable resource for every American household.

Acknowledgments

A nursing textbook reflects the personal ideas, experiences, and convictions of its author, combined with the accumulated knowledge of many other people. It is implicit that there is nothing new or original in the subject matter, all of which is a part of basic nursing knowledge and skill.

We are indebted to many for the advice and suggestions offered in the revision of this textbook but especially to the following members of the Home Nursing Textbook Advisory Committee: Otis L. Anderson, M.D., American Medical Association; Elsie Berdan, U.S. Public Health Service; Lillian Chabala, American Physical Therapy Association; Dr. William H. Creswell, Jr., National Education Association; Marie Grant, U.S. Public Health Service; Dr. Edith S. Greer, U.S. Office of Education; Mrs. Eleanor Hawley, Children's Bureau; Cornelia Knight, American Nurses Association; Dr. Mary Louise Paynich, American Public Health Association; Claire F. Ryder, M.D., U.S. Public Health Service; Mrs. Kathleen Newton Shafer, former associate professor, Cornell University-New York Hospital School of Nursing; Catherine M. Sullivan, formerly of the Office of Civil and Defense Mobilization; Carroll L. Witten, M.D., American Academy of General Practice; and Evelyn Zetter, National League for Nursing. Members of this committee helped in planning the format of the book and in evaluating and selecting areas of content for inclusion and later read the manuscript for accuracy and validity of the subject matter.

Representatives of the Children's Bureau, Department of Health, Education, and Welfare, gave advice and counsel on the parts of the book relating to mothers and children, chiefly chapters 6 and 7.

We are particularly indebted to the American Public Health Association and to the Communicable Disease Center, Public Health Service, Department of Health, Education, and Welfare, for the data on selected communicable diseases included in chapter 5. The material as it appears in the textbook was compiled from an APHA publication, *Control of Communicable Disease in Man,* and was reviewed and edited by medical and nurse epidemiologists of the Communicable Disease Center in Atlanta, Georgia. The proposed immunization schedule in chapter 5 was compiled from the 1961 report of the Committee on the Control of Infectious Diseases of the American Academy of Pediatrics and from the Public Health Service's 1961 report of the Surgeon General's Committee on Poliomyelitis Control. This schedule as it appears in the textbook was reviewed and approved by epidemiologists at the Communicable Disease Center and by a physician in the Public Health Service.

Suggestions for material included in chapters 8 and 9 on the aged and the care of the patient with a long-term illness were made by Kathleen Newton Shafer, author of *Geriatric Nursing,* published by the C. V. Mosby Company in 1961. The procedure for preparing hot compresses was a suggestion of Mrs. Shafer. Medical and nursing representatives of the Office on Aging, Public Health Service, Department of Health, Education, and Welfare, reviewed these sections of the textbook and made many valuable criticisms and suggestions.

Special mention and thanks are given to Mrs. Thomas F. Callaghan and her son, Kevin, of Springfield, Virginia, who were the models for nearly all the illustrations of mothers and babies.

Gratitude and special thanks are due the thousands of Red Cross home nursing instructors, many of them volunteers, whose experience in nursing services programs throughout the years enabled them to make suggestions that have been included in the present book. Both national and chapter Red Cross nursing personnel took a lively interest in the planning of the revision and contributed valuable ideas concerning its content and format.

Appreciation is expressed to the many people at national headquarters who assisted in the preparation of the manuscript and especially to the Office of Research Information for help in obtaining reference materials from the Library of Congress, the National Library of Medicine, the Medical and General Reference Library of the Veterans Administration, and from other sources.

Corliss Williams, R.N., M.A.

Washington, D.C.
June 1963

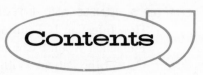

Contents

SECTION I
HOME NURSING INFORMATION

SECTION II

HOME NURSING PROCEDURES

SECTION I

Home Nursing Information

HOME NURSING IS A FAMILY AFFAIR

Nearly every family at some time faces the problem of caring for someone sick or injured. Today, self-help and family help in nursing care take on new meaning in view of the many demands upon physicians and nurses, the steady increase in the aging population, the early dismissal of hospitalized patients, and the growing emphasis on home care programs for the patient with a long-term illness. In addition, the necessity to prepare the family and, in a broader sense, the community to take care of disaster-caused injuries and illnesses has increasing importance in a world grown smaller in time and space. For all these reasons, responsible adults and their teen-age sons and daughters need to learn the skills and to acquire the knowledge that will enable them to give care to the sick at home when it becomes necessary.

What is a "home nurse"? As the term implies, a home nurse is a person who gives nursing care to someone sick at home. That person can be any or each of the members of the family, depending on the circumstances. The word "nurse" is derived from the Latin *nutrire*, which means to *nourish*, to *protect*, to *sustain*, and to *give*. Since all these meanings are attributes of motherhood, what is more natural than to think first of mothers as home nurses, for it is they who most often have responsibility for the care of the sick at home.

Mothers themselves, however, sometimes become ill, and then it becomes the responsibility of someone else to be the home nurse. Frequently, too, the responsibility for patient care must be shared so that it does not become a burden to any one person. Perhaps it is the father, an older son or daughter, or grandmother who helps out when sickness occurs. The home nurse can be anyone who has the know-how and the desire to give nursing care to the sick at home.

Nursing has many qualities, but its chief characteristic is service

1

to others given with the desire to alleviate pain, to bring comfort to mind and body, and to help the sick regain health. Knowing how to recognize the signs of illness may avert serious complications of illness that may occur if the patient is neglected. The home nurse who knows how to guard against the spread of disease protects herself and her family from infection. Knowing how to give simple, basic nursing care to the sick can shorten illness and make the patient more comfortable while he is in bed. The more skillful the home nurse is in taking care of the patient, the less disturbing the illness is to him and to the other members of the household as well.

Another dividend of knowing how to take care of the sick is the self-confidence it gives to the home nurse. Knowledge and practice help the home nurse to become competent, and competence makes the care of the patient easier and lessens the time for her. Sick people are quite perceptive and quickly recognize and respect skilled nursing care. Also they are very sensitive to the attitudes of others, which is reflected in the quality of the care they receive. Sick people are more likely to cooperate and to accept care that they cannot give to themselves if they have rapport with the person who is caring for them.

Everyone wants to be independent and should be encouraged to do whatever he can for himself, but there are times when illness makes it necessary to rely on others. This situation is particularly true for older people, who may feel that because their illness makes them relatively helpless they are a burden. The more skillful the care given, the easier it is for the patient to accept, because the home nurse appears to use so little effort. In a broad sense, having the knowledge and skill to give competent home nursing care and to work knowingly with the doctor makes the home nurse a member of a larger health team whose objective is optimum health for the patient, the family, and the community.

PREPARING TO BE A HOME NURSE

Red Cross home nursing instruction is offered free to everyone who needs and wants the training. The course is based on two premises: one, that care of the sick and injured at home is primarily a family responsibility; and, two, that in the event of a major disaster basic nursing skills can be readily adapted to the care of a great number of casualties.

Home nursing instruction provides an opportunity to learn how to carry out the doctor's orders when caring for the sick at home, how to adapt nursing skills in an emergency, and how to make the best use of time, energy, and available equipment. The course includes the procedures used most frequently in caring for the sick at home and in helping professional nurses to care for the sick or injured in a shelter, an emergency hospital, or other medical facility when a disaster has occurred.

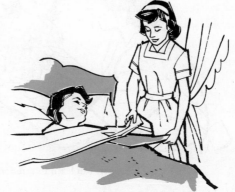

The comfort of the patient is directly related to the nursing care that he receives.

The instructions given in this textbook assume that any care given the patient, other than emergency first aid, is ordered by a physician and that the general nursing care of the patient is under the supervision of the attending physician or a registered professional nurse. Following a natural disaster, and particularly in the event of an enemy-caused disaster, medical and nursing assistance may not be immediately available, and survival may be dependent upon the ability to help oneself. Preparedness for any kind of disaster includes knowing how to help oneself and one's family and neighbors and implies a willingness to give assistance to others when the need arises. Self-help and mutual aid are primary objectives of Red Cross and civil defense disaster preparedness programs and are citizenship responsibilities of all the people.

The time to learn home nursing skills is now. Illness occurs at any day or hour, and it is far better to be prepared to provide the needed care than to have to say later: "I wish I had known this when my mother was ill"; or "It would have been so helpful to know how to do this when my husband got hurt." How to perform simple nursing skills should be learned before illness or accident occurs.

During the emergency period following a disaster much ingenuity may be needed to improvise equipment and to provide the necessary nursing care to the ill and injured. People who have taken the Red Cross home nursing course would be needed to help give nursing care, for they would be prepared to work under trying conditions with only limited guidance and supervision.

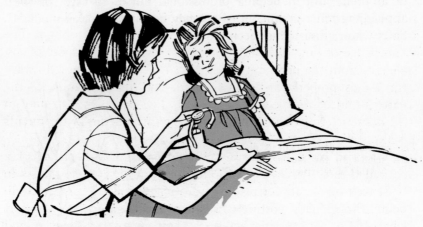

Teenagers can learn to care for the sick at home.

Home nursing instruction is of especial value to young adults of high school and college age. This instruction not only prepares young people to assist in an emergency at home or in the community but also gives them some understanding of nursing skills that they will need as parents. Home nursing instruction also helps them to gain an insight into what it means to be a nurse. Participation in such training and the opportunity to assist in caring for an ill person may be determining factors in choosing a nursing career.

NURSING CARE OF THE SICK AT HOME

Nursing care should be planned around the needs of the patient. Such factors as age, sex, the presence of physical handicaps, and the patient's attitudes and feelings about his illness will affect the amount and kind of nursing care he needs. However, of primary consideration are the diagnosis and the severity of the illness as well as the general physical condition of the patient at the time he became ill. Any nursing care plan must be flexible so that it can be adjusted to meet changing circumstances that inevitably occur. The patient's condition may change from day to day, resulting in the need for different treatment, diet, or nursing care. Or, emergencies may occur that make it necessary for the home nurse to modify household routines that affect the care of the patient. The ability to adjust to events and to meet change with calmness and resourcefulness is an important responsibility of the home nurse.

4

No two illnesses are exactly alike, and nursing care must be given differently in different situations. There are, however, several nursing fundamentals that should be observed in the care of any ill person. The first of these is *safety*, and this essential applies to the home nurse and the family as well as to the patient. Safety is of primary importance in the prevention of disease. The knowledge of how to handle soiled articles, how to dispose of discharges from the nose and the throat, and when and how to wash the hands properly are all safeguards for the protection of the patient and of the people about him. The necessity for safety in the administering of any drug and in the carrying out of treatments is implicit.

A second nursing fundamental is *comfort*. The comfort of a patient is directly related to the nursing care he receives and is to be strived for because it promotes his recovery and feeling of well-being. Proper body posture is an important ingredient of comfort whether the patient is in bed, in a chair, or up and about. Good posture is equally important for the home nurse. If she uses proper body mechanics in her work, she is more comfortable, exerts less strain on joints and muscles, and will be less fatigued.

A dry, clean, well-made bed and the support of pillows contribute to the patient's comfort and are essential to necessary rest and sleep. Comfort that fosters the patient's remaining in one position for too long can, however, be harmful. Unless forbidden by the doctor, sick people should move about in bed, because moving helps them to maintain muscle tone, to get needed exercise, and to avoid deformities and contractures of the joints. It is important in the rehabilitation and recovery of the patient, particularly the elderly person, to let him do as much for himself as he possibly can.

Another fundamental is *economy*, which in nursing care is related to the best and most efficient use of energy, time, money, and household equipment. The home nurse saves energy by using correct body posture. She saves steps and time by planning a work schedule and by collecting needed equipment before starting a task. Meal planning and volume shopping for groceries and staples save her time and money. The use of improvised nursing equipment and the care given to home appliances and household articles help her save money and materials.

Another essential of nursing care is *effectiveness*. As with other tasks, there is more than one way to perform the nursing skills. The test of any method is its effectiveness. The home nurse should ask, "Does it work? Is there a better way that is safe for the patient and for me? Will it save time, money, and equipment?"

Finally to be considered are *order* and *appearance*. A disorderly room can be an annoyance to both the patient and the home nurse. The patient's room should be uncluttered, with the furniture placed to make it easier to care for the patient. There is no need to strip the room of the personal belongings and decorations that lend it charm and attractiveness.

Appearance and grooming are directly related to the personal hygiene of the patient. To be freshly bathed and be clothed in clean and attractive garments and to have one's hair combed and brushed and cosmetics wisely applied not only result in greater comfort for the patient but help to build his morale.

Closely related to the nursing fundamentals, and probably the most important ingredients of patient care are common sense and good judgment. When illness occurs in any family, living arrangements usually have to be adjusted to the new circumstances. Frequently, this readjustment calls for an appraisal of household tasks to see which can be eliminated or streamlined in order to find added time for the care of the patient and to assure that no one person has too much to do. The home nurse who includes each family member in helping to keep the household on an even keel is not only practicing good management but using good psychology as well.

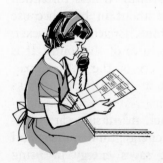

The doctor depends upon accurate and complete reporting by the home nurse.

PATIENT'S DAILY RECORD

One of the most important duties of the home nurse is to keep for the doctor a daily record of the patient's condition. An intelligent, orderly report of the care given by the home nurse under medical direction helps the doctor to make a diagnosis of the illness, to prescribe for it, and to judge the patient's progress. Information on how the patient feels, behaves, and reacts to treatments and about what was done for him, when it was done, and any other pertinent observations should be included in the daily record.

The doctor should write his orders for the patient so that there can be no misunderstanding about his intent. These orders can be written on the patient's illness record or on a separate piece of paper. If the doctor gives instructions on the telephone, they should be recorded by the person who talked with him, and the written record should be signed by the doctor on his next visit. The home nurse then enters on the record the exact time she carried out the doctor's instructions and the results of her action. She must not trust to memory to provide the doctor with an accurate report. Any change in the patient's condition should be reported, because this information may have great significance to the doctor in planning his care and treatment.

When more than one person is giving nursing care to the patient, a daily record is particularly necessary to avoid confusion and mistakes in carrying out the doctor's orders and to safeguard both the patient and the home nurses.

A sample form for keeping the daily record, with typical entries filled in, appears on the following page. The report usually includes the symptoms observed, food eaten, medicines and treatments given, temperature, pulse, and respiration, amount and nature of rest and sleep, bowel movements and urine output as well as the home nurse's impressions of the patient's progress. The date and the hour of each notation should always be recorded. Because the daily record is important to the doctor and to the patient— even though it may seem to be just one more chore for the home nurse—it should be brief, clear, and accurate.

FAMILY HEALTH RECORDS

Another responsibility of the home nurse is to keep family health records. Basic health facts about individual members of the family are often needed for various purposes. For example, they are necessary to complete school records, insurance forms, and the family doctor's medical record. Family health records should be kept in chronological order, accurately, and up to date if they are to be valuable. They differ from, but are related to, the patient's daily record. While the daily record is a detailed report of one illness, the family health records should contain summaries of all illnesses incurred.

Accurate information about all injuries and illnesses, X rays, routine physical examinations, records of immunizations, blood type, operations, and periods of hospitalization should be entered

7

Daily Record — Jane Jones

Date and Hour	Temperature Pulse and Respiration	Diet, Medicine, and Treatment	Bowel move-ment	Urine	Remarks
March 3 2 p.m.	100.8 – 88–20				Complains of sore throat, headache, aching joints and muscular pains.
3 p.m.		1 large glass lemonade			
4 p.m.				✓	Up to the bathroom. Doctor visited.
5 p.m.		#32520 1 Tablet / 1 cup hot tea / 1 cup soup			Had to be urged to eat. Headache not so severe.
5:30 p.m.		1 serving vanilla ice cream			
6 p.m.					
9 p.m.	100.2 – 80–20	#32520 1 Tablet		✓	Less pain and discomfort.
March 4 7:30 a.m.	99.6 – 86–22			✓	Slept fairly well. Awoke several times. Throat sore and now stopped up.
8 a.m.		#32520 1 Tablet / 1 large glass orange juice / 1 cup hot coffee			

The patient's daily record.

in the record. Because many families change doctors when they move, and there may be times when medical information is needed from a former physician, the names of attending doctors should be included in the record. Dental care and the names of the dentists should be part of the record too.

The American Medical Association has published a family health record in booklet form that many physicians provide their patients. Some insurance companies have similar booklets that may be obtained from their offices or agents. However, the importance of the family's health record is the information it contains, and any durable notebook can be used for the record keeping.

SUGGESTED STUDENT ACTIVITIES

1. If you have ever been a patient in a hospital, give your class an account of your experiences. How can those experiences help you in learning activities that you need for home nursing?

2. At the end of this unit of study organize, with the instructor's help, a panel discussion or debate on the topic "Every high school student should take a home nursing course."

3. Write or describe to the class an account of a device, an implement, an arrangement of utensils or furniture that has proved to be an outstanding saver of time and energy for you.

4. Make a list of the qualifications that would make one especially suited to care for a sick member of the family.

5. Report to the class on where to get information about how to organize a future nurses' club in your school.

6. Obtain from your state university the list of requirements for admission to its school of nursing. Discuss with your school's counselors how to earn credits in the required subjects.

2

PUBLIC HEALTH IS EVERYBODY'S BUSINESS

Just as each family is composed of individual members who together form a unit, so each community is made up of all the families and homes within its boundaries. A community has a legal and moral responsibility to develop measures for the conservation and promotion of the well-being of its citizens. It is therefore concerned with the health of all the men, women, and children in all the families of the city, village, or rural area.

The state of well-being of the community is known as public health. Experience has shown that to achieve successful community health protection there must be organized efforts toward disease prevention and health promotion. There must be trained public health workers, adequate funds to carry out a program, and favorable public opinion toward the goals of health officials. There must be a sanitary code that guarantees a clean, safe, and sanitary environment in the community. There also must be laws and regulations to implement the control and prevention of communicable disease. Education of the individuals who compose the community is the foundation of community health. When people understand the importance of health they are willing to build the social structure necessary to provide health protection for the community.

In the United States as in many other countries, the health of the people is primarily an individual responsibility. What the individual or the family does to promote its own health is the most important action in the protection of the health of the entire community. While advancement in personal health is an individual matter, behavior that is harmful to the public's health or that results in an additional burden and expense to the public is a matter of general concern. Government has the legal and moral

10

responsibility to protect the health and well-being of the nation's citizens. To meet this responsibility, the government has developed a complex network of health organizations ranging in size from that of a local health department in a small town to that of the United States Department of Health, Education, and Welfare. The job of these agencies is to spread knowledge of the cause, prevention, and cure of disease, both chronic and acute, to all the people and to increase the competence of the community and individuals in coping with their own health problems.

To know how public health agencies are organized and how they operate it is necessary to understand two underlying principles of public health administration. First, the official health department has a direct responsibility to protect the health of the people. As communities grow in size and population, certain features of public health work require collective or official action that is beyond the ability or the means of the individual. For example, the maintenance of a safe public water supply and the assurance of a pure milk supply are problems too big for any one person to solve. Other features of public health work, such as the control of communicable diseases, require direct and full cooperation between public authorities and private individuals. The health officer or the private physician cannot prevent poliomyelitis or diphtheria unless parents cooperate by having their babies and young children protected.

The second broad principle to be understood is the inherent right of government to establish rules to protect the health of the community against an individual who presents a health hazard to the group. The use of quarantine or of arrest for health violations is enforced under the laws and regulations that apply this principle to protecting the public's health. For example, a patient with active tuberculosis can be compelled to accept hospitalization for the protection of his family and his neighbors. Typhoid carriers can be prevented from accepting employment as food handlers because of the danger they would be to the health of many people.

In general terms, the federal government has authority and responsibility in three broad areas of public health: a general concern for the health of the people of the nation; the prevention of the spread of disease from one state to another; and the prevention of the introduction of disease from outside the United States. To carry out these responsibilities, the government studies national and international health problems and conducts studies and research on the incidence, transmission, and prevention of

11

diseases. It helps control the transmission of disease from state to state by regulating the movement of infected persons, animals, and goods, particularly foods and drugs. Quarantine stations to control the entrance of disease from abroad are located at all international seaports and airports. Before goods or people may enter the country, they must have health clearance by the port authorities.

When states need health guidance and assistance from the federal government this help may be given in a variety of ways. Some states have insufficient funds to provide a satisfactory health program without federal aid in the form of grants of money. Some states have unusual disease problems, such as malaria, occupational diseases, or industrial pollution problems, and need the assistance of expert personnel with special training. What these experts do to help depends on the circumstances. They may act as consultants in planning programs, train local health personnel on the job, or actually work as additional health personnel on loan to the local health agency. The ultimate purpose of federal assistance to the states is to raise standards and to strengthen the departments of health so that they can gradually assume all responsibility for an ongoing public health program that will meet the needs of the people.

FEDERAL HEALTH AGENCIES

Health activities of the federal government are carried on chiefly by or under the supervision of the Department of Health, Education, and Welfare. This department coordinates and directs all federal health and welfare activities. Since 1953 the administrator has been a member of the President's Cabinet, with the title of Secretary of Health, Education, and Welfare.

The United States Public Health Service is an agency within the Department of Health, Education, and Welfare and is under the direction of a surgeon general, who holds the highest public health position in this country. The organizational structure of the Service has changed over the years, but its purposes remain broad enough to meet changing health needs of the nation. Its responsibilities are to conduct and support research in health and the allied sciences, to provide, on request, consultative services in health matters to health agencies, to furnish medical and hospital care for designated beneficiaries, and to act as the responsible federal agency in dealing with other nations of the world in international health matters.

The National Institutes of Health, a division of the Public Health Service, is the principal federal agency engaged in the conduct and support of medical and health related research. It is one of the largest research centers in the world, conducting within its own facilities studies of every major problem affecting community and national health. Among its many activities, it supports health or health related scientific research at universities, medical schools, and other institutions, aids applicants eligible to pursue a research career, and provides funds to assist in building and equipping of research facilities in the health science field. In addition to conducting studies and promoting programs focused on the conquest of disease and the improvement of human health, the National Institutes of Health is responsible for administration of controls designed to insure the purity, safety, and potency of all sera and vaccines used for the prevention and treatment of disease.

The Children's Bureau, also an agency of the Department of Health, Education, and Welfare, was established in 1912 as a result of the findings and recommendations of the first White House Conference on Children held in 1909. The Children's Bureau is concerned with all aspects of the growth and development of children, the problems of illness, maternal and child health, and all social and environmental factors affecting their welfare. It collects, analyzes, and interprets statistical data concerning children and youth and develops materials and standards to be used by persons or agencies responsible for the health care or protection of mothers and children. The Bureau also gives technical assistance to improve the conditions of childhood and administers the financial aid that the federal government appropriates each year for the health and welfare of children. Its services have expanded through the years, always with the aim of improving the health and welfare of children.

The publication of health education materials by the Children's Bureau has reached into millions of homes, and one pamphlet, *Infant Care*, first printed in 1914, rates as a best-seller. Over the years more than 43 million copies have been distributed. It is available in the United States in both English and Spanish editions and has been translated into 11 languages for use abroad.

STATE HEALTH DEPARTMENTS

Every state has a state health department, with its authority vested in the power of the state to enact legislation for public safety and health. The local units of government within the state have only those powers that are granted to them by the state. In this country the states have sovereign power in health matters and the authority of the federal government rests in those areas in which the state has no authority, chiefly in the handling of interstate or international health problems. Because each of the 50 states has its own laws, there is no uniformity in the organization and administration of state health units, although there is similarity among them.

Usually, each state has a separate division of public health with a full-time administrator. This official may be an appointee of the governor or he may be selected by the state board of health. The state board of health is an advisory body, and its members are appointed by the governor of the state. The board acts in an advisory capacity in determining general policies of the health department, in formulating legislation, and in approving the budget. Local health ordinances may be stricter than a state law or regulation, but they may never be less so.

LOCAL HEALTH DEPARTMENTS

The local health department is the agency created by town, city, or county government to preserve and protect the public health. It is supported by local and state taxes or by grants of money from federal funds, and its activities are supervised by a group of local citizens usually called the board of health. The demands of the citizens of a community for services and the moral and financial support they are willing to provide largely determine the quality and quantity of local health services. Also necessary are local action and understanding of the needs of the community.

The offices of the health department are quite often located in the municipal or county building with other city or county departments of government. In a large city this department may be housed separately, with branch offices or health centers located in appropriate places. In rural areas or small towns the health department may have its offices at the community hospital, particularly if it is owned and operated by the county or town. All responsible citizens should know where the office of the local health department is located and what health services are available to them.

An important responsibility of the health department is to give leadership in the health efforts of the community. Because the local health officer is in a strategic position among the representatives of other health and welfare agencies in the community, he has the opportunity to guide and coordinate their activities. Duplication of health services can be eliminated and programs strengthened by pooling the efforts of all agencies involved in any aspect of public health.

In general, all health departments have the same broad responsibilities. Under the laws of the state or local government some of their services are mandatory. There are also permissive services, which are less necessary but still desirable services to offer if the budget permits, trained personnel are available, and the community supports the program. To a large extent, the breadth and quality of the program are determined by the amount of money available to the health department.

The services offered will vary according to the health needs of the communities and their ability to employ personnel to carry out the programs. In metropolitan areas the available health resources are numerous, and many specialized services can be offered. Here, too, are facilities for the study, diagnosis, and treatment of nearly every known physical ill or disability. On the other hand, in rural and less thickly populated areas, while services are organized as they are in the cities they are usually limited. Cooperative arrangements with health departments of nearby counties or cities can help to supplement their services and personnel.

All health departments are required to keep vital statistics—a function that is sometimes called the bookkeeping of community health. These statistics include records of births, deaths, and all reportable illnesses. The control of communicable diseases, including seeing that immunization programs are carried out, is another of their responsibilities. The health department is also required to control hazards to health from food and water by the inspection and licensing of dairies, restaurants, and food processing plants.

In some communities the health supervision of school children, which includes health inspection and a physical examination, and the counseling of children and their parents are functions of the local health department. However, depending on the administrative structure of the municipal or county government, this responsibility may belong to the department of education. Other services offered by health departments are diagnostic and treatment clinics, clinics that provide health supervision for well infants and children, prenatal and postnatal care, classes for expectant parents, and dental care, especially for school children.

An important permissive service of the health department is

health education. Health information is extended to the public through radio, television, newspapers, moving pictures, exhibits, pamphlet material, and discussion groups. The goal is to spread knowledge that will motivate the people to take the action necessary to improve community health.

Nearly all health departments employ one or more public health nurses. These nurses are all registered professional nurses, and about 25 percent of them are college graduates with special education in public health. Public health nurses make home visits to give nursing care or to teach someone else how to do it and how to maintain the health of the well members of the family. They serve as health counselors and are a source of information on health subjects and on available community services. Public health nurses also work in clinics, teach home nursing classes, direct school and industrial health programs, and supervise the care of patients in nursing homes.

Although the future activities of health departments cannot be entirely predicted, shifts in their purposes and programs during the last decade indicate growing attention to new public health problems. With the increased numbers of older people among the general population, the care of the aging and of the patient with long-term illness have become major public health problems. While the provision of medical and nursing care for the patient is a family responsibility, how the family's needs are met in regard to the aging and the long-term ill will be largely determined by what the community has to offer in the way of health programs for these groups and by what federal and state funds are available to assist local health departments in implementing their programs.

In addition to hospitalization, new types of assistance may have to be provided that will directly affect the programs and functions of local health departments. The training and supervision of personnel and the licensure of facilities for the care of the aged and of the long-term ill are likely to be prerogatives of the health department. Among the services to be expected in more and more communities are foster homes for the elderly, homemaker services for handicapped, ill, or old people, convalescent and nursing homes, and home care programs that include medical supervision and nursing care of the sick.

Another problem affecting the public's health is that posed by thermo-nuclear radiation. The use of radioactive materials for peaceful purposes entails some danger in accidental release of energy, and the problem of fallout from nuclear weapons presents incalculable danger. The safe disposal of radioactive waste materials is itself a health problem. While this problem today is chiefly one of research at the federal level of government, it can be foreseen as a future responsibility of local health departments.

Also, the heavy population shifts from the country to the city and its suburbs, as shown in the most recent census, has created problems affecting the health of all the people in the community. The disposal of human waste and sewage and the provision of adequate amounts of safe water to supply a population becoming more and more urban are immediate problems of great magnitude that health departments have yet to solve. On the positive side, however, the urban community has an abundance of health facilities available to its residents. Its hospitals, laboratories, clinics, physicians, dentists, and public health nurses are only a short travel distance away from any person and are available to everyone. In addition, the voluntary health and welfare agencies that provide specialized services, particularly for the sick at home, are likely to be found in urban areas.

VOLUNTARY HEALTH AGENCIES

In nearly every community there are nongovernmental or voluntary agencies that supplement the work of the health department. The voluntary public health agency is as American as apple pie. It is typical of the character of the country and of people helping people in trouble. A review of the history of American voluntary agencies usually reveals that each was started to meet a special need of a group of people. In pioneer days the greatest concern of such agencies was to care for the sick and for the indigent. When the founding fathers of the United States made no constitutional provision for a department to provide for the public's health, it was the voluntary agency that first filled this gap.

Private gifts supported the efforts of the pioneering health and welfare agencies, and in general that holds true for the voluntary health agency today. Contributions by people in the local community, endowments, bequests, and, in some instances, fees collected by the agency for its services are the primary source of revenue. Now that many of these voluntary agencies have become national in scope there are some that conduct annual national fund drives, with part of the locally contributed funds going to support the national organization. Administration, policy making, and education usually stem from the national offices, with direct service to people a function at the local community level.

17

Citizen groups represent the voluntary agencies at both the national and the local level. They serve in an advisory or in an administrative capacity to assure that the services given meet the needs of those to be helped. Such voluntary organizations as the American Public Health Association, the American Cancer Society, the National Foundation, and the American National Red Cross are examples of agencies that have made significant contributions to the development and progress of public health in this country. (A list of other representative health and welfare agencies is contained in the appendix.)

Almost all voluntary agencies have well-defined programs of service and health education designed to inform and guide the public in promoting and maintaining health. The program of the agency or its field of interest determines the emphasis it gives to specific health problems. Its interest may be, for example, heart disease, tuberculosis, cerebral palsy, cancer, or slum clearance. Collectively, voluntary agencies make their influence felt in the enactment of social security legislation, minimum wage laws, housing, health care for the aged, and health insurance, all of which are related to the health of the public.

Although today government carries most of the load of public health services, the voluntary agency is still needed to carry out experimental programs and to assist and supplement the health education of the nation's people. Another contribution of the voluntary agency, and perhaps its most important public health function, is to assist government agencies in setting and maintaining high standards of service to people.

INTERNATIONAL HEALTH AGENCIES

Rapid means of travel from one part of the world to another has brought special recognition to the need for international health agencies. Contagion does not recognize national boundaries, and since certain less frequently encountered diseases, such as plague and yellow fever, exist at all times in some place in the world, there must be international concern for health and agencies that are prepared to cooperate in the eradication and control of disease.

The oldest international health agency is the Pan American Health Organization. This agency was established by the American Republics in 1902 as the Pan American Sanitary Organization. Its origin lies in agreements made in 1887 among Argentina, Brazil, and Paraguay in attempting to regulate the spread of yellow fever between their countries. The headquarters office, located in

Washington, D.C., is one of the regional offices of the World Health Organization. Since 1924 the activities of the Pan American Health Organization have been increasingly devoted to providing technical assistance to underdeveloped countries, to receiving and disseminating epidemiological information, to financing fellowships on health, medical, and nursing education, and to promoting cooperation in medical research.

The World Health Organization organized in 1948 is one of the specialized agencies of the United Nations. Through this organization the public health and medical professions of more than 100 countries exchange their knowledge and experience and work together in an effort to achieve the highest possible level of health throughout the world. The organization is not concerned with problems that individual countries or territories can solve with their own resources. Instead, it focuses on those problems that can be satisfactorily solved only through the cooperation of all or certain groups of countries. For example, the eradication of malaria and the control of cholera, plague, yellow fever, and smallpox are international problems.

Progress toward better health throughout the world also demands international cooperation in other activities. Much of the organization's resources is devoted to giving guidance and other assistance in maternal and child health, nutrition, nursing, and environmental health. Assistance is provided through grants of money and the professional education and training of personnel within the country being helped. The strengthening of local health services in underdeveloped countries unites these efforts with those of more advanced countries to form a common front against disease.

The League of Red Cross Societies is a federation of Red Cross, Red Crescent, and Red Lion and Sun societies throughout the world. Founded in 1919, the League constantly pioneers to discover new and better ways of promoting the health and welfare of humanity. It strives through the member societies to teach people in every land how to improve their health. The League fills gaps in existing health services of national Red Cross societies and gives them further aid when requested. Through its Nursing Bureau and its Health and Social Service Bureau the League provides health education materials, grants scholarships and fellowships, and conducts seminars or training courses for the instruction of health workers of Red Cross societies. In disaster, the League helps to meet the health needs of stricken people by sending trained personnel, equipment, and supplies provided by Red Cross societies around the world. Also, in cooperation with the World Health Organization, the League is often asked to recruit personnel from member societies to help carry out health programs and to meet crucial needs for trained personnel in disaster areas.

SUGGESTED STUDENT ACTIVITIES

1. Write to your local or state health department for available pamphlets on personal health and home nursing. Report, or arrange with the instructor to have some of your classmates report, on what was learned from the pamphlets.

2. Make a list of free and inexpensive materials concerning personal health or home nursing that are available from organizations and agencies, such as:

American National Red Cross

American Medical Association

A life insurance company

U.S. Department of Health, Education, and Welfare

Obtain a copy of as many different items as possible for class use.

3. Invite a representative of your health department to speak to your class on the responsibilities of the department for the improvement of health conditions in the community. Discuss with him the responsibility of each citizen to improve community health.

4. Report on the work done and projects being carried on by the health department in your community.

5. Find out what voluntary health agencies exist in your community and what services they render.

6. Invite a public health nurse to speak to you about her work.

7. Discuss with your local health department regulations regarding examination of food handlers in a school cafeteria. What are the regulations? What are the health department requirements for the washing of dishes, glasses, and cutlery in a school cafeteria?

8. Arrange with the instructor to hold a panel discussion on the advantages and disadvantages of social security legislation on health care for the aged.

9. Offer to help one of the voluntary health agencies in your community collect funds or otherwise promote its activities. Report to the class what impact this experience had on you.

3

FOOD AND NUTRITION

From earliest times man has realized that providing food for himself and his family is one of his major tasks. He soon recognized that food sustains life and that a full stomach brings happiness and contentment. For a long time, however, he did not understand the relationship of food to health. It has been largely in the present century, through the tireless work of men and women engaged in scientific research, that man has come to appreciate the body's delicate and efficient mechanism and has learned something about the physiological processes by which the body makes food into bone, blood, brain, and brawn.

The human body in its functioning is far more amazing than the finest watch or the most intricate machine. There is, however, a striking similarity between the body and a machine. Human bodies need fuel just as machines require fuel or other sources of power. Every breath taken, every beat of the heart, every movement of the body requires energy. Food supplies fuel to yield this energy. The remarkable difference between the human body and a machine is the way in which the body can repair its own worn parts. When a machine needs a new part or needs an old part mended, it must remain idle until the damaged part is repaired or replaced by a mechanic. In contrast, the human body is able to repair itself to a large degree.

The substances of which foods are composed are called nutrients. Each of them is needed by the body and each has its own special function to perform. The most familiar of the nutrients are proteins, fats, carbohydrates, vitamins, and the many mineral elements, such as calcium, iodine, and iron. These are the materials by which the body meets its needs for building and repairing tissues, providing heat and energy, and regulating its physiological

21

functions. Whether well or ill, the body must have these sub-stances. The choice of food should therefore be regulated first of all by the body's needs. This does not mean that preference, custom, convenience, availability, and cost must be set aside and the diet limited to a few foods. On the contrary, if the food needs of the body as well as the composition of the different commonly used foods are understood, it is easy to plan meals that are both adequate and varied.

No single food can be depended upon to furnish enough of all the nutrients required for health. The problem in planning meals for each day is therefore to choose those foods that together will supply all the nutrients needed to build, maintain, and repair the body structure, to regulate the many body processes, and to provide sufficient energy for the activities of the body.

Sometimes illness occurs because of a serious lack of one or more of the specific nutrient substances that the body must have to function properly. More often the person who for sometime has had an inadequate diet does not become critically ill or even sick enough to go to bed. He may simply feel run down, tired, and unable to work. On the other hand, the person who is selecting his food wisely and is enjoying what he eats has a good chance of feeling and keeping well.

CHOOSING FOODS FOR HEALTH

How can one know that the foods selected are the best for the health of the family? The planning of meals that will include the right combination of foods can be simple when a general pattern is developed and followed.

ESSENTIAL NUTRIENTS

One good pattern to follow in the selection of foods is given in *Food for Fitness, A Daily Food Guide.** This guide classifies foods into four basic groups: the milk group, the meat group, the bread-cereal group, and the vegetable-fruit group. Foods chosen from each of these groups provide the essential nutrients for a good diet. Since each group offers a great variety of foods, it is easy to include in the daily meals family favorites, economy foods, and foods available only at certain times of the year. The foods that are grouped together have essentially the same nutrients but they vary in nutrient value per serving. Fruits and vegetables, for

* *Food for Fitness, A Daily Food Guide,* Leaflet No. 424, U.S. Department of Agriculture, 1958.

22

FOOD FOR FITNESS

A Daily Food Guide

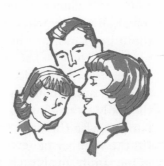

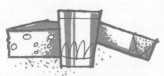

MILK GROUP

Some milk for everyone

Children......3 to 4 cups

Teen-agers....4 or more cups

Adults........2 or more cups

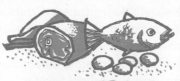

MEAT GROUP

2 or more servings

Beef, veal, pork, lamb,
   poultry, fish, eggs
As alternates - dry beans,
   dry peas, nuts

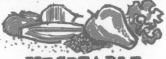

VEGETABLE FRUIT GROUP

4 or more servings include -
A citrus fruit, other fruit or vegetable important for vitamin C
A dark-green or deep-yellow
  vegetable for vitamin A -
  at least every other day
Other vegetables and fruits,
  including potatoes

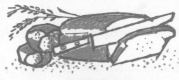

BREAD CEREAL GROUP

4 or more servings

Whole grain, enriched,
or restored

Plus other foods as needed to complete meals and to provide additional
food energy and other food values

Adapted from *Food for Fitness, A Daily Food Guide,* issued by Department of
Agriculture, Agricultural Research Service.

23

example, provide almost all of the daily requirement for vitamins A, C, and niacin but are quite low in calories. The citrus fruits and tomatoes are the main source of vitamin C. Breads and cereals, on the other hand, are high in calories and are therefore the main source of energy. The meat and dairy groups provide a very high percentage of the daily requirement for protein, calcium, iron, thiamin, and riboflavin. The milk group is the primary source of the daily calcium requirement. The homemaker should become familiar with the daily food guide and follow its recommendations for the number of servings from each food group to be provided in the family meals each day.

Studies of buying and eating habits have shown that the milk and the vegetable-fruit groups must be carefully checked by the person responsible for family meal planning and preparation since these are the groups most often neglected in the diet of people living in the United States.* Foods most often omitted are the dark leafy green and the yellow vegetables and the fruits rich in vitamin C.

Milk can be provided in the diet in many ways. Many people never tire of drinking it plain. It can be served on cereals and used as the base of soups, sauces, and gravies and in making puddings, breads and cakes, and ice cream and cheese. Another way to increase the intake of milk is by the addition of dried skim milk to foods as they are prepared. Children should have a daily allowance of from 3 to 4 cups of milk, teenagers should have 4 or more cups a day, and adults 2 or more. The expectant mother should have at least 4 cups a day, while the nursing mother needs an additional 2 cups.

Everyone should have four or more servings daily of fruits and vegetables, including potatoes. One of the fruits should be high in vitamin C. Many people get the necessary amount of this important vitamin in the fresh citrus juice or fruit served with breakfast. Melons and berries are good sources of vitamin C, are relatively inexpensive in season, and are usually well liked.

The dark green leafy vegetables and the yellow vegetables provide vitamin A, which is important in growth, tooth formation, vision, and resistance to disease. A cooked vegetable is usually a part of the main meal of the day and, with the wide variety of vegetables to choose from, meals need not be repetitious. Raw vegetables in salads or as finger foods and cooked vegetables in combinations or in stews all count toward the day's quota of vitamin A.

---

* Agnes F. Morgan and Lura M. Odland, "The Nutriture of People," *Food*, The Yearbook of Agriculture 1959, pp. 186-224.

ESSENTIAL MINERALS

About 15 different minerals are essential to the functioning of the body systems, and all of them can be obtained from food or drink. The three most likely to be in short supply in the diet are calcium, iron, and iodine, sometimes called the critical minerals.

Calcium is one of the chief minerals in bones and teeth. About 99 percent of all the calcium in the body is in the bony structure, while the remaining quantity is in the soft tissues and body fluids. Calcium is essential to nerve function, blood clotting, and the normal contraction and relaxation of muscles. Vitamin D and phosphorus are essential to the utilization of calcium by the body. Phosphorus is found in abundant supply in many foods. Calcium is found in milk and dairy products, green leafy vegetables, dried peas and beans, and seafoods.

Iron is one of the minerals needed by the red blood cells, which carry oxygen from the lungs to each body cell. A shortage of iron may result in nutritional anemia. Liver is an outstanding source of iron. This important mineral is also found in eggs, dried fruits, seafoods, leafy green vegetables, and whole grain cereals and bread.

All living tissue contains many different minerals, some of them in such small quantities they can be barely detected. These minerals have come to be known as trace elements, and their presence, even in minute amounts, is essential to nutrition and biological function. Iodine, one of the trace elements, is an essential part of the thyroid hormone and is of great importance in regulating the rate of body functions. In certain geographical areas throughout the world, the soil lacks iodine, with the result that nutritional goitre has become a public health problem. This deficiency usually can be overcome by the use of iodized salt, which is often recommended by physicians.

Fluorine, another trace element, seems to increase resistance to tooth decay. It is found in varying amounts in water, and studies have shown that in those communities where it is present in the drinking water, dental decay rates are significantly lower. For this reason, many municipalities now add minute amounts of fluorine to their water supply.

MEAL PLANNING

Planning good meals for the entire family, whether sick or well, is well worth the time and thought it takes, not only because appetizing meals are popular but also because food is important to the maintenance of good health. Good food is not always the most expensive food. Proper preparation and the judicious use of imagination in seasoning with herbs and flavoring can make inexpensive foods attractive and enjoyable as well as nourishing. The art of being a good cook is an asset to any homemaker.

A reliable cookbook will help every woman who keeps house to prepare nutritious and appetizing meals. When she makes a new dish or is learning to cook, she should try to follow very carefully the directions given in the cookbook. After she becomes skilled at cooking, she can afford to take "a pinch of this" and "about so much of that" in preparing a particular food. But until her hand and eye are trained, she may ruin much good food by careless mixing of ingredients and improper methods of cookery.

Modern cookbooks can be found in wide variety, ranging from those that offer recipes for the person who lives and eats alone to those that have quantity cooking recipes for 50 or more people. Cookbooks are specialized in other ways too. Some give recipes from New England, the Southwest, and other sections of the country; others feature Chinese, French, Italian, and other national foods, and still others contain recipes for foods prepared with herbs, wine, or spices. Picture cookbooks give step-by-step illustrated directions for both simple and complex recipes.

There are also cookbooks designed to meet special dietary needs. These, for example, contain recipes for the preparation of the diabetic, sodium-restricted, low fat, high protein, and weight reduction diets. Recipes for the patient who is on a liquid diet are distributed by the manufacturers of several brands of blenders.

FOOD FOR THE SICK

Food is an important part of medical treatment for the patient. While it is the doctor's responsibility to decide what kind of food the patient may have, it is the home nurse's responsibility to see that the food served him retains its nutritive value. She must also see that the food is so well prepared and attractively served that the patient will want to eat. Some patients will need help in feeding themselves, and this assistance should be provided as necessary. The home nurse should observe and report to the doctor the amount of food eaten by the patient, any variations in his appetite, and any gain or loss in his weight.

If the doctor does not specify, he should always be asked what kind of diet the patient may have. In some instances the doctor will simply say, "A regular diet; give him anything he wants to eat." He means, of course, that the patient may be offered food at regular meal times and that his favorite foods may be included. Because water is as important as food in illness, it should be offered frequently unless the doctor orders otherwise.

When one is weak and hungry, waiting for food is extremely trying. If the stomach is entirely empty, its walls touch, causing pangs of hunger. To avoid distress from hunger on the part of the patient, the home nurse should see that he is fed at regular intervals and that his meals are prepared on time. If the patient is not able to go to the table, his tray should be prepared and given to him before the family eats and while the food is hot and most palatable. When the patient is allowed to have a light or a full diet he probably can eat many of the same foods that are prepared for the family. Preparing identical menus for the patient and the family eliminates additional work for the home nurse. Always every effort should be made to see that the atmosphere at mealtime is as pleasant as possible.

Since its appearance may affect the appetite favorably or unfavorably, the tray should be pleasing to the eye. Dishes should be attractive and related to the size of the tray. The tray cloth and the napkin should be spotless. Paper tray covers and napkins are convenient, inexpensive, and disposable. Different kinds of decorated or colored napkins provide an element of interest and color that is pleasing to adults as well as to children. The practice of placing a fresh flower or a little surprise on the tray may help to make mealtime an occasion to which the patient looks forward with pleasure.

Because the sight, aroma, and taste of food that one enjoys aid the digestion, the foods served the patient should be those that he likes, if the diet allows them. Care should be taken to make sure that each food is sufficiently seasoned, tastes good, and is as appetizing and attractive as possible. Fresh, colorful foods should be selected, and vegetables should be cooked in as small an amount of water as possible and served at once. Liquids served hot must be only pleasantly hot so as not to burn the lips and tongue.

Before the tray is brought into the sick room, the patient should be allowed to use the bedpan, if desired. He should have an opportunity to wash his hands and face so that he can be clean and refreshed for his meal. Then the room and bed should be put in order, the backrest or pillows adjusted to his comfort, and the bed table arranged comfortably and conveniently. The patient who is calm and relaxed will have less difficulty in digesting his food.

The cooperation of the patient is essential if there are any limitations on his diet. Any questions he may have regarding a special diet ordered for him should be answered if at all possible. If certain foods are restricted, he will accept their elimination more readily if he knows something about the damage such foods might do to his body, or, on the other hand, the benefits to be gained by strict adherence to the diet. This is particularly true for the patient on a sodium-restricted or a diabetic diet.

The average person prefers to feed himself, but helpless and weak patients or small children must be assisted. (See "Feeding the Helpless Patient," chapter 13, pages 233-235.) The tray should be placed where the patient can see his food, and the food should be given to him in small bites, alternating various foods as he would do if feeding himself. Unless he is weak, he may prefer to hold his bread and butter and eat it when he wishes. Usually he will wish to wipe his own mouth. If the patient is too ill to help himself, the home nurse can feed him, using a glass or cup, a spoon, or a drinking tube. The patient's head should be allowed to recline in a comfortable position; the neck must not be bent forward because it will interfere with swallowing.

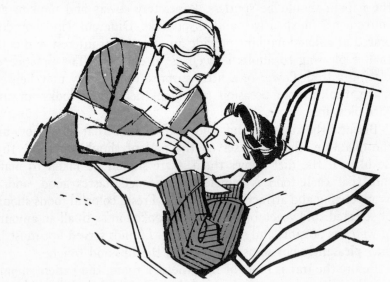

When helping the patient to drink from a cup, support his head.

The kind and the amount of food eaten should always be noted on the patient's record so that the doctor may determine whether the patient is taking enough nourishing food.

A patient who has an injury or illness that merely keeps him from exercising and has no effect on his appetite may eat more than he needs. As a result, he may put on too much weight and also may become constipated. To correct constipation, the doctor may order foods for the patient that have a high roughage content to aid elimination and he may greatly increase the amount of liquids—especially fruit juices—the patient is to receive. He may also ask that the high calorie foods, such as fats and sweets, be given sparingly so that the patient will not gain too much weight.

THE DOCTOR'S DIET ORDERS

It is best to ask the doctor to write all his orders, including the kind of diet the patient may have. The home nurse has many responsibilities and should not rely on memory in carrying out the doctor's orders. When the doctor prescribes a liquid, soft, light, or full diet there should be clear understanding of what foods may be included. Since food is an important part of the treatment in many illnesses, the doctor's instructions as to diet should be followed with as much care as those given for medicine.

When a special diet has been ordered, the home nurse may need assistance in planning meals that not only meet the patient's needs and the family's food habits but are also within the limits of the food budget. Special diets need not be expensive. When the patient is hospitalized and plans are being made for him to come home or if he is receiving treatment in the hospital's outpatient department, a conference usually can be arranged with the hospital staff dietitian or the clinic nutritionist to discuss meal planning, methods of preparing special foods, and the substitutions that can be made to meet individual food preferences. The doctor will give advice and will know best where to obtain additional counseling if it is needed. He may be able to recommend authoritative books on nutrition available at the local library. The public health nurse, because of her knowledge of food and nutrition, may also be called on for assistance. An excellent general reference book is *Food*, the 1959 Yearbook of Agriculture.

KINDS OF DIET

When the doctor prescribes a liquid, soft, light, or full diet, there should be a full understanding of what foods are included.

Liquid Diet

A liquid diet is the regular diet liquefied to make it smooth in

29

texture and easy to digest. The full liquid diet permits the use of any foods in natural fluid form and any that will liquefy at body temperature. It is fairly easy to plan an adequate liquid diet from the four food groups. Although bread is not used in liquid form, cereals may be made into gruels by cooking, straining, and adding milk or water. Potatoes and other vegetables may be pureed and used in thin milk soups. Fruits also may be cooked and mashed or put through a sieve. The juices of fresh vegetables, such as tomatoes and carrots, and of canned vegetables may be chilled or heated and served as broths, as may fish and meat stocks and beef juice.

In some acute illnesses, the liquid diet may be restricted for a short time to clear broths, bouillons, and plain jellied consommes, thin gruels, strained fruit juice or lemonade, plain gelatin dessert, and ices and sherbets made without milk. The addition of energy foods, such as honey, sugar, hard candies, and carbonated beverages may make the diet more appealing, especially to children. Egg albumin in water or fruit juice and plain tea or coffee are usually permitted.

Soft Diet

The regular diet modified so that it is smooth, easy to digest, and leaves little residue in the digestive tract becomes a soft diet. Liquid foods and those solid foods that contain no tough skins, fibers, or seeds are included. Fruits and vegetables are cooked and pureed, and meats, when allowed, are usually limited to broiled or roasted tender chicken, lamb, fish, scraped beef, and sweet-breads. All raw, coarse, and fat-rich foods, concentrated sweets, spices, and condiments are restricted.

Light Diet

The light diet is the regular diet modified to make food easier to digest. All foods are plainly cooked, and smaller servings are given. Rich gravies, salad dressings, and other fat-rich foods, raw and coarse vegetables and fruits, spices, and concentrated sweets are limited.

Regular or Full Diet

In the regular or full diet, also called the general diet, meals are planned in accordance with the four food groups previously discussed. The full diet for a convalescent may include all foods except fried foods, gas-forming vegetables (cabbage, onions, cauliflower, turnips), rich pastries, and concentrated sweets.

The regular diet that has been modified to eliminate irritation to the digestive tract is known as a bland diet. The modification may be in consistency, in flavor, or in the way the food is cooked. Consistency is changed by eliminating all indigestible tough skins and fibers, connective tissue, and seeds. The diet can be modified in flavor by eliminating spices, condiments (except salt), flavoring extracts, vinegars and wines, and other highly flavored foods. Simple, well-cooked foods should be used in the bland diet. Raw foods are eliminated. Juices and cereals are strained, and vegetables and fruits are usually mashed or sieved after cooking. Fried foods, very hot and very cold fluids, carbonated and alcoholic beverages, and concentrated sweets are omitted.

MODIFYING A REGULAR DIET TO MEET SPECIAL NEEDS

The special or modified diet is an adaptation of regular diet in that the foods are modified in nutritional value, physical consistency or texture, flavor, ways of preparing and serving, or by a combination of these factors. Many times diets can be adapted by making one or more simple changes in regular family meals.

If a family member is suffering from a disease in which diet is a prominent part of the treatment, it is important to follow the diet exactly as the doctor prescribes it. Since food helps the body to make repairs and thus to hasten recovery, the modified diet must meet the usual nutritional needs and the extra needs of the illness and convalescence, must tempt the patient's appetite, and be easily digested. The good convalescent diet is always planned around the same protective foods that make for an adequate diet. In illness caused by infection and injury, the requirement for ascorbic acid (vitamin C) is increased since it favors resistance to infection and promotes the healing of wounds. In fever, the need for calories, ascorbic acid, and thiamine (vitamin B) is greater.

The following tables will be helpful. Table I* lists the foods usually allowed the hospital patient for whom a liquid, soft, light, or general diet has been ordered. Table II* suggests pattern menus containing foods that can be modified for the patient on one of these diets. Table III and Table IV suggest pattern menus for a day's family meals at two cost levels. These menus illustrate what foods from the family meals may be served to the convalescent patient who is on a liquid, soft, or full diet and how these foods may be modified to meet his special needs.

---

* Adapted from Lenna F. Cooper, Edith M. Barber, Helen S. Mitchell, and Henderika J. Rynbergen. *Nutrition in Health and Disease*, pp. 223-224.

TABLE I

Foods Allowed on Convalescent and General Diets

Type of Food	Full Liquid Diet	Soft Diet	Light Diet	General Diet
Fruits	Fruit juices, strained	Fruit juices Cooked and canned fruits (without seeds, coarse skins, or fibers) Bananas	All cooked and canned fruits Citrus fruits Bananas	All
Cereals and cereal products	Gruels, strained Infant cereals in milk	Cereals: dry or well cooked Spaghetti and macaroni, not highly seasoned	Same as soft diet	All
Breads	None	Enriched white and whole wheat Soda crackers	Same as soft diet	All
Soups and broth	Broth Strained cream soups	Same as liquid diet	All	All
Meat, fish, and poultry	None	Tender chicken Fish Sweetbreads Ground beef and lamb	Tender steak and chops Lamb Veal Ground or tender beef Bacon Chicken Sweetbreads Liver Fish	All
Eggs	Eggnogs	Soft-cooked eggs	Same as soft diet	Eggs cooked all ways
Dairy products	Milk, sweet and acid Cream Milkshakes Butter and margarine	Milk, sweet and acid Cream Butter and margarine Cottage and cream cheese Cheddar cheese used in cooking	Same as soft diet	Milk, sweet and acid Cream Butter and margarine Cheese, all kinds

TABLE I (Cont.)

Type of Food	Full Liquid Diet	Soft Diet	Light Diet	General Diet
Vegetables	Strained Vegetable-beef soup Blended vegetable juices Tomato juice Creamed vegetable soups	Cooked: asparagus; peas; string beans; spinach; carrots; beets; squash; potatoes: boiled, mashed, creamed, scalloped, baked Salads: none	Same as soft diet

Salads: tomato and lettuce | All, including salads |
Desserts	Ices Ice cream Plain gelatin Junkets Thin custard	Ices Ice cream Cereal pudding Custard Gelatin Simple cake Plain cookies	Same as soft diet	All
Beverages	Tea, coffee, cocoa Coffee substitutes Milk and milk beverages Carbonated beverages	Same as liquid diet	Same as liquid diet	All
Sweets	Honey Syrup Sugar dissolved in liquids	Same as liquid diet	Same as liquid diet	All

TABLE II

Typical Menus for Convalescent and General Diets

Full Liquid Diet	Soft Diet	Light Diet	General Diet
Breakfast			
Orange juice, strained	Orange juice	Orange	Fresh pear
Strained oatmeal gruel with milk or cream	Oatmeal with milk or cream	Oatmeal with milk or cream	Oatmeal with milk or cream
Coffee with cream and sugar	Soft scrambled eggs	Soft scrambled eggs	Scrambled eggs
	Buttered whole wheat toast	Buttered whole wheat toast	Buttered whole wheat toast
	Coffee with cream and sugar	Coffee with cream and sugar	Coffee with cream and sugar
10:00 a.m.			
Eggnog			
Lunch			
Strained cream of pea soup	Cream of pea soup with crackers	Cream of pea soup with crackers	Cream of pea soup with crackers
Plain gelatin with whipped cream	Macaroni au gratin	Macaroni au gratin	Macaroni au gratin
	Buttered beets	Head lettuce salad with French dressing	Head lettuce salad with Russian dressing
	Bread: white or whole wheat	Bread: white or whole wheat	Bread: white or whole wheat
	Butter or margarine	Butter or margarine	Butter or margarine
	Plain gelatin with whipped cream	Fruit gelatin	Fruit gelatin
	Tea with cream and sugar	Tea with cream and sugar	Tea with cream and sugar
3:00 p.m.			
Malted milk or buttermilk			
Dinner			
Broth with rice, strained	Strained vegetable soup	Vegetable soup	Vegetable soup
Ginger ale with ice cream	Ground beef	Roast veal	Roast veal
Coffee with cream and sugar	Mashed potato	Mashed potato	Mashed potato
	Buttered carrots	Buttered carrots	Buttered broccoli
	Bread: white or whole wheat	Tomato salad with French dressing	Tomato salad with French dressing
	Butter or margarine	Bread: whole wheat, rye, or white	Bread: whole wheat, rye, or white
	Vanilla ice cream with chocolate sauce	Butter or margarine	Butter or margarine
		Peppermint stick ice cream	Peppermint stick ice cream
9:00 p.m.			
Hot cocoa	Milk	Milk	Milk

34

TABLE III

Meals at Low Cost Level

Sample Family Meals for a Day	For Adult on Full Liquid Diet	For Small Child on Full Liquid Diet	How to Modify for Full Liquid Diet	Soft Diet
Breakfast Sliced oranges Oatmeal Toast with jelly Coffee Milk (for children)	Orange juice Oatmeal gruel Coffee with cream and sugar	½ cup orange juice ½ cup oatmeal gruel Full glass milk	Squeeze oranges; strain juice Strain oatmeal through sieve; add milk to thin Serve with 3 tbsp. cream or milk and ½ tbsp. sugar	Orange Oatmeal Toast with jelly Coffee Milk (for children)
10:00 a.m.	Frosted milkshake	Frosted milkshake (1 cup, scant)		Frosted milkshake (if desired)
Lunch Potato soup Peanut butter sandwich Cole slaw Fruit gelatin Milk	Potato soup Plain gelatin Milk	½ cup potato soup ½ cup plain gelatin ½ cup milk	Put cooked potato through sieve; thin soup to desired consistency with rich milk, stock, or vegetable water Omit fruit from gelatin mold	Potato soup Poached egg on toast Fruit gelatin Milk
3:00 p.m.	Fresh fruit ade with ginger ale	Fresh fruit ade with ginger ale (1 cup, scant)		Fresh fruit ade with ginger ale (if desired)
Dinner Tomato juice Beef stew (carrots, potatoes, tomatoes, celery, peas) Canned peach and cottage cheese salad Bread, butter or margarine Soft custard Plain cookies Coffee	Tomato juice Strained beef broth Soft custard Coffee	½ cup tomato juice ½ cup strained beef broth ⅓ cup soft custard	Just before thickening stew, remove enough broth for patient; strain, reheat, and serve Vegetables may be sieved and added Soft custard is different from firm custard It is really a cooked eggnog that liquefies at body temperature	Tomato juice Beef stew (carrots and potatoes only) Peach and cottage cheese (no lettuce) Toast and butter or margarine Soft custard Plain cookies Coffee or milk
8:00 p.m.	Hot cocoa	½ cup hot cocoa		Hot cocoa (if desired)

35

TABLE IV

Meals at Moderate Cost Level

Sample Family Meals for a Day	For Adult on Full Liquid Diet	For Small Child on Full Liquid Diet	How to Modify for Full Liquid Diet	Soft Diet
Breakfast Grapefruit juice Cream of wheat Soft-cooked egg Toast, butter or margarine Coffee with cream and sugar Milk (for children)	Grapefruit juice Strained cereal gruel Coffee with cream and sugar	½ cup grapefruit juice ½ cup strained cereal gruel Milk (full glass)	Strain juice Strain cream of wheat and thin with milk to desired consistency	Grapefruit juice Cream of wheat Soft-cooked egg Toast, butter or margarine Coffee with cream and sugar Milk (for children)
10:00 a.m.	Eggnog or malted milk	Eggnog or malted milk (1 cup, scant)		Eggnog or malted milk (if desired)
Lunch Cream of tomato soup Macaroni and cheese Tossed green salad Vanilla ice cream with sliced peaches Beverage	Cream of tomato soup Vanilla ice cream Strained orange juice Tea with sugar and cream	½ cup cream of tomato soup ⅓ cup vanilla ice cream ½ cup strained orange juice Milk (1 cup, scant)	Strain juice	Cream of tomato soup Macaroni and cheese Vanilla ice cream with peaches, canned or slightly cooked Milk
3:00 p.m.	Ginger ale ice cream soda	Ginger ale ice cream soda (1 cup, scant)	Pour ginger ale over scoop of ice cream in tall glass; stir briskly	Ginger ale ice cream soda (if desired)
Dinner Jellied consomme Swiss steak Mashed potatoes Stewed tomatoes Hearts of lettuce, dressing Bread, butter or margarine Caramel junket Beverage	Jellied consomme Chilled tomato vegetable juice Plain junket Milk	½ cup jellied consomme ½ cup chilled tomato vegetable juice ⅓ cup junket	A variety of canned consommes are available. All need chilling for about 4 hours to set. Heat and serve as broth in winter	Jellied consomme Swiss steak Mashed potatoes Toast, butter or margarine Caramel junket Coffee, tea, or milk
8:00 p.m.	Hot milk	Hot milk (1 cup, scant)	Heat milk or chill juice, depending on the weather	Hot milk (if desired)

FEEDING THE PATIENT ON A LIQUID DIET

A liquid diet is often prescribed for the patient who is acutely ill, who is suffering from some gastro-intestinal condition, who has had surgery, or who for some reason is unable to swallow solid food. To satisfy nutritional requirements of the body, the patient on a liquid diet should be offered frequent feedings.

Fruit juices, tea or coffee, carbonated drinks, strained soups, milk, eggnogs, thin custards, and ice cream are included in most liquid diets. Because sugar is a good source of energy, the doctor may request that certain drinks be sweetened. Gruel can be made by cooking cereal thoroughly, straining, and diluting with water or milk to make it easy to drink. Salt and butter or margarine may be added to make it more flavorful if the patient prefers. Flavorings such as vanilla and nutmeg are frequently added to milk or eggnog to make it more appetizing.

As the patient progresses toward recovery, the doctor may order a soft diet which will include buttered toast, breakfast cereals except bran, soft-cooked eggs, strained or pureed vegetables, and baked or mashed potatoes. As the patient improves, his meals gradually change from liquid, to soft, to light, and eventually to the general diet.

When the patient has a fever, body protein is destroyed in greater than normal amounts and the body's need for fuel is increased above normal requirements. For these reasons, the doctor may order, whenever he considers it wise, a diet that contains additional carbohydrates and protein for extra fuel and body building material.

FEEDING THE CONVALESCENT

Human beings require adequate amounts of all nutrients to maintain health, and hunger and appetite are the factors that encourage one to eat. Frequently the person who is beginning to convalesce has lost his appetite, and it is hard to find foods that he will enjoy. Eating is usually a pleasant experience, particularly if the food is appetizing, served in a manner that has eye appeal, and if it smells good. Most people dislike eating alone. If it is possible for the patient to eat at least one meal a day with the family, the social atmosphere will usually stimulate his appetite. It will still be the responsibility of the home nurse to see that the patient gets a well-rounded diet that contains the essential foods, including milk, fruits, cereals, vegetables, and meat or a protein substitute for meat. Within the limits of the diet ordered by the doctor, cater to the likes and dislikes of the patient as far as possible.

If the patient has had a severe illness, he may be able to tolerate only small amounts of food at a time and will have to have food more frequently. Midmorning, midafternoon, and bedtime nourishment should be offered unless it appears to complicate matters further by decreasing the amount of food eaten at regular mealtimes. Frequently a high caloric diet, one that offers especially nourishing foods, may be ordered if the patient is very weak or has lost a lot of weight. Foods that are rich in fats or very sweet may upset the patient's digestive system. It is better to add nourishment between meals than to attempt to over-feed the patient at regular meal times.

Meats are a good source of protein, but the patient's appetite for meat may be so poor that other sources, such as milk, must be increased. To increase the protein without adding bulk, dried skim milk may be added to many foods. To meet the higher energy requirements, increase carbohydrates by adding sweets to the diet, such as jelly, jam, strained honey, and sugar.

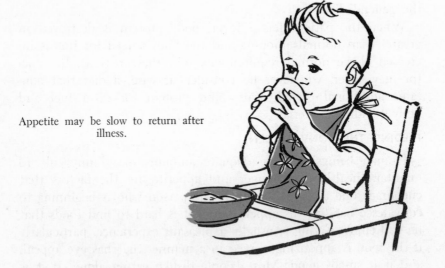

Appetite may be slow to return after illness.

FEEDING THE SICK BABY OR CHILD

When children are sick, they are apt to be fussy about food, so it appears sensible not to be too insistent about their eating, and to offer small amounts of food. A child not acutely ill will appreciate food served in unusual ways and on different china with colorful napkins and tray covers.

The doctor will prescribe the diet for a sick child. If the patient has a fever, he usually loses most of his appetite and is apt to reject solid foods. Vomiting occurs with many illnesses, particularly in the beginning, and even fluids may not be tolerated by a sick child. If vomiting occurs, one should wait a while and then offer small amounts of cool boiled water, cracked ice, ginger ale, or fruit juice. If these are tolerated, fluids should be offered about every half-hour. It is difficult to make a rule about giving milk to sick children, for certainly it is one of their basic foods. If milk can be taken without vomiting, it is usually the right food to offer because of the nourishment it supplies.

The child who has been ill for several days usually has lost some weight and parents may be overly concerned by this. Appetite may be slow to return, and undue urging to eat may cause the child to turn away from foods he normally enjoys, thus creating another problem. Most babies and children are the best judge of when and how much they should eat. The best course to follow is to offer small portions of the liquids and solids that the child wants and enjoys, and wait for his appetite to return. One should keep in touch with the doctor and consult him if the child persists in not eating.

FEEDING THE AGED AND THE PATIENT WITH A LONG-TERM ILLNESS

Although the nutritional needs of people remain the same throughout life, the caloric requirement and probably the total amount of essential foods become less with increasing age. It is important for the older person's diet to be fully adequate so that his body is supplied with all the essential nutrients. His meals usually can be chosen from the food prepared for the family unless the doctor has ordered a special diet. Eating is often one of the principal pleasures left to the older person, and as nearly as possible he should be given foods to which he is accustomed. However, if he is overweight he should be encouraged to cut down on the amount of food eaten and to avoid high-calorie foods. He should try to keep his weight near or below the average standard established for his height and his age.

Meals offered to the ill or aged may meet all nutritional standards; but unless they are eaten, they fail to meet the person's needs. If, for example, the patient refuses to drink milk or to eat citrus fruits, or, because of poor dentition, is unable to chew meat, then his meals must be modified. Milk may be included in combination with other foods; citrus fruit may be acceptable as juice, either plain or mixed with a blander fruit juice; and meat may be ground or chopped before or after cooking.

The atmosphere at mealtime is of great importance. If at all possible, the patient should get out of bed. Whenever possible he should eat with other members of the family so that mealtime becomes an interesting, companionable experience. Needless to say, taste, odor, and appearance of food influence appetite.

SUGGESTED STUDENT ACTIVITIES

1. Cut from magazines pictures of foods for a soft diet that illustrate the part that color, variety, and essential food groups play in a satisfactory diet. Arrange the pictures on paper as you would on a serving tray.

2. Prepare a complete list of all the food that you eat (at and between meals) for three consecutive days, including Saturday and Sunday. Could your diet have been improved? If so, how?

3. If possible, visit a model dairy and observe the homogenizing of milk, and also enrichment of its vitamin content.

4. From what source(s) may films on nutrition be obtained? Arrange to view some of these films and then discuss what you have seen.

5. Prepare a report on food fads and fallacies.

6. Prepare a 1-day diet for a baby, a high school boy or girl, a young adult, and an older adult. Why did you suggest the various foods?

7. Arrange with your instructor for a demonstration of correct methods of cooking food to preserve its vitamins and minerals.

8. Suggest ways to include milk in the diet of a person who dislikes it.

9. Arrange a tray for a convalescent patient on a regular diet. If facilities are available, actually prepare the meal.

10. Arrange with the home nursing instructor to invite the home economics instructor to speak to the class about diets for the healthy, as well as the sick, and appetizing ways to serve food.

11. Describe to the class how cooking food influences digestion. If possible, demonstrate the process.

4

RECOGNIZING ILLNESS

The nursing care required by a sick person is directly related to the nature and severity of his illness. The symptoms of illness are the home nurse's guide to what needs to be done for the patient until the doctor gives specific instructions. The better informed the home nurse is, the more likely it is that her judgment will be right.

The ability to observe and to weigh the evidences of illness increases with practice and experience. Judgments made by the home nurse are influenced by her knowledge of the patient's personality and the individual manner in which he reacts to illness and to anxiety or stress. Her observations combined with factual information, such as temperature or pulse rate, are essentials that assist the doctor in planning the care and treatment of the patient.

Some of the symptoms of illness are subjective (evident only to the sufferer), while others are objective (evident to someone else). Since babies and small children are not able to describe their feelings, parents or the home nurse in the family must learn to recognize the location of pain or discomfort in the child by his behavior. Many symptoms of illness can be detected only by scientific laboratory procedures, but even laboratory tests do not always provide sufficient evidence for the doctor to make the right diagnosis. Therefore, the results of such tests together with the sick person's description of his pain or discomfort, the history of his past illnesses, and the observations and judgments of the home nurse must be studied before a diagnosis is made. Also, in making a diagnosis the doctor depends as much on the absence of certain signs as on the presence of others. For all these reasons, the keen observation of symptoms is an important responsibility of the home nurse. Frequently, the earlier the symptoms are noticed and the sooner the patient is placed under medical care, the more rapid will be his recovery. However, children and many adults who know that their physical condition is being carefully watched are likely to exaggerate every little ache or pain. Usually they do not intend to mislead but are only unconsciously attempting to get satisfaction from special attention. If possible, symptoms of illness should be observed without the patient's knowledge and without too much obvious concern so that his interest or anxiety may not be aroused.

SYMPTOMS OF PHYSICAL ILLNESS

The symptoms of physical illness described below are not presented in the order of their frequency or of their importance because people react differently to illness. Nor is the severity of a symptom a true guide to its importance, for a mild symptom may precede a serious illness.

General Appearance

The total process by which the home nurse evaluates the condition of the patient includes the impressions that she has of changes in the patient as they contrast with his pre-illness appearance. Perhaps the simplest explanation is to say that the nurse decides how the patient is by his general appearance, by those things one can see as well as those things one senses. The relationship of the home nurse to the patient is a face-to-face relationship. It follows therefore that judgments about illness are based on what can be seen in the patient's face, his expression, his movements, and what he says as well as how he says it.

The Face

The appearance of the patient's face often gives a clue to the nature of his illness and to how much he is actually suffering. The facial expression may be drawn and haggard, alert and anxious, or dull and listless. The face may seem swollen or puffy about the eyes or it may be flushed or pale.

The eyes may seem heavy or unusually bright, and the sclera or whites of the eyes may be yellow or show a yellowish tinge. The eyes may be inflamed, bloodshot, or unusually sensitive to light. Because some diseases are characterized by disturbance of vision, the doctor should be told whether the patient complains of spots before the eyes, of halos around lights, of seeing double, or of not being able to see clearly.

The Nose and Throat

A running nose, sneezing, coughing, hoarseness, difficulty in breathing, and sore throat are all symptoms of the common cold. They may also mean the onset of influenza, poliomyelitis, pneumonia, sinusitis, and, in fact, any disease of the respiratory tract. When these symptoms are accompanied by fever and if they persist, they are a matter of concern, and the patient should be given medical attention. A chronic cough, hoarseness, and continued difficulty in breathing are especially serious.

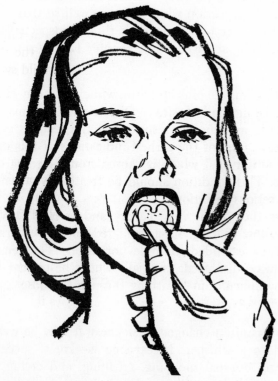

Inspect the back and sides of the throat for redness, swelling, and yellow or gray patches.

A sore throat accompanies many disease conditions, including most colds, coughs, and sinus infections. The most common type of sore throat is that caused by an infection characterized by an inflamed, raw throat with or without whitish patches. Abscessed or infected tonsils usually cause pain and difficulty in swallowing. A sore throat is an important symptom in the diagnosis of several communicable diseases. Severely sore and swollen throats, painful throat conditions that persist and are accompanied by fever,

43

throats that show yellow or grayish patches, and throats that are raw and bleeding should be reported to the doctor immediately.

Any person with a sore throat should keep away from others, go to bed if he has a fever or any patches in the throat, drink plenty of fluids, eat a light or a soft diet, and get plenty of rest. The toilet articles and dishes he uses should be kept separate from those of others until communicable disease is ruled out.

So many of the early signs of illness include a sore throat that it is wise to know how to inspect the throat easily, quickly, and skillfully. It is good practice for parents to accustom their children to throat inspection when they are well so that they will be less likely to object to having their throats inspected when they are ill. (See "Throat Inspection," chapter 12, pages 185-186.)

The Mouth

Healthy gums are pink and firm, while unhealthy gums may be swollen, bleeding, and sensitive. Disease of the gums, the lining of the mouth, and the bony sockets of the teeth is called periodontal disease. One of the earliest indications of this disease may be "pink toothbrush," which is caused from bleeding of the sensitive gums. This condition should be treated by a dentist before it leads to serious infection.

In illness the tongue may be dry and cracked, have a heavy white or yellow coating, be a vivid red and have a raw appearance, or when extended, tremble noticeably. The sense of taste is nearly always disturbed, especially when the patient has a high fever or any difficulty in breathing through the nose.

The Voice

The voice is often changed in sickness; it may be weak, hoarse, or reduced to a whisper. In extreme weakness, speech may be difficult. Any unusual moaning, groaning, and crying should be noted as an indication of some disturbance.

The Skin

The entire surface of the body should be observed for discoloration, swelling, itching, rash or eruptions of any kind, or breaks in the skin. Sometimes there is a puffiness of the skin under the eyes or swelling around the wrists or ankles. Any of these symptoms should be reported to the doctor. The skin acts as a protective covering for the body and as a barrier against disease, and any break in it may serve to permit the entrance of bacteria.

In the skin there are two kinds of glands, the sebaceous or oil glands and the sweat glands. The oil secreted on the skin makes it soft and pliable. Very dry skin is subject to abrasions and breaks in the surface through which infection can enter. The sweat glands normally produce about a quart of perspiration a day. They are part of the excretory system of the body and help in the removal of water and waste products. They also aid in maintaining the water balance of the body and normal body temperature. Heat noticeably increases the activity of the sweat glands, as do tension, nervousness, and extreme emotional upset. Excessive perspiration usually occurs in the hands and the axillae or arm pits and on the face and the feet.

Appetite and Hunger

Appetite is an emotional reaction to the stimulus of an empty stomach, and hunger is the physical response. When the stomach is empty, it is shrunken, and the contracted muscles of its walls irritate the nerve endings, causing the sensation of hunger. After eating, the walls of the stomach are stretched and its nerves are soothed so that one is no longer hungry. Any food that is ingested will suffice to destroy hunger because of its mechanical action, but appetite makes some foods more appealing than others. Appetite is also a sensory response to the desire to repeat a previously enjoyed experience. The sight, taste, smell, and even the texture of foods in the mouth are all part of remembered pleasurable experience and sometimes are the stimuli that cause one to eat after hunger is appeased.

Loss of appetite usually accompanies illness. Therefore, the amount and kind of food eaten as well as the amount of water and other liquids taken by the patient should be recorded for the doctor. Occasionally, sick people have strong cravings for certain foods or will develop enormous appetites.

Children may have the desire to eat unusual things such as dirt, plaster, paint, hair, or grass. This condition is called *pica*. This craving may be a physical response to supply some body deficiency or it may be an emotional reaction to deep-seated problems. In any event, it is a fairly serious abnormality and should always be called to the attention of the doctor.

Weight

Continued loss of weight in either adults or children in the absence of dieting is usually a sign that something is wrong. It may be caused by disease, disordered functions of the internal organs, emotional tension, or an insufficient amount or the wrong kind of food. A definite gain in weight may also indicate a change in the physical condition. Because nearly everyone loses weight in a severe illness, it is of special importance that nourishing foods be provided the ill person to protect the body from too great a weight loss.

Sleep

A person in bed all the time may not need as much sleep as when he is up and about, but sleep is nature's way of resting the mind and the body and is essential in both sickness and health. Some of the body changes that occur during sleep are not entirely understood, but sleep comes primarily as a result of lessened activity of the nervous system. Breathing slows down and may be irregular; heart action is decreased, sometimes as much as 20 beats a minute, and is accompanied by a lowering of the blood pressure; muscles relax; and the energy requirements of the body are lessened. The amount of sleep needed varies with age. An infant will sleep from 18 to 20 hours a day, children from 12 to 14 hours, and adults from 7 to 9 hours. Old people sometimes sleep no more than 5 hours at night because they take cat naps during the day.

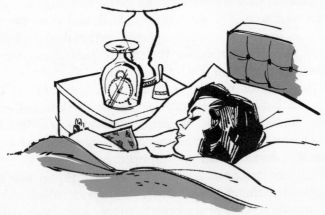

Sleep is nature's way of resting the mind and the body.

Because of the restorative nature of sleep, the number of hours a sick person sleeps should be recorded as accurately as possible. Too little sleep may be a result of discomfort or tension and should be noted. Information from the patient about his sleeping is not always reliable. When one is ill, a short period of wakefulness may seem much longer than it really is, especially at night when others in the household are asleep. The character of the sleep should be observed: whether the patient is quiet or restless, sleeps for short periods of time and wakes often, or sleeps unbrokenly for several hours. Naps also should be noted, because the person who naps during the day may not sleep as long at night as he ordinarily would.

General Malaise

A feeling of vague general discomfort, weakness, and fatigue is known as malaise. It may be present at the beginning of an illness and usually accompanies convalescence following a serious illness. At the start of an illness, malaise may be accompanied by such symptoms as headache, sore throat, and fever. Infection will often increase the feeling of exhaustion, which may be the result of toxins produced in the body by the infectious micro-organisms, for these poisons are more powerful than the body wastes accumulated during normal activity. Bed rest is essential when infection is present because fatigue lowers resistance to disease.

Another kind of physical fatigue occurs in the patient who is confined to bed for some time. Lack of exercise causes loss of muscle tone and strength, and it may take several days of activity before the feeling of weakness and fatigue disappears.

Children may show illness in much the same way as an adult or the onset of their illnesses may be entirely different. (See "The Sick Child," chapter 7, pages 108-110.) However, irritability, unwillingness to play, refusal of food, crying, and whining may be the child's way of showing malaise. The wise mother learns to know her children, for each child will be different in the way he behaves when he is ill. Children are sensitive to suggestion, and the mother who is apprehensive and alarmed creates similar feelings in the child. Asking a child if he has a pain in his ear, for example, may give him the idea that he is supposed to answer yes, and the attention he receives may be so gratifying that he feigns earache. Here again, common sense and judgment are invaluable assets for parents as well as for the home nurse.

Fever

Feeling chilly alternating with feeling hot may mean that fever is present. The skin may be hot and dry. Usually some loss of appetite, considerable thirst, and general discomfort accompany fever.

47

Fever is a sign that something is out of order in the body, although sometimes a person may be ill but still be without an elevation of temperature. A change from the normal body temperature has been used by doctors for years as a basis for judging whether a person is sick, for diagnosing and treating illness, and for noting the progress of the patient's recovery from illness. Frequently, one of the first questions asked when illness occurs will be, "What is the temperature?" It is therefore desirable for every family to own a clinical thermometer and to know how to use and care for it. (See "Care and Use of the Clinical Thermometer," chapter 12, pages 186-193.)

Usually the temperature is taken by mouth, although it may be taken in the rectum or in the axilla. For infants and very young children, for the unconscious, for very sick patients, and for those unable to keep the lips closed, either the rectal or the axillary method should be used.

Temperature should be taken:

• Whenever a person complains of feeling ill or shows signs of illness
• During illness, once or twice a day, at the same time each day, usually in the morning and evening or whenever the doctor orders (Temperature may be taken as often as every 4 hours or only once a week, depending on the condition and age of the patient.)
• Whenever there is a sudden change in the patient's condition, such as a chill, restlessness, or pain
• Whenever there is headache, pain in the chest or the abdomen, sore throat, chills, vomiting, diarrhea, or skin rash

Fever, in combination with the symptoms mentioned above, may mean the presence of serious illness or of conditions needing immediate attention. A person with a head cold or with a cough and who has a mouth temperature of more than 99.6° Fahrenheit should not go to work or to school but should remain at home away from others, preferably in bed. A person with a fever, together with other symptoms of illness, needs medical care.

Unless the doctor has requested it, the patient should not be awakened to have his temperature taken. For accuracy, there must be a wait of not less than 15 minutes between the time a temperature is taken and the time the patient has had a hot or a cold bath, has taken hot or cold food or drink, or has been smoking, because temperature in the mouth under these conditions will not be the same as the actual body temperature. After at least another 15 minutes the temperature should be taken again to verify the accuracy of the first thermometer reading. A rectal temperature is not to be taken immediately after an enema or when the rectum is full of fecal matter.

Pulse and Respiration

The pulse rate, even of persons in good health, varies with the individual. Age and sex account for some of the wide variations. A child's pulse rate, for example, is faster than that of an adult. The average rate for a man is about 70 beats per minute, while for a woman it may be as much as 90. The rate may increase for many reasons, such as fever, exercise, eating, fright, emotional tension, and extreme heat or cold. It decreases when a person is resting or asleep or is emotionally depressed.

The pulse may be felt most easily where a large artery is near the surface; this may be at the wrist, at the ankle, at the throat, or at the temple. The inner side of the wrist above the thumb is the place most often used to count the pulse because it is usually the most convenient. The pulse should be counted after the patient has been resting quietly, or if the patient is a child, when he is asleep. A watch or a clock with a second hand is needed to count the pulse.

Respiration is usually faster if the patient has a fever. Because the rate of breathing can be voluntarily controlled, the patient should not know that his respirations are being counted. In addition to the rate or number of times the patient breathes each minute, the doctor will want to know anything unusual about the respiration, such as difficult or painful breathing. (See "Counting Pulse and Respiration," chapter 12, pages 193-194.)

Pain

Pain is an important symptom in illness and should never be disregarded. *It is a warning that something is wrong.* Because pain cannot be measured, the home nurse or the doctor must rely entirely on the patient's description of its intensity. Some patients overemphasize minor pains, while others disregard severe ones. Some people have high pain thresholds and others have low ones, which means that different people can tolerate different degrees of pain. The aged, for example, are much less sensitive to pain than younger people; therefore, when they complain of pain, the complaint has great significance. Older people quite often have some degree of discomfort at all times and are inclined to minimize pain. The doctor must draw his own conclusions

49

about its significance after considering other symptoms and using his personal knowledge of the patient's behavior pattern. Frequently the alert home nurse has come to know the patient's habitual responses to pain and is well able to judge their significance. The report to the doctor should include the location, onset, and duration of the pain; when the pain is most severe; whether it is relieved or increased by physical acts, such as eating or changing position, or by a new interest; and the patient's description of the pain as dull or sharp, stabbing or throbbing, intermittent or continuous, slight or severe.

Pain in the abdomen or the stomach may be caused by improper eating or by food poisoning or it may be from appendicitis or some other acute and serious condition in the abdomen. Abdominal pain caused by poisoning from spoiled or contaminated food is commonly accompanied by nausea and vomiting and by diarrhea. If abdominal pain is not relieved promptly by rest and by withholding food, the patient should be seen by a doctor. *Do not give a laxative or an enema. Do not apply heat.* Abdominal pain accompanies so many serious conditions that it should always be reported to the doctor and the patient observed carefully.

Nausea and Vomiting

If nausea and vomiting are accompanied by severe cramps or abdominal pain, the doctor should be notified because the patient may have appendicitis, a bowel obstruction, or another serious illness. Vomiting, if caused by indigestion, tension, or mild food poisoning, usually brings its own relief. The color, general appearance, and amount of material vomited should be observed. If vomiting is continuous, severe, and accompanied by blood, either bright or dark red, or if the material has an offensive odor, a report should be made at once to the doctor and the vomitus saved for him to see.

Bowel Movements

In sickness the number and frequency of bowel movements and their color and consistency should be noted. The normal color of feces is brown or yellow and the consistency is somewhat soft. Changes in the consistency or in the color of the stool if continued for several movements or if accompanied by other symptoms should be noted and reported to the doctor. The stool should be saved for him to see. The doctor may order a laboratory examination of the stool to determine the cause of the illness. If the stool is found to be infectious it must be carefully disposed of to prevent the spread of the disease to other members of the family. The doctor will give instructions for its disposal.

Diarrhea, which is characterized by frequent watery or slimy stools, may be caused by an infection, by poisonous or undigested food, or by emotional strain. It is sometimes caused by a disease process in which there is irritation of the mucous membrane, as for example, colitis and cancer. In babies and small children, diarrhea is usually the result of improper feeding or of consuming unclean water, milk, or other food. Diarrhea is nature's effort to remove the substances that do not agree with a person after they have passed from the stomach into the intestines. It may have serious results because it exhausts the patient and dehydrates his body tissues. Severe or persistent diarrhea should be reported to the doctor. Widespread epidemics of this illness have been prevented by prompt diagnosis of individual cases.

First relief measures for both children and adults in severe cases of diarrhea are to withhold food and to give only boiled water until a diagnosis can be made and treatment instituted. After the diarrhea has stopped, a liquid or a soft diet should be given until bowel movements are again normal. The patient should be kept quietly in bed until all symptoms have subsided.

Urinary Disturbances

The inability to urinate, pain or burning sensation when voiding, incontinence, the presence of blood in the urine, and too frequent urination are all critical symptoms and as such should be considered danger signals. The amount of urine, whether more or less than usual as well as any change from the usual amber color and any deposit of sediment after the urine stands should be carefully noted.

SYMPTOMS OF MENTAL ILLNESS

The symptoms of mental ill health may be evident to both the sufferer and the observer, neither of whom, however, may recognize the signs as anything serious. Because the onset of symptoms may be insidious and change may occur gradually, true mental illness may be quite advanced before it is detected. For these reasons, and because mental illness requires tactful and skillful treatment, medical consultation should be sought as soon as any concern is felt about the behavior of the individual.

Undesirable behavior symptoms that should be a warning when

they continue are anxiety, depression, brooding, inability to concentrate, sleeplessness, and lack of interest in friends, family, job, or accustomed recreation. Obsessions or fixed ideas, fears that are baseless, headaches not attributable to usual causes, and physical complaints of an imaginary nature are rather common symptoms of mental illness. Other observable symptoms of mental ill health are oversensitivity, reluctance to mingle with others or to go to new places, confusion as to one's identity or that of others in the family or to one's surroundings, recurrent daydreams or hallucinations of an impossible nature, and resentment toward a person without apparent cause. Any suicidal threat is an undesirable behavior symptom that should never be disregarded.

Some mental conditions of temporary nature, disappearing as the patient recovers, may accompany illness or result from the use of certain medications. The mental condition of the patient who has a high fever or of one who has a severe infection of any kind should be carefully watched. The very ill patient may become delirious (a temporary state of mental excitement) or he may become disoriented (not know where he is) and try to get out of bed. Because such a patient is not responsible for what he may do, he should never be left alone. The elderly patient, especially, may be confused, delirious, or disoriented because of medications that have been given. Sedative drugs are particularly likely to cause such symptoms.

It is believed that many types of mental illness are buried deep in the patient's past experiences and that the causes usually date back to the person's early childhood and his relationships with his parents. It is not always possible to understand fully the deep-seated causes without long treatment, and the family doctor or the psychiatrist needs the cooperation of the family in learning all he can about the patient. Attitudes of others toward the patient are particularly important in the treatment of mental disorders. Fortunately, mental illness and emotional disturbances are recognized as health problems that can be treated.

The line dividing the mentally well from the mentally ill is a fragile one, and it is not readily discernible because there are many degrees of mental health and many causes for mental ill health. Everyone at some time exhibits unhealthy behavior traits, but most people are able to get along with most others most of the time without undue guilt feelings and can meet the problems of everyday living. (See "Mental and Emotional Attitudes," chapter 8, pages 126-128.)

REPORTING SYMPTOMS TO THE DOCTOR

In reporting symptoms to the doctor, the home nurse should describe the character of the illness, the complaints of the patient, and her observations on the following signs and symptoms:

- The degree of severity, the duration, and the location of any pain and how the pain is affected by a change in body position or by eating. The pain may be a dull ache or it may be acute, shooting, or stabbing
- The temperature and the pulse rate
- The location, color, and amount of any bleeding
- The color and character of the stools, the vomitus, the sputum, the urine, or other body discharges. If a discharge is unusual in appearance, a sample should be saved in a covered container for the doctor to examine
- The patient's behavior, how he says he feels, and the length of time any unfavorable condition has been noticeable
- Any other unusual condition noted, such as a rash, a discoloration of the skin, or a swelling of any part of the body
- Any first aid or treatment given to relieve the patient

SUGGESTED STUDENT ACTIVITIES

1. Practice taking the temperature, the pulse, and the respiration of a friend or a classmate for 1 week. Keep a record and then plot the data on a graph. What do you notice?

2. Weigh yourself at the same time each week for 1 month. What does your weight record show?

3. Describe how you feel when you are angry. How can anger affect physical health?

4. Consult books from a library and prepare a paper on the functions of the skin.

5. List several factors that may cause fatigue. Why is exercise, either mental or physical, that is extended to the point of fatigue a poor practice?

6. With another student, role play the following situation for the class: You are a mother, and your classmate is a babysitter who has not been in your home or with your children. What signs of illness do you consider are important enough that you would want her to telephone you? Give her the necessary instructions.

7. Discuss ways in which an infant or an adult shows that he has pain. Cite examples in your own experience that show the significance and the importance of pain.

5

ILLNESS AND INFECTION

Fears and superstitions about the cause of illness have ancient roots, but the prevention of illness is a relatively modern concept. It is becoming more and more apparent that prevention of disease, both the common communicable diseases and the degenerative diseases of old age, depends primarily on the efforts of the individual to protect and to promote his own health.

Today more than ever before medical science knows what causes illness. Through research and experimentation, ways have been found to prevent, alleviate, and cure many diseases, and this knowledge has brought many changes in the treatment of illness and infection. Advances have been made especially in treating the acute communicable diseases, many of which are rapidly made noninfectious by drug therapy. Thus, periods of illness are shortened and the possibility of infection caused by exposure to the patient is reduced.

Along with modern measures in effect to prevent and control the spread of disease are some centuries-old ones that have been retained because of their effectiveness—for example, quarantine and community sanitation, which are mentioned in the Bible. Because most infection is spread from person to person, control is most effective when the infected person protects others by simple measures of personal hygiene. Hand-washing, covering the mouth and nose when coughing or sneezing, and the safe disposal of secretions from the nose and mouth are easy but very effective safeguards to others. A chart will be found at the end of this chapter with detailed information about many of the communicable diseases prevalent in this country. The chart presents factual information in brief form about the way the listed communicable diseases are spread, how they may be prevented, and some of their symptoms and possible complications.

HOW INFECTION IS TRANSMITTED

Organisms that cause disease may enter the body either directly by way of contaminated water or foods, or by being breathed in with air containing bacteria-laden dust, or indirectly through contact with material contaminated by body discharges. Every communicable disease comes from a person, an insect, or an animal capable of spreading infection directly or indirectly. Infected wounds and the discharges of the nose, the mouth, the bowels, and occasionally the bladder may carry disease germs. In some diseases the infection is carried in the blood stream. Milk that has not been pasteurized or boiled may transfer such diseases as undulant fever and tuberculosis. The bite of an infected flea may cause plague, while the sting of an infected mosquito may cause malaria and the bite of an infected animal may cause rabies.

Infection can also be transferred by a human carrier, a well person who carries the agent of disease in his body but who has no apparent symptoms of the disease himself. Such a person may have had the disease at some previous time and have recovered or he may be suffering from a mild form of the disease without showing the characteristic symptoms. The diseases most often carried in this way are diphtheria, scarlet fever, typhoid fever, and epidemic diarrhea of the newborn. The human carrier serves as a host to the disease-causing organisms that have taken up temporary or permanent residence in his body and are harmless to him because his body defenses are able to keep them under control. It is the transfer to another person who has no immunity and whose body defenses may be less able to ward off illness that makes the carrier of disease a public health menace.

Since disease germs can live indefinitely in the mucous membranes of the nose and the throat or in the intestinal tract of healthy people and may be harmful if transferred to others, everyone should consider himself a possible carrier and should develop health habits that protect himself and those about him. Young children and sick or aged people, who may not have the ability to resist disease, are especially in need of protection.

The regular observance of simple personal hygiene practices, such as bathing, getting enough rest and sleep, and eating adequate amounts of body-building and protective foods, strengthens body resistance and lessens the danger of infection and disease.

55

Good hygiene habits are more than good manners; they are an obligation to one's family and one's community.

When a person coughs or sneezes and sprays the discharges from his nose and throat into the air, or even when he talks and laughs, tiny droplets of saliva are expelled. Another person who is near enough may become ill if he breathes in the droplets of infectious material. Some disease organisms die quickly when exposed to light and air, while others may live indefinitely, even through a drying process. A person should hold a handkerchief or tissue over both his nose and his mouth when sneezing or coughing. If the sneeze comes unexpectedly before he can cover his nose and mouth, he should turn his head away from other people. A person should not stand close to someone else when talking or laughing. Droplets from an explosive laugh or sneeze may carry 6 or 8 feet; they cannot be escaped at 12 inches. Coughing and sneezing are the most common ways of spreading communicable diseases.

Because the hands are in frequent contact with the nose and the mouth, they are often a means of carrying germs from one person to another. Using another person's drinking glass or eating from his fork or spoon, sharing foods, such as an ice cream cone, an apple, or a lollipop, and kissing are especially dangerous practices in spreading disease. Little children should be taught health practices early, particularly the importance of hand-washing, keeping the hands away from the face, and using a handkerchief.

As protection against communicable diseases, everyone should carry out the following precautions:

- Avoid contact with people who are suffering from communicable diseases.
- Use disposable handkerchiefs that can be safely destroyed after use, especially with a cold, a discharging nose, or a cough.
- Cover the nose and the mouth when coughing or sneezing.
- Keep the hands away from the face, especially the mouth and the nose. Turn the head to avoid droplets if someone coughs or sneezes.
- Always wash the hands before eating and before preparing or handling food, after handling soiled articles, and after going to the toilet.
- Wash the hands before and after giving care to a sick person to avoid carrying disease to or from the patient.
- Keep personal articles, such as toothbrushes, hairbrushes, and combs, clean and reserved for one person's use.
- Use safe water, milk, and other foods. Keep milk and perishable

foods refrigerated. Cover unrefrigerated foods to keep them clean.

- Use clean glasses, dishes, and eating utensils and do not touch the parts that come in contact with the mouth, such as the rims of cups and glasses, the bowls of spoons, and the tines of forks.
- Make every effort to maintain health at a high level by eating the right kind and quantity of food and by getting an adequate amount of sleep, rest, sunshine, fresh air, and exercise.
- Obtain protection against the diseases for which there are known immunizing agents.
- Treat with suspicion any illness that starts with such symptoms as headache, fever, nausea, sore throat, discharging eyes or nose, stiff neck, sneezing, aching, and a feeling of being "all in."

Many of these symptoms are common in cases of communicable disease. If they occur, keep the person away from others, put him to bed if possible, and have him see a doctor if the symptoms do not abate promptly.

PROTECTION AGAINST COMMUNICABLE DISEASE

Human beings are not susceptible to some diseases caused by organisms that affect other animals because the human body does not provide the proper environment for the growth of such organisms. The resistance that man has to these diseases is called *natural* resistance. The newborn infant may be naturally immune to some diseases for some time after birth, depending in part on whether the mother has immunity or is resistant to the diseases.

Another kind of resistance or protection is developed by frequent exposure to disease germs or by exposure to small numbers of germs over a long period of time. This is the kind of resistance that some adults have built up against diseases that are common among children. It is known as *acquired* resistance.

It is well known that people develop immunity to some diseases by having the disease itself. This immunity varies from one person to another, in some cases lasting a relatively short time and in others for a lifetime. An attack of whooping cough or smallpox usually makes an individual immune to that disease for life, although second attacks do sometimes occur. This is known as *active* immunity and is the result of the body defenses producing specific substances in the blood serum known as antibodies, which act to overcome the disease-causing microbe and its products. Some diseases, particularly the streptococcal infections, produce toxins (powerful poisons) that are absorbed into the blood stream. The body defenses produce an antitoxin, which is a type of antibody but specific to only the one disease that it is combatting.

Gamma globulin is a protein blood fraction that carries antibodies. It is sometimes used to provide *passive* immunity. Because gamma globulin acts quickly, it is given after a known exposure to disease, but protection lasts only a short time, generally from a few weeks to a few months. It is used for protection against measles, for protection after exposure to infectious hepatitis, and after exposure to or during an epidemic of poliomyelitis.

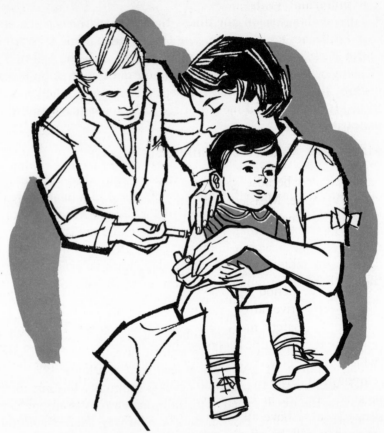

Protect children against the diseases for which there are known immunizing agents.

Another way to obtain protection against certain communicable diseases is by *artificial* immunity or protection. Scientists, in addition to discovering how the body defends itself by the production of antibodies, have discovered additional ways to protect against disease. The way in which smallpox is controlled is a case in point. Successful vaccination against smallpox will usually provide protection for several years but should be repeated at intervals. If given during infancy, it is usually repeated before the child enters school. Some universities and colleges require vaccination again before entrance, and it is done routinely upon induction to the armed forces. Many countries require arriving travelers to present evidence of a recent smallpox vaccination or of a previous attack of smallpox. The fact that the United States is among these countries means that almost without exception all people from the United States who travel outside the country (except to U.S. territories and possessions and Canada) are vaccinated against smallpox before their departure. Presence of a vaccination scar is not evidence of permanent immunity, and a second "take" produces a second vaccination mark. Because immunity does not last, a person should be protected by revaccination when indicated.

The need for immunization of very young children against communicable diseases is great because the death rate and the incidence of complications within this age group is high. Doctors advise that infants be protected against smallpox, diphtheria, poliomyelitis, whooping cough, measles, and tetanus during their early months because any natural immunity or resistance is lost after this time. Measles vaccine has only recently been tested, approved, and made available. Many doctors advise routine protection against other diseases also, such as scarlet fever and typhoid fever. In addition, booster doses of some immunizing agents are given at specified times on the advice of the doctor.

Because a period of time is required for the immunization to become effective after vaccination or inoculation, it is a preventive and safety measure to have children protected routinely and not to wait until they have been exposed to a disease against which they could have acquired immunity. It cannot be overemphasized that the precautionary measures that are available against diseases in every community in this country should be carried out. Above all, *immunizations should be kept current* so that they will be effective when they are needed to protect the individual against communicable disease. When an emergency occurs, immunizing materials may not be available, and there may be no authorized person to administer them. Immunization should be done early; after exposure may be too late.

The immunization schedule that follows is based on current practice and recommendations of the American Academy of Pediatrics and the Public Health Service and is presented as a guide.

SUGGESTED IMMUNIZATION SCHEDULE

Disease	6 weeks to 2 months	Months			Years							
		3	4	12	2	4	6	8	10	12	14	16
Diphtheria [a]	x	x	x	x	x			x [b]		x [b]		x [b]
Pertussis [a]	x	x	x	x	x							
Tetanus [a]	x	x	x	x	x			x [b]		x [b]		x [b]
Smallpox [c]				x		x						
Poliomyelitis [a] (See Note)	x [d]	x [d]	x [d]	x [d]	x [d]	x	x [d]	x	x	x	x	x

[a] May be given separately or together.
[b] Persons 8 years of age and over should receive "adult type" antigen.
[c] Revaccination is recommended every 5 years, before going abroad, and in the presence of an epidemic.
[d] Immunization schedule for the use of inactivated vaccine, recommended by the Surgeon General's Committee on Poliomyelitis Control, January 1961.
Note. Oral poliovaccines, such as the Sabin vaccine, have been approved after extensive investigation. They are available and may be used in place of inactivated vaccines, such as the Salk vaccine. The interval between administration and subsequent booster doses is determined by the doctor.

CARE OF THE PATIENT WITH A COMMUNICABLE DISEASE

The nursing care of the patient with a communicable disease does not differ from that given any patient. The extra burden for the home nurse is in preventing the spread of the infection to other members of the family and in protecting the patient against other infection. In most instances all of the family has been exposed to the disease before a diagnosis has been made, so that isolation (separation from others) of the patient is of limited value. This is especially true of the acute communicable diseases, which are of relatively short duration and are usually most infectious during the onset of illness and before the appearance of recognizable symptoms.

The length and type of illness will largely determine what special protective measures to take. In general, communicable diseases are transmitted by discharges from the nose and throat and the intestinal tract or from open lesions of the skin. Direct contact with discharges from the patient is the greatest source of danger. Therefore, the safe handling and disposal of all body discharges is of primary importance in preventing the spread of the disease. The care of dishes and linens is of less importance, because the usual methods of cleaning them by washing, rinsing, and drying will probably eliminate most of the danger of transmitting infection.

If at all possible, the patient with a communicable disease should have his own room so that he can be kept away from others. The

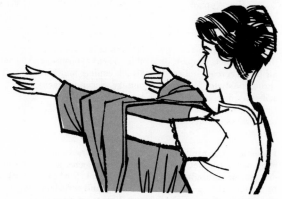

Slip the arms into a pinafore apron without touching the inside of the garment.

person taking care of him should wear a coverall apron, which can be removed when leaving the room. Strict observance of hand-washing after caring for the patient or after handling of soiled articles or body discharges is essential to safety. If other precautions are necessary, the doctor will give specific instructions.

Although it is almost impossible to carry out strict isolation techniques in the home, exposure of the family should be as limited as possible. The safety measures to be observed are:

- Keep the patient away from others if at all possible, either by keeping him in his own room or by placing a screen around him.
- Wash the hands before and after caring for the patient, using soap, running water, and friction.
- Wear a coverall apron when giving care to the patient and re-move it when leaving the patient.
- Provide the patient with tissues for nose and throat discharge and a waste container for soiled tissues.
- Dispose of waste materials *immediately* by burning or by some other acceptable method.
- Handle soiled articles as little as possible. Whenever possible, use tongs, a snap clothespin, or a piece of paper to pick them up.
- Keep the patient's personal articles, such as toothbrush and towels, separate from those of other people.
- Use disposable dishes and other utensils.

CHART OF SELECTED COMMUNICABLE DISEASES

To prevent the spread of infection, any person suspected of having a communicable disease should be kept away from others. Measures for the control of communicable diseases are established either

Disease	How Spread	Prevention	How Long From Exposure to Onset
Chickenpox (Varicella)	From person to person by direct contact, droplet, or air-borne spread; indirectly through articles freshly soiled by discharges from the skin and mucous membranes of infected persons.	No immunization available. Avoid exposure; one attack confers long immunity. Second attacks are rare.	2 to 3 weeks, commonly 13 to 17 days.
Common Cold	Presumably transmission is by direct contact or by droplet spread; indirectly by handkerchiefs, eating utensils, or other articles freshly soiled by discharges from the nose and mouth of infected persons.	No specific prevention. Personal hygiene, as covering mouth when coughing and sneezing and disposal of nose and mouth secretions.	12 to 72 hours, usually about 24 hours.
Diphtheria	Contact with a patient or a carrier or with articles soiled with discharges and secretions from mucous surfaces of nose and throat and from skin and other lesions. Milk has served as a vehicle.	Inoculation with diphtheria toxoid series in early infancy (2 to 6 months of age) with "booster" dose 3 to 12 months later; reinforcing doses essential in preschool life, desirable on entrance to school, and elective in later life. Give exposed adults Schick test to determine susceptibility before immunization. Second attacks are possible.	2 to 5 days, sometimes longer.
Dysentery (Shigellosis)	By eating contaminated foods or drinking contaminated water or milk and by hand-to-mouth transfer of contaminated material; by flies; by objects soiled with stools of a patient or a carrier.	No immunization. Avoidance of known sources of infection; personal cleanliness; good sanitation.	1 to 7 days, usually less than 4 days.
Gonorrhea	Almost wholly by sexual intercourse. In the newborn, by transfer from the mother during birth.	No immunization. Avoidance of contact; use of prophylactic drugs in the eyes of the newborn. One attack does not protect against subsequent infection.	Usually 3 to 9 days, sometimes longer.

by law or by regulation in the various states and communities. Every individual is responsible for cooperating with local health authorities in preventing the spread of disease.

Common Symptoms	How Long Communicable	Some Possible Complications
Acute onset, with slight fever. Small reddish pimples followed or accompanied by blisters, usually more abundant on the covered than on the exposed parts of the body, that cause itching.	Probably not more than 1 day before or more than 6 days after rash (eruption) appears. One of the most contagious of the communicable diseases.	Complications rare. Skin lesions may become infected and may leave pitted scars.
Tickling, dry sensation in the throat; rarely fever; malaise; chilliness; cough and runny nose.	1 day before onset and about 5 days afterward.	Sinusitis; bronchitis; laryngitis; pneumonia; middle ear infection.
Inflammation of the nose, throat, and tonsils, with grayish white patches in the throat; an acute infection accompanied by fever.	Variable; until the germs have disappeared from secretions and lesions; usually 2 weeks or less, seldom more than 4 weeks.	Damage to the heart; pneumonia.
Frequent stools; abdominal cramps; fever.	As long as the stools contain the infecting agent as shown by laboratory tests; sometimes several weeks.	Often recurs. Rarely fatal.
Thick, yellow, purulent discharge from mucous membranes of the genital tract or of the eyes; usually burning and pain on urination.	For months or years unless treated with specific drug therapy, which ends communicability within hours or days.	Few complications when treated early. Can cause sterility, pelvic inflammatory disease, and blindness.

Disease	How Spread	Prevention	How Long From Exposure to Onset
Hepatitis, Infectious	Probably through intimate person-to-person contact; respiratory spread possible; also through transfusion of whole blood, blood serum, or plasma; by contamination of syringes and needles with traces of blood from such persons; contaminated water, food, and milk.	Good sanitation and personal hygiene, with particular emphasis on disposal of stools; proper technical procedures to prevent transmission by blood or blood products; administration of immune serum globulin to contacts.	Variable; from 10 to 40 days, commonly 25 days.
Impetigo Contagiosa	By direct contact with moist discharges of skin lesions or indirect contact with articles recently soiled with discharges; also, contact with others whose skins, noses, or throats are contaminated or infected.	No immunization. Reinfection possible.	From 2 to 5 days, occasionally longer.
Influenza	By direct contact, through droplet spread, or by articles freshly soiled with nose and throat discharges of infected persons.	Immunity to a specific influenza virus may last for several years after attack, but because there are many strains of influenza viruses, there may be frequent attacks of the disease. Vaccines are effective when they closely match the prevailing strain of virus. Inoculation after exposure is useless.	24 to 72 hours.
Measles, German or 3-day (Rubella)	By droplet spread or direct contact with infected persons; indirect contact with articles freshly soiled with discharges from nose and throat.	Immune serum globulin (gamma globulin) provides irregular protection; recommended for adult female contacts with no history of having had rubella who are within first 4 months of pregnancy. Deliberate exposure of girls in good health before puberty recommended by some authorities.	14 to 21 days, usually 18 days.

Common Symptoms	How Long Communicable	Some Possible Complications
Fever; loss of appetite; nausea; malaise; and abdominal discomfort; usually followed by jaundice.	Unknown; possibly several months. Greatest communicability from a few days before to a few days after onset, usually not exceeding 7 days.	Fatal cases rare. Relapses may occur, or the disease may become chronic, resulting in liver damage.
Blisters, which later become crusted, commonly on face and hands.	As long as the sores are unhealed.	Occasional secondary infection of the sores.
Sudden onset; fever for 1 to 6 days; chills; discomfort; aches or pains in back, legs, or shoulders; sore throat; runny nose; cough.	Probably limited to a brief period before onset and 1 week after.	Pneumonia. Deaths concentrated among the old, especially those with long-term illness, among women in late pregnancy, among infants, and among those whose acute illness is neglected.
Few symptoms; mild cold symptoms may be present. Slight fever; almost always enlargement of lymph nodes behind the ears and back of neck; rash that may resemble that of measles or scarlet fever.	For at least 4 days from onset of cold symptoms and probably not much longer, the exact period unknown. Highly communicable.	Usually none; serious for women during early pregnancy; may cause congenital defects in the baby if the mother contracts disease during early pregnancy.

Chart of Selected Communicable Diseases (continued)

Disease	How Spread	Prevention	How Long From Exposure to Onset
Measles (Rubeola)	By droplet spread or direct contact with infected persons; indirectly through articles freshly soiled with nose and throat secretion; in some instances probably airborne.	Experimental measles vaccines are under study. No immunization at present. Administration of gamma globulin within 3 days after first exposure will prevent the disease in most instances and modify it in others. One attack usually confers immunity. Babies of immune mothers usually immune during first few months of life.	About 10 days from exposure to initial fever; about 14 days until rash appears; as long as 21 days if gamma globulin or convalescent serum has been given.
Meningitis, Meningococcal (Cerebrospinal Fever)	By direct contact with infected persons; droplet spread; human carriers.	No immunization. Avoid contact with infected persons and droplet spread. Prevent overcrowded living conditions; stress personal cleanliness.	Varies from 2 to 10 days, commonly 3 to 4 days.
Mononucleosis, Infectious	Unknown, but believed to be from person to person by way of nose and mouth discharges.	No immunization; the degree of immunity conferred by an attack is unknown.	Unknown, seemingly varies from 4 to 14 or more days.
Mumps	By droplet spread or direct contact with infected persons; indirectly through articles freshly soiled with the saliva of such persons.	Effective vaccines available but of limited value because immunity probably does not exceed 2 years. Vaccine has value in selected groups of susceptibles, for example, the military.	From 12 to 26 days, commonly 18 days.

Common Symptoms	How Long Communicable	Some Possible Complications
Fever, runny eyes and nose, and eruption in the mouth, followed by a characteristic dusky-red, blotchy rash on the face, body, and extremities.	During period of runny eyes and nose; usually about 9 days, and from 4 days before to 5 days after rash appears.	Middle ear infection; pneumonia. Infants and children under 3 years of age are particularly susceptible.
An acute bacterial infection with sudden onset, fever, intense headache, nausea and vomiting; frequently a rash of small, round, purplish-red spots; dizziness, stiff neck, delirium, and coma.	Until germs are no longer present in discharges from nose and throat of infected persons. Usually disappears in 24 hours after appropriate treatment.	Spread of the infection to the brain tissue; pneumonia; middle ear infection; mastoiditis; chronic heart damage.
An acute infection with varying symptoms. Onset may be gradual or abrupt. Loss of appetite; irritability; nausea and vomiting; sleepiness; chills; fever; enlarged lymph glands of the neck; enlarged spleen; in some cases a rash or jaundice. Symptoms may subside in a few days or last for months.	Undetermined.	Pus may form in glands; nephritis; meningitis, or encephalitis. Prognosis is excellent; death rarely occurs.
An acute viral infection with sudden onset, fever, swelling, and tenderness of the salivary glands.	From about 7 days before distinctive symptoms and persisting as much as 9 days thereafter, or until swelling of the glands has disappeared.	Inflammation of the ovaries or testicles in adults; middle ear infection and sometimes permanent deafness. Meningitis or encephalitis is common. Children under 12 usually free from complications.

Chart of Selected Communicable Diseases *(continued)*

Disease	How Spread	Prevention	How Long From Exposure to Onset
Poliomyelitis	By direct contact or droplet spread of nose and throat secretions of infected persons; stools of infected persons; contaminated milk.	Active immunization by inoculation of Salk vaccine or by administration of oral vaccine reduces the risk of paralytic disease and increases resistance to infection. Passive protection with gamma globulin may prevent only an occasional case in an exposed family; in instances of known single exposure, may have considerable value if given within 2 days after exposure. Immunization of infants can begin at 2 months of age. Second attacks are rare and presumably due to infection with a different type of poliovirus.	From 3 to 21 days, commonly 7 to 12 days.
Rheumatic Fever	Unknown; attacks are usually precipitated by streptococcal infection.	No immunization; disease recurs. Individuals known to have had rheumatic fever or convalescing from that disease should receive prophylactic drugs for long periods thereafter to prevent recurrence.	Symptoms appear about 2 to 3 weeks following a streptococcal infection.
Ringworm	Direct contact with infected persons or animals, especially dogs, cats, or cattle. Sources of infection are such materials as the backs of theater seats, barber clippers, hats, or clothing contaminated with hair from infected animals or persons.	No immunization; repeated attacks are common. Effective control of animal ringworm is essential in control of infection in man.	10 to 14 days.

Common Symptoms	How Long Communicable	Some Possible Complications
An acute illness, with fever, malaise, headache, and stiffness of neck and back. Temporary or permanent paralysis may occur.	Greatest in late incubation and early days of acute illness, virus being present in throat secretions and feces; persists in feces for 3 to 6 weeks, but spread of infection after the acute stage is rare.	Pregnant women are highly susceptible. Paralysis of varying severity of affected parts of the body.
Fever, rapid pulse, unexplainable nosebleeds, pallor, loss of appetite, weight loss or failure to gain weight, fatigue, restless sleep. Heat, swelling, and tenderness of joints with pain on movement.	Not known to be communicable; the associated streptococcal infection has usually become non-communicable by the time rheumatic fever develops.	Serious damage to the heart.
Infection begins as a small pimple and spreads outwards, leaving scaly patches of baldness on the scalp. On the body, infection shows a characteristic ring-shaped lesion. On the feet, there is scaling or cracking of the skin, especially between the toes, or blisters containing a thin watery fluid.	As long as lesions are present and live spores are present on contaminated materials.	Occasional secondary infection of the lesions.

Chart of Selected Communicable Diseases *(continued)*

Disease	How Spread	Prevention	How Long From Exposure to Onset
Scabies (Itch)	By direct contact and from undergarments or sheets freshly contaminated by infected persons.	Avoid contact with infected persons; cleanliness of body, garments, and bedclothes.	1 to 2 days; several days or even weeks may elapse before itching is noticed.
Scarlet Fever*	Contact with acutely ill or convalescent patients or carriers. Discharges from nose, throat, or purulent lesions; objects contaminated with such discharges. An outbreak may follow the ingestion of contaminated food or milk.	No immunization; avoid contact with infected persons. Pasteurization of milk.	Usually 2 to 5 days.
Smallpox	Contact with persons sick with the disease. Contact need not be intimate; airborne transmission may occur over short distances. Spread by nose and throat discharges or by material from skin lesions.	Vaccination at about 3 months of age and on entering school; when faced with unusual exposure, as in travel to regions where disease is prevalent; when exposed to disease. Revaccination is recommended every 5 years.	From 7 to 16 days, commonly 12 days.
Syphilis	By direct contact (sexual intercourse, kissing, fondling of children) during primary and secondary syphilis. Source of infection is exudated from early lesions of skin or mucous membrane of infected persons. An infected woman may transmit syphilis to her unborn child.	No immunization; one attack does not confer immunity. Best measures are health and sex education, preparation for marriage, premarital and prenatal examinations as part of general physical examination.	10 days to 10 weeks, usually 3 weeks.

* Scarlet fever and streptococcal sore throat, erysipelas, puerperal fever, cellulitis, mastoiditis, osteomyelitis, otitismedia, peritonitis, and various skin and wound infec-

Common Symptoms	How Long Communicable	Some Possible Complications
Penetration of the skin visible as pimples and blisters or as tiny linear burrows containing the female mite and her eggs. Primary symptom is itching at site of lesions, especially at night. Lesions commonly occur on finger webs, inner surface of wrists, the elbows, axillas, around the waist, and lower portion of the buttocks.	Until mites and eggs are destroyed by treatment.	Occasional secondary infection of the lesions.
Acute onset with high fever, sore throat, strawberry tongue, nausea and vomiting; fine rash, which blanches on pressure, appears on neck and chest in about 24 hours. When the rash subsides, the skin begins to peel; in severe cases, the hair may be shed.	In uncomplicated cases, during incubation and illness, approximately 10 days. In untreated cases, from 2 to 3 weeks; for months in carriers. Adequate treatment eliminates possibility of transmission within 24 hours.	Middle ear infection; damage to the heart and kidneys; inflammation of the glands in the neck is common.
Sudden onset with fever, chills, headache, severe backache, and prostration. Temperature falls in 3 to 4 days and rash appears, finally forming scabs that fall off in about 3 weeks.	From first symptoms to disappearance of all scabs and crusts, usually 2 to 3 weeks. Most communicable in early stage of the disease.	Secondary infection of the skin with subsequent septicemia; pneumonia; laryngitis; pleurisy; emphysema (air in tissues); middle ear infection; occasionally kidney damage.
Primary lesion (chancre) at the point of contact, which will heal without treatment; a secondary eruption involving skin and mucous membranes; latent period may last for years with occasional relapses and appearance of lesions. In congenital syphilis, only the late manifestations, such as the listed complications occur.	Variable and not definitely known. Adequate treatment usually ends infectivity within 24 hours.	Sterility; abortion or miscarriage; damage to the heart; blindness; deafness; paralysis; insanity.

tions are all caused by the same strain of Group A hemolytic streptococci. The same principles of control hold generally for the group.

Chart of Selected Communicable Diseases *(continued)*

Disease	How Spread	Prevention	How Long From Exposure to Onset
Tetanus (Lockjaw)	Tetanus spores, found in soil, street dust, and animal and human feces, enter the body through injury, usually a puncture wound. These spores may also enter the body through burns and trivial or unnoticed wounds.	Routine immunization with tetanus toxoid in infancy and early childhood, with reinforcing doses at intervals no longer than 5 years. An attack does not confer immunity. In the absence of active immunization, tetanus antitoxin provides passive protection to injured persons.	Commonly 4 days to 3 weeks; longer periods have been noted.
Tuberculosis (Pulmonary)	Infection usually results from continued and intimate exposure to infected persons with active disease. Coughing or sneezing by a patient whose sputum contains the tubercle bacillus releases a cloud of highly infectious droplets. Bovine tuberculosis transmitted by ingestion of unpasteurized dairy products from infected cows.	Isolation and treatment of active cases; examination of contacts and suspects; X-ray screening of adults in communities where the frequency of tuberculosis is known to be excessive; pasteurization of milk and the elimination of tuberculosis among dairy cattle; BCG vaccination for uninfected persons subject to unavoidable, heavy exposure.	From infection to primary phase lesions, about 4 to 6 weeks; from infection to progressive pulmonary tuberculosis may be years, with first 6 to 12 months most hazardous.
Tularemia (Rabbit Fever)	By bite of infected flies or ticks; by handling infected animals; or by fluids from infected insects or animals; by ingestion of insufficiently cooked rabbit meat; drinking contaminated water.	Killed vaccines are of limited value. Avoid bites of flies and ticks and handling animals in areas where disease is prevalent. Avoid drinking raw water where disease prevails among wild animals. Permanent immunity usually follows recovery.	From 24 hours to 10 days, usually 3 days.
Typhoid Fever	Direct or indirect contact with infected persons or carriers. Principal vehicles of spread are water and food contaminated with feces or urine of infected persons. Contamination is usually by hands of a carrier or of an undiagnosed case. Flies may also play a part in spread.	Immunization with typhoid vaccine; periodic reinforcing injections desirable, commonly once in 3 years. A high degree of immunity usually follows recovery from the disease.	Variable; average 2 weeks; usual range 1 to 3 weeks.

Common Symptoms	How Long Communicable	Some Possible Complications
Painful muscular contractions of neck, jaw, and trunk muscles. Stiffness increases until jaws become locked; the head is drawn backward. Slight stimulation of patient causes convulsions and extreme pain. Usually low fever; difficulty in swallowing and breathing is common.	Not directly transmissible from person to person.	Rare under proper treatment and prevention; probably fatal if not treated promptly.
Primary infection usually goes undetected, but resembles the common cold. Course of disease varies widely. Earliest symptoms usually fatigue, weight loss, loss of appetite, chronic cough, fever, night sweats.	As long as tubercle bacilli are being discharged by the patient. Commences when a lung lesion becomes open and continues until healed or death occurs. Some patients intermittently infectious for years. Coughing habits and hygienic practices of patient influence his degree of infectiousness.	Pleurisy, with or without effusion; meningitis; infection of gastrointestinal tract when sputum is swallowed; infection of the lymph system; rectal fistulae and abscesses; tuberculosis of the kidney.
Nausea and vomiting; chills; fever; an ulcer usually appears at the site of infection and lymph glands in the area become tender, swollen, and commonly suppurate. Acute symptoms subside in 2 to 3 weeks, but recovery may take 2 to 3 months.	Under natural conditions not directly transmissible from person to person. Infectious agent may be found in the blood of man during the first 2 weeks of the disease and in lesions up to a month and some times longer.	Pneumonia; meningitis; encephalitis.
Fever; headache; constipation more commonly than diarrhea; abdominal tenderness and distention; rose spots on the trunk.	As long as typhoid bacilli appear in excreta; usually from second week throughout convalescence; thereafter variable. From 2 to 5 percent of patients become permanent carriers.	Hemorrhage or perforation of the intestine; peritonitis; blood clot in a vein; early heart failure; bedsores; bronchitis and pneumonia.

Chart of Selected Communicable Diseases *(continued)*

Disease	How Spread	Prevention	How Long From Exposure to Onset
Undulant Fever (Brucellosis)	Contact with infected animals, animal tissues, or secretions, and by ingestion of milk or dairy products from infected animals.	Immunization by vaccination not widely accepted; its effect is controversial. Search for and elimination of infected animals, meat inspection, and pasteurization of milk and dairy products are common preventive measures.	Highly variable and difficult to ascertain; usually 5 to 21 days; occasionally several months.
Whooping Cough (Pertussis)	By direct contact with infected persons, by droplet spread, or indirectly by contact with articles freshly soiled with discharges from the nose and throat.	Immunization of all susceptible preschool children. Vaccines may be used alone or in combination with diphtheria and tetanus toxoid. Immunization can be started at 1 to 2 months of age. A single reinforcing dose at 1 to 2 and again at 4 to 5 years of age; and additionally if there is a known, direct contact with a case in the family.	Commonly 7 days; almost uniformly within 10 days and not exceeding 21 days.

SUGGESTED STUDENT ACTIVITIES

1. Draw a floor plan of your own bedroom. Suggest any changes that could be made easily if the bedroom were to be used for a sick room.

2. If possible, arrange to visit a hospital and observe methods used to sterilize instruments and dressings. Report your observations to the class.

3. List several communicable diseases, giving their symptoms and treatments. Why is it important to have some knowledge of the different types of communicable diseases?

4. Compare your immunization record with that suggested in this chapter. Are there any deficiencies in your protection? If so,

Common Symptoms	How Long Communicable	Some Possible Complications
Onset may be acute or gradual, with fever, headache, weakness, profuse sweating, chills, and generalized aching. The disease may last for several days, many months, or occasionally for several years. Recovery is usual, but disability is often pronounced.	Rarely communicable from man to man; the infectious agent may be discharged in urine and other excretions for long periods of time.	Heart damage; chronic arthritis; pneumonia; habitual or occasional abortion; mastitis; inflammation of the ovaries in women, of the testes in men.
Acute bacterial infection involving the respiratory tract, and characterized by a typical "whooping" cough, lasting 1 to 2 months. Beginning symptoms like those of the common cold.	From 7 days after exposure to 3 weeks after onset of typical paroxysmal cough.	Pneumonia is usually the chief cause of death from this disease; bronchiectasis; emphysema; middle ear disease; brain damage; hernia; convulsions.

discuss them with your physician and get his recommendations. Outline the plan for your protection suggested by your physician.

5. If you have access to a microscope, look at some different bacteria to see how scientists learn to recognize the nature of a disease by the appearance of the causative organism.

6. Make a list of what every person can do to protect himself against injury or illness.

7. Obtain from the local health department its regulations for the control of communicable diseases. Ask a health department representative how regulations now differ from regulations of 25 years ago.

6

MATERNITY CARE

Having a baby is a natural physiological process for women; with proper care and preparation, it is a safe and satisfying experience. Although childbearing is a normal function of women, it involves all the body systems and processes, whose delicate balance can be upset by the additional work they are called on to perform. Ideally, preparation for motherhood begins in childhood with health supervision, good nutrition, dental care, and the building of healthy attitudes.

The objective of medical care during pregnancy is to keep both mother and baby in the best possible physical condition and to carry the mother-to-be safely through the pregnancy and a normal delivery as well as to insure her speedy postnatal recovery. Medical supervision during pregnancy is thus preventive in nature, and the doctor watches over the expectant mother, alert to her progress and her well-being. Pregnancy is a different experience for every woman, and though a woman may have several pregnancies, no two will be exactly the same. The mother will be sensitive to these differences, and they need cause her no concern. It is the way nature operates.

Preparing for the baby's arrival is a family affair. It is of equal importance to both parents. Particularly at the coming of the first baby, the husband and the wife need to plan together for changes and adjustments that are going to take place in their lives, although the full impact of the differences will not really be apparent until after the baby has come. Thinking ahead about some of the ways in which life is going to be different for each of them should make the adjustment easier.

It is well for both parents to make the first visit to the doctor together and for both to attend parents' classes on baby care when they are available so that both may learn and have similar experiences. Generally, it is the new mother who is apt to be overanxious about caring for the baby, but as she becomes acquainted with the baby and his ways and more skillful in doing things for him, she relaxes and can enjoy being a mother. This concern sometimes makes the father feel that he is being neglected and is loved less than before the baby came. If the responsibility of taking care of the baby is shared by the parents, the baby becomes theirs in the truest sense.

When there are other children in the family, they too must be prepared for the arrival of the new brother or sister. To tell children about the expected birth too far ahead of time makes the waiting period long, for even a month or two seems a long time to little children. It should be kept in mind that, even with the most thoughtful preparation, the new baby may likely be the cause of some jealousy among other children in the family, though it may not show up in ways that can be readily recognized. Some young children betray their insecure feelings by reverting to more babyish ways of acting. Any oddities of behavior in the new baby's brothers and sisters should be considered as possibly the result of their getting less attention than before the baby came and should be treated with patience. It is usually the parents' thoughtlessness or extra busyness that brings about such behavior. It pays to take special pains to give more, rather than less, loving care to other children on the arrival of a new baby. Even though the parents may have less time to give older children, the quality of the attention may be made to count. After the baby comes, a mother can read to an older child while she nurses the baby, and if the older child is big enough and mature enough, he can often assist with caring for the baby. Fathers, too, may help by giving more time to the older children, who frequently regard the attention as an indication that they are "growing up."

MEDICAL SUPERVISION

Plans should be made to obtain medical supervision early in pregnancy. Women may go to their private physicians, and there are many hospitals and health departments that have free or part-pay clinics where excellent obstetrical care can be obtained. In addition, the service of the public health nurse is available, and she will be able to answer many questions of expectant parents. By the end of the third month the doctor can determine whether pregnancy has occurred and will be able to advise the mother-to-be about future care.

Pregnancy is divided into three periods of 3 months, each of which is known as a trimester. The woman under medical supervision is observed throughout her pregnancy for development of the baby and for the signs related to her condition. Usually the doctor will want to see her at least once a month during the first two trimesters and then more frequently during the last one.

Each trimester marks a milestone in the development of the baby and presents certain changes in the mother both physically and emotionally. During the first trimester it is not at all unusual for the expectant mother to be moody or depressed and to have mixed feelings about her pregnancy. At times she looks forward to the happiness of having the baby, and at other times she may feel unhappy because she senses that a baby is going to bring many changes in her life that she is reluctant to accept. This, too, is the time, if it occurs at all, when the mother will have "morning sickness," with the unpleasantness of nausea and vomiting. Sleeping more than usual is common during the first trimester for sleep and rest are nature's way of aiding the body to make many adjustments to pregnancy. During the second trimester, the mother usually feels fine and she anticipates the coming of the baby with much happiness. By now she usually has proudly confided her secret to family and friends and is busy getting ready for the new baby. As the mother-to-be enters the last trimester of pregnancy, time seems to slow down and tasks take longer to perform. Fatigue is more apparent and physical activity is more limited in scope because of the increased size and weight of the growing baby. Frequent rest periods, an afternoon nap, and moderate exercise become the routine. Soon the baby will arrive.

The expectant mother may have a family physician who is experienced in obstetrics. This is an advantage, because the previous knowledge the doctor has of her, when she comes for consultation about her pregnancy, provides him with a basis for comparison of any changes that occur as the pregnancy continues. On the other hand, a woman may need help in finding a doctor who practices obstetrics. There are several ways to get the information. She may ask the family physician to suggest someone. The local or state health department, the local or state medical or obstetric society, or a hospital will provide a list of names, usually three, from which a doctor can be chosen.

It is a great comfort to be able to ask the doctor for answers to questions that are bound to arise. No written word can possibly cover all the individual questions, whether before the coming of the first baby or a later one. So much is constantly being added to medical knowledge that even a woman who has borne a child quite recently may find that there are new ways of increasing her safety and comfort and the well-being of the baby. The physician and the nurse, in a private office or in a clinic, are ready to help with problems whether they are financial, medical, or other. All these matters are important and affect the ability of the mother to be calm and relaxed. Things to be discussed with the doctor and any questions that have arisen since the last visit should be written down. A list of this sort saves time and assures that nothing important is forgotten.

An excellent source of information for parents-to-be is *Prenatal Care*, a pamphlet published by the Children's Bureau, which contains detailed information about pregnancy, childbirth, and care of the baby. Another Bureau publication, *When Your Baby Is on the Way*, is a picture leaflet on the care of the mother before the baby is born. Designed for quick reading, it covers the most important points in good maternity care.

Classes for parents are held in many communities. These may be conducted by the health department, the visiting nurse association, the Red Cross chapter, or a hospital. Also, some obstetricians hold classes for their patients. The value in attending these classes is the opportunity to discuss freely and openly with other members of the group the attitudes that most people experience in becoming parents and to get additional information from the instructor or the group leader. Most young parents of today recognize the importance of knowing about the physiology of pregnancy and the physical changes that will occur. Quite often prospective parents are interested in the period of labor and delivery because many of their fears concern this part of having a baby. Finding that they have the same feelings, apprehensions, and desires as other parents is comforting and reassuring.

THE OBSTETRIC PHYSICAL EXAMINATION

The mother in her first pregnancy may not know what to expect when she goes to the doctor to be examined. Every doctor will be sure to carry out the following routines:
- Take a medical history.
- Take blood for laboratory examination.
- Make an evaluation of the pelvis.

- Examine the urine.
- Take blood pressure and check body weight.
- Check the heart and lungs.
- Examine the body.
- Recommend dental examination and correction of defects.

The medical history of the expectant mother, as well as that of other members of the family, is of importance to the doctor in evaluating her health status. He will want to know about previous illnesses, what communicable diseases she has had, what ones she is protected against, and any surgery or serious accidents she may have had. This is done to disclose any adverse factors that might influence the successful progress of pregnancy. Although all pregnant women should have good prenatal care, there are certain ones among them who need extra attention. These include women who have diabetes, tuberculosis, heart disease, or have Rh incompatibility. Very young women, those near the end of the childbearing period, and anyone who has had a previous complicated pregnancy also require careful observation and supervision.

A sample of the blood will be taken by the doctor to determine the blood type of the mother and whether she is Rh negative or Rh positive, to tell how long it takes the blood to clot, to measure the iron content, and to determine whether she may have syphilis.

Determination of the Rh factor is important to the baby, but the publicity about it has produced fear out of proportion to the actual danger. Most people are Rh positive. If both parents are Rh positive or Rh negative, there is no problem for their children. The difficulty may arise when the mother is Rh negative and the father is Rh positive, for some or all of their children may be Rh positive. During pregnancy, blood from the Rh positive baby may pass through the placenta into the mother's blood stream, stimulating the mother's body to form antibodies against the Rh positive factor. If the antibodies pass through the placenta from the mother to the baby, they are capable of destroying the Rh positive cells in the baby's body. Most Rh negative mothers have Rh positive babies without ever becoming sensitized. This situation never occurs in the first baby unless the mother has been sensitized by a prepregnancy transfusion of Rh positive blood. However, once an Rh negative mother has had an Rh positive baby who has been affected, there is a strong probability that her future Rh positive babies may also be affected. Early knowledge of the existence of the Rh factor complication gives the doctor the information he needs to follow a required course of action. With methods of treatment available today, almost all "Rh babies" are saved.

Knowledge of the hemoglobin content of the blood tells whether the mother has anemia. The function of the red blood cells is to carry the hemoglobin, which takes oxygen to the tissues and removes carbon dioxide. Knowledge of the clotting time of the blood helps the doctor prepare against the possibility of hemorrhage. Should the mother have syphilis, she must receive prompt treatment. Congenital syphilis does not appear in the baby if the mother has adequate treatment before the fifth month of pregnancy.

Evaluation of the pelvis, the basin-shaped cavity formed by the hipbones and the end of the spine, is made to make sure that its size and shape are adequate for passage of the baby through the birth canal. The doctor may use X ray to take more accurate measurement, but this is done late in pregnancy when the baby's head has nearly reached its maximum size before birth. Pelvic X rays are not always done, but are valuable when needed.

Urine is tested for sugar, albumin, and waste materials that show whether the kidneys are functioning properly. The examination of urine is a sensitive test, quickly and easily done, and provides a good index of how the mother is tolerating the increased stress of her pregnancy. Urine analysis is usually done at each visit to the doctor.

Measuring blood pressure is another routine but significant procedure done at each visit to the doctor to provide information about the circulatory system. A rise in blood pressure is a diagnostic sign that in pregnancy sometimes indicates an early toxemia, the presence of waste materials in the blood.

Special attention should always be given to the nutritional status of the mother to insure adequacy of the essential nutrients needed for her and the growing baby and to regulate weight gain as much as possible. Gain in weight is gradual, with the greatest and most rapid increase coming during the third trimester. Some women may lose weight in the early weeks of pregnancy. How much the pregnant woman should weigh is an individual matter that depends on her weight at the beginning of pregnancy and on what her doctor determines is best for her. Most of the weight gain during pregnancy is temporary, made up of the weight of the growing baby, the fluid around the baby, and the increased tissue in the uterus and the breasts.

Tests for tuberculosis may be made during early pregnancy. The pregnant woman with tuberculosis has a much better chance of carrying her baby to term without spread of the disease in her lungs or harm to the baby if the doctor has current accurate information and if she is receiving adequate medical care.

The breasts will be examined for any abnormalities. Lumps in the breast are not unusual during pregnancy, but only the doctor can determine whether they are of medical significance. The breasts should be kept clean. Should there be a watery solution from the nipples during late pregnancy, it should be gently washed away; the doctor will recommend any special care or treatment. As the breasts become larger in preparation to nurse the baby, they become heavier; extra support may be needed early in pregnancy. A larger brassiere will be needed, with wide adjustable straps and cups large enough to support the breasts without undue pressure. The doctor frequently will give suggestions for the type of brassiere to be worn.

Throughout pregnancy the doctor will pay attention to the feet and legs, observing for swelling and varicose veins. Generally varicosities are caused by pressure of the enlarging uterus on the large blood vessels that supply blood to the lower extremities. Varicose veins sometimes require treatment. The symptoms are dull aching pains, a sense of weight or heaviness, fatigue, sometimes itching, and the outward evidence of the enlarged veins, which are readily seen. Frequent rest periods, particularly with the feet elevated on a stool or a chair when sitting, or on pillows when lying down, usually bring relief from discomfort. One should not cross the legs when sitting and should avoid wearing tight clothing or garters, which restrict the free flow of blood from the legs.

SIGNALS OF POSSIBLE DANGER

The woman who understands and knows what changes she may expect during her pregnancy is better able to recognize the unfavorable changes that are danger signals. If she has had good care throughout pregnancy, she is less likely to develop any complications. Complications of pregnancy are comparatively rare. The doctor should be notified at once and the patient put to bed to await instructions from him if any of the following symptoms should occur:
- Vaginal bleeding or spotting
- Puffiness of the face, hands, or legs
- Persistent and severe headaches
- Blurred vision
- Chills and fever

FOOD FOR THE EXPECTANT MOTHER

The diet of the expectant mother is of special importance because it should supply generous amounts of protein, minerals, and vitamins to protect the mother's health and to build new tissue for the mother and the baby. Good nutrition is an important factor in the development of the baby and equally important to the mother during and following pregnancy. During pregnancy the growth of the baby and of the tissue in the mother's breast and uterus causes a significant increase in protein requirements. Since the mother's blood volume increases during pregnancy and protein is an important blood component, additional reserves of protein are needed to provide a safety factor in preparation for delivery. Also, protein is highly concentrated in the colostrum, the fluid secreted from the mammary glands immediately preceding and following the baby's birth. It is therefore essential that the expectant mother eat the foods rich in protein and in the important minerals and vitamins to protect her health and provide food for the baby.

Gain in weight is one of the general indications of the mother's nourishment and is one of the observations that the doctor makes regularly as a measure of her progress. An excessive gain or loss in weight indicates maternal liability to disease and is a hazard to the unborn baby. Weight gain will, of course, vary from one woman to another because of many individual differences, but the average is from 16 to 20 pounds. If weight gain is restricted too severely, there is some danger that the baby will be born prematurely.

The woman who is well nourished before pregnancy and who eats an adequate diet during this period, with enough of the foods rich in protein, calcium, and vitamin C, is not only more likely to remain in fine health but also has a better chance of giving birth to a normal healthy baby. Milk is a rich source of calcium and contains high quality protein. Dry skim milk and evaporated milk used generously to drink or in preparing cooked foods will add calcium and protein of low cost and high value to the diet. An advantage of skim milk is that it contains no fat, which may be restricted by the doctor if the mother needs to watch her weight. The expectant mother should also eat the foods that are rich in iron, such as eggs, liver, lean red meats, dark green leafy vegetables, and the whole-grain breads and cereals.

It should be remembered that the foods needed by the expectant mother are a balanced normal diet *plus the following additions each day*: from 2 to 4 cups of milk, 1 serving of citrus fruit or tomato, and 1 serving of a food high in protein, such as lean meat, liver, fish, eggs, beans, and cheese. After the baby comes, the nursing mother requires *in addition to her normal diet* 4 cups of milk, 2 servings of citrus fruit or tomato, 1 serving of meat, eggs, cheese, or any protein-rich food, and 1 serving of a dark green leafy vegetable. A recommended food guide follows.

Recommended Food Guide During Pregnancy and Lactation*

Period	Food Pattern			
	Milk	Citrus Fruit or Tomato	Lean Meat, Fish, Poultry, Egg, Beans, or Cheese	Dark Green Leafy Vegetable
Pregnancy	1 quart	2 servings	3 servings	1 serving every other day
Lactation	3 pints	3 servings	3 servings	1 serving daily plus 1 additional serving every other day

*The food groups in the chart are those high in calcium and other minerals, vitamins, especially vitamin C, and protein. In addition, everyone needs food from the bread and cereal group, some fats and sweets, and other fruits and vegetables to make the diet appetizing.

During the first trimester, the expectant mother's calorie requirements are about the same as they were before pregnancy. Weight gain is not desired during this period unless the individual was below the desired weight at the beginning of pregnancy. During the second and third trimester, the needs for proteins, minerals, and vitamins increase gradually, with the increase greatest for calcium, protein, vitamin C, and riboflavin. The need for calories may increase during the third trimester, when an extra allowance may be necessary; this is the period of rapid growth of the baby. Most doctors guard weight gain very carefully during the last trimester. The quality of the diet is most important and those foods containing essential nutrients should take precedence in the daily diet.

The recommendations for food for the expectant mother are general. The food needs of every prenatal should be considered individually, because her requirements will depend on her nutritional status at the time of conception, her normal food pattern, and what the doctor recommends as necessary to meet the changing needs of both the mother and the growing baby. There is a close relationship between nutrition and the outcome of the pregnancy, the survival of the baby, and the mother's ability to nurse him. Therefore, a diet that meets adequate nutritional standards contributes to health, makes premature birth less likely to occur, and provides a better nutritional start for the baby.

SUPPLIES FOR THE BABY

The layette for the baby should be simple. Clothing should be light in weight, suitable to the climate and season of the year, and nonirritating to the skin. Garments should be loose to allow freedom of movement and to make them easier to put on and remove. Labels should be examined to learn how the articles should be laundered and how durable they are. Clothing that is easy to launder and that requires a minimum of care should be selected. It is a needless expense to buy very small clothing because the baby soon outgrows it. If this is not the first baby, there are many items of used clothing and equipment that can be used for the newcomer. Often the baby receives clothing as gifts.

When making purchases, costs should be kept within the family budget. Whether some articles might be made better and cheaper than to get them ready-made should be considered. For example, four crib blankets can be made from one large blanket, usually at a considerable saving.

The supplies procured should be kept to the minimum. The following list covers the essentials:
- 3 or 4 dozen diapers
- 3 or 4 shirts, size 2
- 3 or 4 crib blankets
- 4 to 6 receiving blankets at least 36 inches square
- 5 or 6 protective pads of cotton material about 18 inches square to put under the baby
- 1 waterproof sheet or mattress cover to protect the crib mattress
- 4 to 6 crib sheets
- 3 or 4 nightgowns
- 2 or 3 lightweight sweaters
- 3 or 4 waterproof pads about 12 by 18 inches to protect clothing when holding the baby
- 2 dozen large safety pins
- A bassinet or crib

- A bathtub
- A diaper pail
- 3 or 4 bottles and nipples to give water and orange juice

EMERGENCY DELIVERY

Occasionally a baby is born before a doctor or a nurse can arrive, or there may be an unavoidable delay in getting to the hospital. Only in exceptional circumstances, however, is an untrained person required to assist with the delivery. The important action to be taken is the safe handling of the baby so that he breathes and so that he and his mother are protected against infection. Fortunately, only a small fraction of all births present any problem. When a problem does occur, every effort must be made to provide the best medical and nursing care available.

Labor is the work the uterus does to allow the baby to be born. It is a well ordered, routine procedure. At the first indication that labor has begun, the doctor should be notified. The onset of labor is usually indicated by discomfort, caused by the contractions of the uterus, that starts in the lower back and radiates to the lower abdomen. There is usually a vaginal discharge, either of mucus or of blood-tinged fluid, which is a sign that the cervix or mouth of the uterus has begun to dilate in preparation for the baby's birth. The appearance of a watery fluid indicates the rupture of the membrane or the bag of waters in which the baby is enclosed. This fluid may appear early and has no effect on the length or difficulty of labor. However, should this occur *before* the onset of labor and *before* the baby is due, the doctor should be notified and the patient put to bed pending further instruction from the doctor. Usually the contractions in the first stage of labor are mild and irregular at first, probably 20 minutes apart and lasting as little as 10 seconds. If this is the first baby, delivery is not imminent and there is time to spare to get ready.

The second stage of labor, when the baby is being moved through the birth canal, may last a short time or for several hours. There are frequent strong contractions of the uterus, 5 minutes or less apart, and the mother pushes and strains to help the baby through the birth canal. There is little to be done at this time except to reassure the mother and to make her as comfortable as possible.

Most babies are born head first, and the body follows with much less effort on the part of the mother. When no doctor or nurse is present, whoever is helping with the delivery should support and hold the baby as he is being born so that he does not drop into the fluid expelled with him. Occasionally the baby is born in the membranous sac in which he has been growing. If so, the sac should be quickly broken or torn and the baby should be taken out of it so that, when he takes his first breath, he does not get fluid in his lungs. Most babies cry and begin to breathe immediately. All of them have some fluid in the mouth and in the nose and throat passages that must be drained out. The best way to do this is to hold the baby for a few minutes by the feet, head downward, head and shoulders supported. As the newborn baby is very often slippery, care must be taken in handling him. The following procedure is recommended:

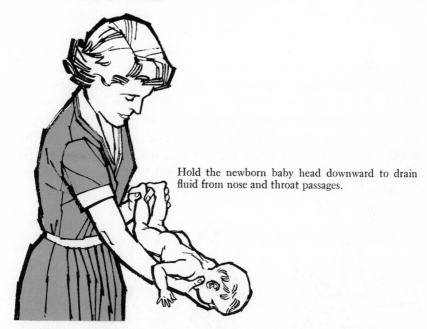

Hold the newborn baby head downward to drain fluid from nose and throat passages.

- Grasp both the baby's feet with one hand, placing a finger between the ankles.
- Support the baby's head, face down, with the other hand and let his chest rest on the wrist and the forearm, the thumb and little finger part way around his neck. If necessary, the baby's mouth can be held open with the index finger.
- Handle the baby gently and use no rough slapping or shaking to get him to breathe. If he does not cry and breathe without assistance, mouth-to-mouth resuscitation may be necessary. (See "Artificial Respiration," chapter 17, pages 294-297.)

- Wrap the baby loosely in a towel or receiving blanket.
- Place him on his right side, with head lowered and facing away from the mother's face, across her abdomen, to wait for the final stage of labor.
- Keep the hands off the mother's genitalia, away from the birth canal, and off the umbilical cord to lessen the danger of infection.
- Do not pull on the cord at any time.

The third stage of labor is the expulsion of the placenta, which usually occurs from 5 to 30 minutes after the birth of the baby. For a few minutes after expulsion of the placenta the umbilical cord is round and blue. Then it turns pale and becomes thinner as the circulation reverses and blood stops flowing through it. Now the cord can be cut. The placenta, a round flat membrane from 6 to 8 inches in diameter and about the color and consistency of liver, can be wrapped and placed with the baby and the cord can be cut later if the doctor is not present when the baby is born.

If, as might happen in a disaster or other emergency, there is no prospect of having a doctor or a nurse present at the time of delivery, preparations should be made to cut the cord. However, there is no hurry about this, and the safety of the mother and baby should be looked after first. A shoestring or other woven cotton tape or a ¼-inch strong ribbon can be used to tie the cord. It can be cut with scissors, a sharp knife, or a razor blade.

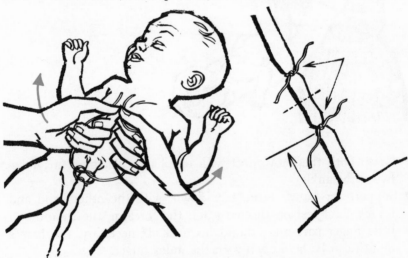

Tieing and cutting the cord.

Tie a square knot in the cord about 4 inches from the baby. Use strong cotton tape or cloth.

Tie a second knot 2 to 4 inches from the first one. Cut the cord midway between the square knots.

Cutting the umbilical cord involves the following steps:

- Boil the cutting instrument and two pieces of tape or ribbon 8 to 10 inches long for 5 minutes in a small covered basin, drain off the water, keep the basin covered, and set aside to cool.
- When ready to tie the cord, wash the hands well.
- With one piece of tape, tie a square knot around the cord 4 to 5 inches from the baby's navel.
- With the second piece of tape, tie a square knot around the cord 2 to 3 inches from the navel.
- Without touching the cutting surface of the knife or scissors, cut the cord midway between the two knotted tapes.
- If a sterile dressing is available, place it over the cord stump and hold in place with a binder around the baby's abdomen.

The baby must be kept warm and protected at all times. After the umbilical cord has been cut, he can be wrapped and placed on his side, head lowered, in his bed. If additional warmth is needed, well-protected hot water bottles can be placed around him outside the blanket. If there is no other means of keeping him warm, he may be placed under the blanket beside his mother, face uncovered so that he can breathe. The mother should be reassured and kept as comfortable as possible.

The person attending the mother following the birth should feel the uterus through the abdominal wall. It should be a hard, firm mass about halfway between the umbilicus and the pubic bone. If the uterus is firm, there is nothing to do except to check regularly. If the uterus does not feel hard, it should be massaged through the abdomen until it contracts and hardens. If the baby is strong enough to nurse, putting him to the breast will cause the uterus to contract and aid in its return to normal size. Putting the baby to the breast has another advantage in that the sucking reflex is usually quite strong at birth and gives the baby practice in nursing. If the mother should continue to bleed from the vagina, elevate her feet and hips higher than her head and treat for shock. Give fluids and keep her comfortably warm.

The essentials to remember in an emergency delivery are:

- Let nature take its course; do nothing to hurry the delivery along.
- Keep hands away from the opening to the birth canal to protect against infection.
- Reassure the mother.
- While the baby is being born, do not push or pull on the baby's head or body.

- Support the baby's head as it emerges to keep it out of blood, fluid, or feces.
- If the baby is born with the membrane intact, tear it open at once so that he can begin to breathe.
- Lower the baby's head, supporting the head and shoulders, to drain fluid from nose, mouth, and throat.
- When the baby has been born, observe carefully to see that he is breathing well.
- Keep the baby warm and handle him gently and safely.
- Place the baby on the mother's abdomen, on his side with head lowered, until the cord can be cut.
- Wait for the placenta to be expelled; never touch or pull on the cord during delivery.

SUGGESTED STUDENT ACTIVITIES

1. Plan a day's diet for an expectant mother and a nursing mother.

2. Using an 18 or 20 inch doll, demonstrate how to handle a newborn baby.

3. Using the list of minimum supplies for the baby, shop for prices and compute the cost of a moderate price layette.

4. If there is a Red Cross or other blood center in your community, arrange with the instructor to appoint three or four class members to visit and report to the class on the collection and use of blood, particularly why so many questions are asked the donors.

5. Arrange to see the Red Cross film *Prescription for Life* and write a brief report on the uses of blood.

6. List the resources your community offers for prenatal and postnatal advice and care for mothers. Are these facilities adequate? If not, how could they be improved?

7. Write an account of what you would tell a five-year-old child to prepare him for the coming of a new baby.

8. Determine whether your birth certificate has been registered at the vital statistics office of the health department. If it has not, what has to be done to get it registered?

9. Make a list of uses for a birth certificate.

7

CARE OF INFANTS AND CHILDREN

Probably no phase of human development has received as much study as the age period known as infancy and childhood, yet it has been only during the twentieth century that spectacular changes affecting children have come about through medical research, experimentation, and increased knowledge.

One of the greatest changes that has occurred is the lowered death rate of both babies and mothers. Not only do they receive better medical care now but also the infectious and communicable diseases that cost so many lives among them can be successfully overcome by immunizing agents and specific drug therapy. Research has found the cause of many diseases and crippling conditions, some of which are preventable. Others can be treated and the patient restored to optimum health.

Parents of today are quite sophisticated. They are much better informed and more health conscious than were parents one, two, or three generations ago. Health education has reached into every community, spread by public health agencies, doctors, nurses, and teachers. Reliable information about health and disease is available to nearly anyone, much of it at no cost. Health pamphlets are available in doctors' waiting rooms, clinics, and hospitals. Libraries generally have a health education section. Daily newspapers, current periodicals, and paperbacks written by reliable authors present a wealth of health information. Excellent materials on the care of infants and children are published by the Children's Bureau of the Department of Health, Education, and Welfare. A basic guide in the care and the growth and development of babies is the Bureau's publication *Infant Care*.

Many people say that all babies look alike. Perhaps to some they do, but each baby is an individual and totally unlike any other human being. Boys are usually a little longer and a little heavier at birth than are girls. The baby's length will vary from approximately 18 to 21 inches and his weight from 5½ to 8 pounds. Some babies appear to have no hair at all; others have hair that is thick and long. Often the hair changes color, being dark at birth and becoming much lighter, even blonde. Sometimes there is fine, downy hair on the back, the arms, and the legs, and occasionally on the face, but this hair usually disappears.

The baby's head is large in proportion to the rest of his body, and at birth it may be somewhat misshapen from being squeezed as he came through the birth canal. This condition usually lasts for only a few days. The baby's head grows very fast before birth to accommodate the brain and the nerve centers which control his development. However, his body will soon grow larger, and he will appear more like a miniature adult. The head continues to increase in size, and by the time the child is 4 or 5 years old, the skull will have approximately 90 percent of its total growth.

The baby develops coordination in his hands before he does in his feet. This head-to-foot development is the result of the maturing of nerve and muscle control from the brain. For example, the ability to perform complex hand activities comes before a child learns to use his feet for dancing or skating.

The growth of a baby is orderly, that is, one stage of development

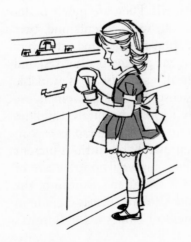

The toddler usually attains the ability to pour water without spilling it before he learns to hop or to skip.

follows another systematically. At birth the baby cannot hold up his head, but, as he develops, the muscles strengthen and the nervous system matures and he can support his head. Soon he can turn over, next he can sit up, then he can stand with help, and finally he can stand alone. These progressions illustrate what is meant by orderly development. Most babies crawl before they walk.

Every baby has his own rate of growth and development, and for this reason should not be compared with another baby. The baby next door may walk at 9 or 10 months, while one's own baby may not walk until he is a year old. Occasionally a baby is born with one or two teeth, but that does not mean that he is more advanced than a baby born without teeth. Whether a baby cuts the first tooth at 2 months or at 6 or 7 months really does not matter. What is important is that both the first and second sets of teeth are already well developed in the jaw and waiting to come through the gums. Almost without exception the first teeth to come through will be the two lower central incisors.

The lower jaw at birth is smaller than the upper jaw bone and proportionately will grow at a faster rate to accommodate the first teeth. At birth the baby's face is rather small and appears even more so because of the relatively large brow. Facial changes will occur until about the teens but are faster in the first few months of life. The mouth and the lips are well developed at birth because they are essential to getting food.

The newborn baby's bones are soft because the mineral content, chiefly calcium, is small and the water content is large. In time, this imbalance reverses, and there is a decrease in water and an increase in minerals. The bony structure of the body will increase in size about 20 times, also changing in chemical composition and in number of bones. Height depends largely on genetic factors, sex, and bone growth. Bone growth is influenced by the supply and utilization of minerals by the body. Studies show that children who have been denied proper nutrients during their infancy and childhood are shorter than those who have had consistently balanced diets. Studies also show that young adults of today are taller than were their parents or their grandparents as young adults, a situation that is a direct result of improved nutrition during the last half century.

The newborn has a large abdomen. One reason for this is that the liver is enlarged because it has been storing up iron. Also, the abdominal muscles are comparatively weak and cannot compress the intestines, which distend with food and gas. The baby, therefore, has a potbellied appearance, which will disappear as muscle strength increases and the abdominal wall tautens as the child begins to stand and walk.

The sensory perceptions of the newborn vary in their acuteness. He can taste and smell and seems to get especially strong feeling sensations through his skin. He gets pleasure from being touched and fondled and yet is extremely sensitive to tension and insecurity in his handling. Much has been written about the trauma or shock that occurs to the baby in being born. He comes from a sheltered, controlled environment whose temperature and fluid support never change into a world that is decidedly different. He is extremely sensitive to heat and cold and reacts sharply to loud noises. At first, the baby cannot see very well, although he is aware of light and darkness and moving objects. Nerves and muscles have to grow and develop before he can focus his eyes on an object.

It is instinctive for the baby to nurse. As soon as his cheek touches the breast, he will turn his head to touch the breast with his mouth and will begin to root in an effort to get the nipple into his mouth. The baby sucks because he is hungry and because he loves to suck. If he does not get enough opportunity at the breast or the bottle, he sucks his fists, fingers, or clothing.

Babies seem to have a built-in clock that tells them when to eat. How they take the feeding will vary from one baby to another. Some of them appear to be famished and can hardly wait to eat and will suck vigorously until satisfied. Others may dawdle and not appear interested. Some babies are agitated and so impatient for food that they scream and squirm, making it more difficult for them to get any food at all. One needs to be patient and to learn how to adjust to the baby's temperament.

THE PREMATURE BABY

The diagnosis of prematurity is based on two circumstances: the weight of the baby at birth and the number of months of development before birth. The normal gestation period is about nine months, or 280 days. The nearer to the end of the gestation period that the baby remains within the uterus, the better is his chance for survival and freedom from handicaps. However, the tremendous medical and scientific advances of the last quarter century have done much to conserve the life of both the immature and the premature infant. The premature baby is immature in the functioning of his organic systems. This may also hold true for the full term infant, particularly if he is a small baby.

94

There are marked individual differences for the premature infant as for all babies. In appraising his condition at birth, such factors as weight, the amount of fatty tissue underlying his skin, his ability to suck, the vigor of his movements, and the efficiency of his respiratory function all influence his ability to survive. His temperature-regulating mechanism is less fully developed, and his digestive system, as in fact everything about him, is unprepared to take over the functions of independent living. But interestingly, as soon as he begins to gain in weight, he seems to be in a hurry to catch up, and before many months it may be difficult to tell that he was born before full term.

Usually there is no difference in the pattern of growth and development of the premature baby except that the progressive stages may be somewhat later than with the full-term baby. The premature baby is therefore often slower in sitting, standing, and walking.

Like all babies, the premature infant needs tender, loving care and attention. At first, because he is so little, parents are likely to be apprehensive about handling him, but by the time he weighs 6 pounds, they consider him to be quite husky and are confident of their ability to give him the necessary care.

The premature baby needs immediate medical attention. If he should be born without the doctor present, the following care is necessary:

- Avoid unnecessary handling.
- Wrap the baby loosely in a soft flannel or wool receiving blanket, with his face exposed so that he can breathe.
- Place the baby in a padded bassinet or basket with one end elevated so that his head is at a lower level than his feet.
- Place well-wrapped hot water bottles around the baby outside the blanket to conserve his body heat. Refill bottles frequently so that an even temperature is maintained.

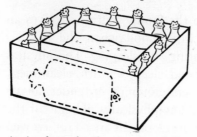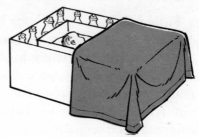

An incubator for the premature baby can be improvised from 2 cardboard cartons, one placed inside the other, and can be warmed with bottles of hot water or heated stones placed between the boxes.

- Take every precaution not to burn the baby's sensitive skin. An improvised incubator can be made by placing the wrapped baby in a padded cardboard carton inside a larger carton and putting hot water bags between the sides of the two boxes. Substitutes for hot water bags, such as heated bricks or stones or glass bottles filled with hot water, can be used in the same manner, allowing the heat from them to radiate around the baby.
- Place a diaper or a soft pad under the baby's buttocks so that it can be changed with a minimum of handling of the infant.
- Withhold food and water for 6-8 hours or until the doctor gives definite instructions for the baby's care and feeding.

If it is possible, the premature baby should be born in the hospital, where there are special facilities for taking care of him. Some hospitals and health departments, particularly those in large cities, have made special provisions for the transport of the premature baby from his home to a hospital.

The premature baby has a better chance for survival in the hospital than at home because his environment can be controlled and advances in modern medical science can be utilized more efficiently. In addition, trained personnel in the hospital know better how to care for the baby. The first few days in the premature baby's life are most important, and every day that he lives increases his chances for survival.

The premature baby who has to remain in the hospital when his mother goes home is a special kind of problem for parents. The anxiety and the separation from the baby are hard to endure. When he is finally ready to come home, parents are likely to be more apprehensive than they should be. This apprehension is a temporary reaction and an experience that is common to parents of all premature babies.

THE BABY'S FIRST YEAR

Fitting the care of the baby into the family routine involves an easy acceptance of the trial-and-error period when the baby is determining his own schedule of eating and sleeping. The physical needs of a young baby are simple. Food, sleep, warmth, cleanliness, protection against infection, and liberal amounts of tender, loving care are about all that are required. The physical well-being of the baby and his emotional growth and development are so interwoven that one cannot be isolated from the other. The baby is born with his personality traits and almost immediately begins to react to his environment. He has two instinctual drives: to seek what satisfies him and to be aggressive and angry when he is frustrated.

Emotional maturity comes with learning experiences, and the baby eventually learns how to gain personal satisfaction and the approval of those who take care of him. Weaning is such an experience. Sucking, it will be recalled, is a pleasure for the baby, and when it is denied him, he is likely to become aggressive. When he is no longer fed from the bottle and takes his food from a cup or a spoon, his mother must give him emotional support and praise him for his accomplishment. The timing of weaning, as of toilet training, is important to assure success for both the mother and the baby. The child must be ready for the new learning and must have emotional support from his mother.

The first social responses to love and affection come early in life, when the baby smiles or stops crying when talked to. Close personal contact is one of the first and best ways of contributing to his security and emotional health. The days of letting the baby cry in his crib are past, and rocking him is back in favor.

Food

It is easier and simpler to breast feed a baby than to give him bottle feedings. Nursing the baby also gives great satisfaction to mothers by adding an opportunity for cuddling and fondling the baby and for talking softly to him to add to his sense of comfort. Even though the mother may not have quite enough milk for the baby at first, she should not give up trying to breast feed him. The act of nursing promotes the secretion of milk, just as apprehension and tension inhibit it. As the baby gets practice in sucking, he helps to stimulate a greater flow of milk. If, however, there is some reason why the baby must be bottle fed, he can do well on the proper formula. It is how his mother feels about formula feeding that is important. If she can be relaxed and confident that she is giving him the best possible care, the baby will be all right.

At one time babies were fed regularly at 3- or 4-hour intervals because experience had shown that regularity in feeding resulted in healthier and happier babies. But regularity and rigidity are two different things, and the baby's hunger is the guide to follow. Until he is several weeks old, a baby cannot take into his small stomach enough food to last very long. Consequently, frequent feeding will be necessary during the early period of his life. By the time he is a month old, the baby usually can wait 3 hours between feedings, and by the time he is 3 months old he will have fairly well regulated his own feeding schedule and will want to be fed about every 4 hours during the day. Parents should recognize that every baby will need his own feeding schedule.

Sleep

Some newborn babies have a way of turning night into day or of being wakeful in the evening hours. Parents who expect irregularity of behavior during the first few months of the baby's life need not be disturbed by irregular behavior and usually find that they can fit the baby's needs to their own requirements and habits. To parents with their first baby everything is different and new, but they should recognize that everyone with a first baby has feelings of uncertainty and that common sense is an excellent guide.

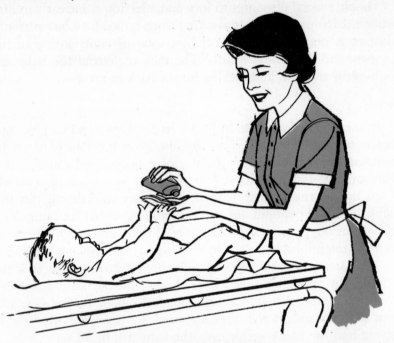

During infancy the baby should have many opportunities to kick and stretch unhampered by clothing.

Physical and Emotional Development

The baby's physical growth is greatest during the nine months before birth, when he develops from the union of two cells to a fully formed baby. During the first year he has another tremendous growth spurt and will probably double his weight in from 4 to 6 months and triple it in from 12 to 14 months. Along with the

98

baby's increase in size comes development of his mind and his body.

The baby's emotional life steadily unfolds. He was born without fear, and careful parents can prevent fear from arising. For example, care should be used when he is bathed so that he does not slip. Also the temperature of the bath water must be right so that the bath is a pleasant and enjoyable experience for him. Anger appears when a baby is frustrated. The fewer and milder the frustrations, the fewer the outbursts of temper. A baby whose hunger and other needs are satisfied with reasonable speed has few occasions for anger. Because dressing and undressing are frustrating to him, as is any restraint, his clothing should be easy to put on and to remove. Any handling of the baby should be done quickly and confidently.

To provide the best opportunity for the baby to develop his capacities, the mother should allow him to have maximum freedom within the limits of safety. In early infancy, he needs plenty of chances to kick and stretch unclothed and should be played with, sung to, rocked and cuddled, and talked to while he is being fed, bathed, and dressed. As the baby grows, his physical environment must be kept free from danger. Toys should be carefully selected. They should be too large to be swallowed, relatively unbreakable, without sharp edges or removable parts, and if painted have nonlead or nonpoisonous paint. A playpen provides a safe place for a baby to crawl and exercise, but there should be nothing placed in it that endangers him in any way. When he crawls or walks alone outside his playpen, loose objects must be put out of reach so that he can explore and experiment safely. Above all, the baby should never be placed in his crib or in his playpen as punishment. The crib is for sleeping and the playpen is for exercise and for play.

The baby whose needs are understood and attended to promptly is being given the foundation for a happy, relaxed, and well-adjusted personality and an orderly emotional development. His parents' expressions of affection and their enjoyment of him will be reflected in his responses and behavior. What and how the baby learns are dependent on his parents' manner and attitude. If they are too eager to see him develop and mature before he is ready, he will feel the pressure and will become frustrated and resistant. Parents should wait until the child shows signs of readiness for new learning and has reached a stage of maturity that will insure success.

When a child is mentally and emotionally ready, he will learn; before that, no amount of urging or prodding does any good. He cannot be toilet trained until his body has reached a certain stage of physical development and growth. Trying to train him too early is as hard on his parents as it is frustrating to him. The mother who is relaxed, confident, and unhurried during the baby's feeding periods will have a child who eats well and enjoys his food. If he refuses food, she should make no issue of it but instead should try to feed him again later. Babies, like adults, are not always hungry and they get tired of certain foods. As soon as the muscles in his hands reach a readiness stage, the child will want to feed himself and he should then be provided with finger foods and a spoon. His untidiness in eating need not cause any concern. He has to learn to feed himself and that takes practice. If his hands are held or if he is fed too long without an opportunity to learn for himself, learning will be delayed. An early start in offering the baby fruit juices,

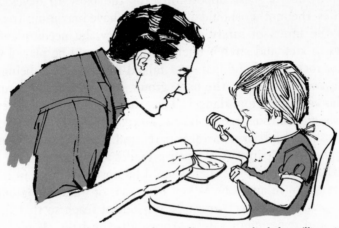

As soon as hand muscles reach a readiness stage, the baby will want to feed himself.

water, and some of his milk from a cup is desirable so that he will have learned how to use this equipment before he is asked to give up sucking on the nipple.

Having a personal physician for continuing medical supervision will contribute to the baby's well-being and to his mother's peace of mind. Immunization and advice about disease prevention may be obtained when visiting the private physician or a well-baby clinic. By following advice on how to care for the baby, the mother learns to know her baby and to judge when it is necessary to call or to see the doctor between regular visits. Learning to recognize symptoms of illness will assist her in knowing how to protect the baby when others in the family are ill.

The parents of a baby should have two goals in mind: first, to have a healthy and happy baby who enjoys his family and is enjoyed by them; and second, to have a baby who progresses from complete helplessness to self-reliance and ability to adjust to others. Responsive and understanding parents will try to provide, to the best of their ability, the emotional climate that helps the child to grow and develop into a well-adjusted adult. The baby must face some restrictions, such as waiting for hot food to cool so that it can be eaten, but the restrictions should be fitted to his abilities.

THE TODDLER

The end of the first year of infancy is a milestone. From then on a noticeable slowing down of growth is apparent, and, while physical growth is still rapid, mental growth is more spectacular and becomes more exciting to watch. The baby's world expands and he begins to explore. This is the time when attention must be given to care of his feet.

Foot Care

Foot care should begin in infancy with the proper fitting of shoes and stockings. Because a young child often outgrows a shoe before he outwears it, parents should be alert to his need for new ones. Shoes should extend about one-half inch beyond the tip of the first or second toe. Socks and stockings for children should

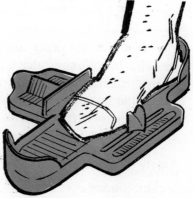

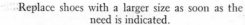
Replace shoes with a larger size as soon as the need is indicated.

extend about one-quarter inch beyond the end of the longest toe when the child is standing. Particular care should be taken that stretch hose are not too short.

Speech and Vocabulary

Speech development as vocal sounds has been going on for many months for the toddler. When he is about 1 year old, he usually

101

begins to master a few words. He is past the babbling stage and is trying to imitate the sounds that have meaning to him. He knows his name and knows the meaning of "no" as being restrictive. Usually by the end of the second year he will have a vocabulary of approximately a hundred words. Talking depends on several factors. His ability to hear and to make what he hears a part of his language is modified somewhat by his temperament and by that of persons around him. The happy, outgoing baby usually talks earlier than the quiet or more placid one. If his mother is tense and silent when caring for him, he is less apt to try to communicate verbally. A child understands words before he is able to say them.

The toddler needs help in acquiring a vocabulary. It is probably instinctive for people to use single words and short sentences with the young child so that he has an opportunity to grasp the meaning. Soon he parrots his mother and associates the word sounds with objects. Nouns, such as cup, milk, mama, daddy, dog, and bed, are learned soonest. There is a sprinkling of action words and verbs, such as bye-bye, up, down, and wait. Naturally, the baby hears much that he does not understand, but this very lack of understanding is a challenge to learn. Nearly all babies mispronounce words when they begin to talk, but their precision in speech gradually improves.

One must recognize that the vocabulary of the toddler is limited and that, unless directions are given clearly and simply, he may become confused. Stress situations, such as a visit to the doctor or the clinic or any other unusual occurrence, may make the baby less able to communicate verbally. He may be unable to tell what it is that frightens him, and at these times especially a child needs understanding and reassurance. To tell him to stop crying or kicking or whatever it is that he does to show stress displays a lack of understanding.

Safety

The toddler is an explorer. He goes from place to place, examining everything within reach and testing it for taste, smell, and touch. He is seldom inactive when he is awake. If his parents understand that this activity is part of his eagerness to learn and evidence of his talents, it is much easier on everyone. Naturally, he must be protected against any harm. For example, much of his mother's time may be spent in the kitchen, and the toddler will want to be where she is. He will make short excursions away but will return frequently to see that she is there. There have been few toddlers who have not opened drawers and cupboard doors to get at the fascinating objects hidden away there. Soaps, detergents, insect poisons, cleaning substances, knives, matches, and even drugs may be in the kitchen, and any of them can be fatal to the toddler. All precautions should be taken to keep these hazards out of his reach.

In spite of wide publicity and efforts to educate parents in accident prevention, accidental deaths still occur among children. For example, there is the hazard of suffocation caused by the child's pulling a plastic clothesbag over his head or the danger of the unused refrigerator stored in the basement or on the back porch without its doors having been removed or padlocked to prevent a child from closing himself in an airtight box.

It is a wise precaution to put the child in his playpen during meal preparation, when his physical presence in the kitchen is a hazard in itself. There is danger that someone may trip over him or, if he gets too close to the stove, that he may be burned by spattering grease or scalded by hot liquid. If the child must remain in the kitchen, care should be taken to turn the handles of pans on the stove to the back so that he cannot reach up and pull the pans off the stove. Since it is natural for him to want to see what is there, the mother should lift him up and allow him to look.

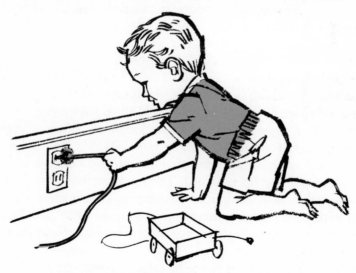

A safety plug over the outlet would remove this hazard.

Electric appliances and electric cords have a fascination for the young child. A parent should guard his own handling of an electrical apparatus so that the child, who is a mimic, never sees an unsafe act. Light bulbs must be kept in all lamp sockets, and unused electric outlets should be covered with adhesive tape or should have safety plugs that the child cannot remove. He should be taught early that he is not to play with electric cords or appliances.

Every room in the home should be examined critically for safety, and hazardous objects should be removed or put where the child cannot get to them. All medicines must be put out of sight and out of reach. Poisonous substances should be stored in a safe place. Bottles and containers that have held substances potentially harmful to the child must be disposed of. It is a poor practice to give him any empty container for a plaything, because he cannot be expected to know whether it once contained a harmful substance.

Frequent inspection of the baby's furniture is needed, and repair should be made promptly if any safety device, such as the safety belts in carriage and stroller, the tray catch on the high chair, and the lock that holds the side of the crib in position, is not in working order. The high chair should have a broad base so that it will not topple. A grab bar is especially helpful to the toddler in getting in and out of the bathtub without assistance. Gates placed at the top and the bottom of stairs prevent falls. The child should be allowed to inspect and to become familiar with everything about him so that his natural curiosity is satisfied. This is the way he learns and develops.

Sleep

Learning to sleep at suitable times and places should be a natural procedure for a child, but sleep can be promoted by providing the right conditions. If it is possible, a child should have its own room where he can enjoy quiet and be undisturbed. While a bassinet has advantages for the very young baby—its very size helps give him a sense of security—a crib that he can use until he is 3 or 4 years old should be his next bed. The mattress should be firm and smooth and have a waterproof covering to keep it clean and free from odor. Firm foam rubber probably makes the best kind of mattress for the crib because it provides body support and promotes proper sleeping posture.

During the second year the baby's sleep pattern changes. Usually the morning nap is eliminated, and the long nap comes after lunch. If the child becomes sleepy before his usual lunch hour, it is wise to feed him earlier. He can then go to bed and sleep well. There is a stage when one nap is not enough and when two naps are not required. The problem can be solved by putting the child to bed earlier in the evening. Parents should expect that his behavior will change from time to time. At about 2 years of age, a child may resist going to sleep, perhaps because of mild anxiety at being separated from his mother. At this stage the child finds innumerable excuses to get his parent back into the room, asking to go to the toilet or to have a drink of water when he really wants neither. If a parent complies, the child does it over and over again. The child should be reminded that he has had his wants satisfied and then he should be left alone. He may cry a little, but his unhappiness will not last long if there is no encouragement to continue.

Toilet Training

Bowel and bladder control comes during the toddler stage. When the child has been weaned, his interests shift to his body and its waste products. He has to learn that his urine and feces are waste materials and are not to be played with. The only way that he can learn socially acceptable toilet methods is by being taught. His readiness depends on the development of his nerves and muscles. Until he has some understanding of the relationship between feeling the need for and going to the toilet, it is a waste of time and emotionally disturbing to the child to try to train him.

During the first year the baby soils and wets his diapers with no restriction and he is completely unaware that he will have to change his ways. An indication of readiness for toilet training is the toddler's awareness that he needs to have a bowel movement. Usually he grunts and strains or pulls at his diaper and in some instances makes verbal sounds that are a sign of his need, all indications for the mother that he is ready for training. Beginning at this time the child should be reminded to go or should be taken to the toilet at regular intervals. His desire for approval and his imitation of his mother are strong factors for success. If he is not the first child in the family, he imitates the older children and does much toward training himself. Self-training usually begins to occur late in the second year, and some children can toilet train themselves in a few days. Of course, the toddler will have lapses and accidents, and his mother's attitude toward this situation as a usual event is important. Children vary so much in their development and in their environment and experiences that what works with one child does not necessarily work with another. The important things are his state of readiness and his parents' attitude of encouragement and approval.

Eating

Eating patterns change too. The toddler no longer needs as much food as in his first year because his growth spurt has slowed down. In addition, his increasing recognition of himself as a person makes him more discriminating about what he eats. He has ideas of his own and forms definite likes and dislikes for foods about which he previously had no marked feelings. Babies less than a year old are usually so hungry that they will eat almost anything offered to them, but the toddler's appetite and hunger are much more variable and his memory is longer. He knows that meals are fairly regular and that he is not going to go hungry.

The toddler stage is the time when parents' feelings have much influence on the child's eating habits and when they need to remember that no child is going to starve himself. Undue pressure to finish a meal creates antagonism and resistance. The child has mixed feelings about wanting to please his mother and about asserting his independence and it is best, therefore, not to make an issue of his refusal to eat. If he is allowed to give up certain foods for a while he will come back to them. To insist that he eat will only harden his dislike. Dr. Benjamin Spock has said: "Feeding problems start more commonly between 1 and 2 years than at any other period. Once a child becomes balky, once a mother becomes worried and angry, the fat's in the fire. The more the mother frets and urges, the less the child eats. And the less he takes, the more anxious the mother is. Meals become agonizing. The problem may last for years." *

Discipline

Discipline is part of the child's learning experience and its primary aim is to help him to learn self-control. The toddler has so many things to learn. His efforts to learn speech so that he can communicate frequently thwart him. Because his span of attention and memory is short, he has to be told over and over. Because his knowledge of ownership is limited, he takes what he wants without heed to the feelings of others. He loves and hates with equal intensity and may bite and claw and kick the playmate with whom he was playing happily a few moments before. The toddler does these things because he has not yet learned the checks and balances of acceptable behavior, has no conscience, and is ruled by the pleasure of the moment. He is still too young to have learned what

---

* *Baby and Child Care*, p. 278.

his mother considers acceptable behavior, but he does recognize that her love and approval are more important to him than doing something of which she does not approve. It is this recognition that gradually teaches him to know what behavior is considered good or bad. The example set by his elders must not be underestimated.

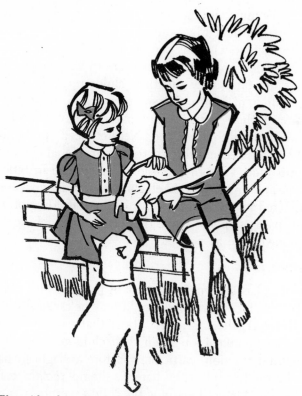

Play with others stimulates the mental, social, emotional, and physical growth of children.

The toddler also learns to know when he is naughty. Although he feels guilty about what he has done, he may go from one irritating act to another if the parent fails to require acceptable behavior. At these times he is really asking for punishment and wants to be halted. He wants to be a good boy, and it is the parents' responsibility to help him learn self-control and keep out of trouble. Rewarding the child's efforts to conform is more successful than punishment. Exerting control is very difficult for some mothers because they can remember how they rebelled at discipline or punishment. However, control must be maintained for the safety of the child and for his emotional growth and to help him achieve socially acceptable behavior patterns. Consistent discipline is an essential factor in child guidance; the toddler and older child need to know what to expect. For children, kindness needs to be combined with firmness and consistency. Discipline should be fitted to the deed and controls changed as the child becomes older and more understanding. Parents must not only protect the child's self-esteem but they must also recognize that his emotional growth and learning are strengthened by positive examples and by rewards for his efforts to become what his parents want him to be.

If parents understand that mistakes are to be expected and that blunders are not fatal, they and their children can be more light-hearted. Children, of course, may sometimes have angry and hostile feelings toward their parents, and parents may sometimes feel hostile toward their children too. Neither need feel guilty over occasional clashes, because the day-to-day emotional climate of the family counts more than the occasional upsets and irritations that loom so large at a single time. Each child is an individual and needs to be considered in that light. To foster the unfolding of a child's abilities, his parents should make the setting in which he develops as free and favorable as possible.

THE SICK CHILD

Every parent has known the anxiety of having a sick child. The first time parents face this experience, it may be especially alarming to them. However, there is never a time that parents do not feel some degree of apprehension when their child gets sick. This is a perfectly natural reaction, particularly before a diagnosis has been made. To be on the safe side, parents should remain calm and should notify the doctor, describing the child's symptoms, and then carefully follow the doctor's instructions.

Familiarity with a child's actions under usual circumstances enables a person to note any change in behavior that may indicate illness. Cranky, fussy, irritable, or whiny behavior does not specifically indicate how the child feels physically. Rather, such behavior is a clue to the probable onset of illness and should be weighed along with physical signs that appear. All parents come to recognize instinctively the changes in the behavior of a child that are signals of underlying discomfort or illness. Aside from the discomforts of his illness, whatever they may be, he is probably anxious about himself. If he is in pain, he dreads more pain and looks forward with no pleasure to any treatment. Recalling numerous admonitions that he will become ill if he does not wear his raincoat in bad weather or if he stays in the swimming pool too long, the child may think of illness as punishment for wrongdoing. From the age of 5 or 6 and on into adolescence children may even associate illness with death because they may have known of someone who died after an illness. Emotional support and understanding are important to the recovery of sick children, and they are entitled to as much explanation as they can understand about what is happening to them and about what the outcome will be.

Acute illness in children is usually abrupt and is announced by a sudden change in behavior and disposition. The child may have nausea, vomiting, and a headache and may refuse to eat. With the onset of infections and communicable diseases, there is usually an elevation of temperature, sometimes to 104° F. or 105° F.

One should remember that body temperature does not remain stable, that it is always fluctuating a little, depending on the time of the day and the amount of physical activity. The younger the child, the more acute is the rise and fall of temperature, because his temperature-regulating mechanism is not well established. The average normal range of a baby's temperature is from 98.6° to 99.6° F. A temperature of more than 99.6° F., if combined with other signs, is considered fever. Temperature generally rises with illness, and the range is usually higher in children than in adults. A sick child may have fever at any time of the day or the night, but his temperature is usually higher in the late afternoon and evening than in the morning.

When a child becomes ill, the general rules that apply for any other sick person should be followed:

- Keep the child as quiet as possible. Rest is important to recovery. The sick baby may need to be held or to be rocked to soothe him until he sleeps.
- Keep other members of the family, especially children, away from the sick child until the illness has been diagnosed. This is only a sensible safety precaution against the spread of possible infection.
- Withhold all food if the child is vomiting or has diarrhea. Offer small amounts of boiled water until vomiting has subsided.
- Let the child's appetite be the guide in offering him food.
- Give no medicine or treatment unless ordered by the doctor.
- Keep for the doctor a record of temperature, nature and fre-

quency of bowel movements and urination, vomiting, food and fluids taken, and duration of sleep.

• Consult the doctor as soon as any unusual symptoms are observed.

THE HOSPITALIZED CHILD

Authenticated studies have shown that hospitalization is a crucial experience for the child between the ages of 18 and 24 months, especially if he must be separated from his parents. Elective surgery can often be postponed beyond this age range, and, if the doctor feels there is no hurry, the probable emotional disturbance of the child is sufficient reason to delay.

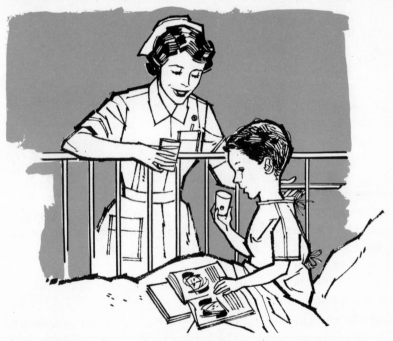

When a child must go to the hospital, he should be told what to expect.

Separation from his mother when he is too young to adjust to separation and change inevitably results in feelings of anger and fear on the part of the child. If undue anxiety is to be avoided, the young child must have the emotional support of his mother, and both of them need understanding and preparation for the hospital experience. The child's parents should explain to him some of the things that are likely to occur in the hospital. Since he has no idea of what it will be like, his imagination may lead him to build up

110

intolerable fear. He should be told what the doctors, nurses, and other hospital workers do and the kind of clothes they will be likely to wear. The child should know that the nurse will probably wake him in the morning to take his temperature and later may give him a bath in bed, and even make the bed with him in it. He should have the reassurance that the nurse will come to him if he calls her when his mother or father is not there. His meals will be served on a tray and will probably be eaten in bed. He may ride through the hall in a wheel chair or on a stretcher and will probably be taken on the elevator to another floor of a hospital for some special examination. He may expect a visit from the laboratory technician, who will prick his finger to get a sample of his blood for examination.

It is important for the child not to be led to believe that there will not be pain or unpleasant experiences in going to the hospital. However, he should not be told everything, for too much knowledge may cause undue apprehension. Calm, matter-of-fact statements help the child accept going to the hospital as another new experience. Most young children adjust very well to hospital life even though they may be uncomfortable.

When a child enters the hospital his father or mother may be allowed to stay with him while he adjusts to his new environment. The strangeness of hospital surroundings is frightening, and the young child is particularly worried about being separated from his parents. A toddler may suffer deeply and lastingly from the hospital experience unless all possible measures are taken to help him feel secure and relaxed. He should have with him a beloved toy or some other familiar possession to lessen his feeling of isolation and strangeness.

The hospital's rules for visiting should be explained to the child. Most hospitals, particularly those for children, encourage parents to visit at any time. When leaving, the parents should tell the child when they will return and then go without prolonged goodbyes. Seeing his parents return reminds the child that although they come and go, he is not forgotten.

Hospital staff members encourage parents to talk freely to them about the child, including his likes and dislikes and how he generally reacts to stress. This information gives them greater understanding of why the sick child behaves as he does. Parents are members of the team that is engaged in restoring the child to health. During their hospital visits they may assist with the child's care, help him to eat, give him his bath, read to him, and hold him in their arms to give him comfort and emotional support. Parents also have an opportunity to talk with the doctors and nurses and can learn how to carry out simple treatments the child may need, how to give medicines that have been ordered, and what reactions can be expected.

Once a child is convalescing, in the hospital or at home, a mother's or a nurse's ingenuity is tested to find interesting but quiet occupations for him. During convalescence is the time to bring out suitable toys, to look for materials with which the child can make playthings, and to bring out the mail order catalogs and colorful magazines for cutouts. An older child may want to learn to knit, to make a puppet, to paint a picture, or to start a scrapbook. Whatever the recreation, it must be chosen with regard for the child's manual ability and interest so that what he creates will give him success and satisfaction. However, the convalescing child must not be allowed to become overtired. The use of radio or television for entertainment should be limited to programs that will not excite or overstimulate. Reading or listening to someone read is a desirable activity. The period of convalescence offers a wonderful opportunity for children to talk about the things that concern them and to bring these concerns out into the open where they can be talked away.

THE HANDICAPPED CHILD

The child who may have to learn to live with a lifetime handicap presents a special problem, for as a rule his needs require skillful handling. Because he must learn to live within the limit of his strength and ability, he must not be coddled or overprotected. However, he must be kept safe and his daily living adjusted to his special needs.

The attitude of his parents is an important factor in helping the child to adjust to and live with his handicap. The parents who feel secure and accept the child's physical appearance and condition will transmit their feelings to the child and he will probably be unaware that he is not like other children. As far as his capabilities permit, he should be treated like any other child. This treatment is what he wants and what best nourishes his emotional growth and development. Although some activities may be out of the question for him, he should be encouraged to play with children so that they become accustomed to each other. Children can be unkind, it is true, but they can also be very understanding and helpful and will usually make allowances for the handicapped child who cannot always keep up with them. If the parents accept the child as he is, his brothers, sisters, and playmates will be likely to do the same.

If guidance with the care of the handicapped is needed, the parent may seek advice from a child psychologist or from a child guidance center. Some children do better in a convalescent or a sheltered home among other handicapped children than at home. Since the circumstances of the handicapping condition differ with every child, no rule can be applied that fits all. The parents' responsibility is to seek the best advice possible, especially if they see that their child is becoming irritable, withdrawn, depressed, or fearful of meeting the problems of everyday life.

In many communities visiting teachers are available for the child confined to bed at home or in the hospital to enable him to continue his studies while convalescing. Special classes for the handicapped may be the answer for children who are not bedfast. A variety of schools, convalescent homes, and boarding homes provide care for crippled children, cardiac patients, the deaf, the blind, children with cerebral palsy, and others. The family doctor and the local or the state health department are able to give information and advice to meet individual needs.

SUGGESTED STUDENT ACTIVITIES

1. If there is a well-baby clinic in your community, obtain permission to visit it while babies are being examined. Make a list of duties that you could assist with at the clinic if you were a volunteer helper.

2. If possible, as a teacher's aide, help with a kindergarten or a first grade group. Report on your duties.

3. If you have no younger brothers or sisters, "borrow" a child for a few hours in order to learn more about children. Make notes and report briefly on what the child did and what he appeared to enjoy.

4. Prepare a list of activities and games that might interest a convalescent child. Specify his age.

5. Consult reports published by large life insurance companies to find mortality rates of infants, adolescents, and young and older adults. What do you think are reasons for the differences in rates of death?

6. Consult several of the books on child growth and development that are available in libraries. Report to the class on the physical, mental, and emotional development of an individual at one of the

following ages: birth to 1 year, the toddler, 4 to 6 years, 6 to 10 years, the preadolescent, and the adolescent.

7. How do the changes in growth and behavior of a child affect the care he should receive? Can adults hasten a child's development?

8. Describe how you might improvise a playpen.

9. Make a list of toys and games suitable for a boy or girl of these ages: 1, 3, 6, and 10 years.

10. Arrange with the instructor to organize a debate on the following statement: It is better for handicapped children, including the mentally handicapped, to be kept at home than to be placed in institutions.

8

THE LATER YEARS

Too many people have stereotyped ideas of what old people are like and what makes them the way they are. They identify the old as rigid, cranky, meddlesome, and forgetful, but these labels are generalizations that may apply to the young as well. The only major difference between old and young people is how long they have lived.

Late maturity can be a satisfactory period of life, with the individual enjoying the warmth of friends, the satisfaction of personal accomplishment, material prosperity, and earned leisure. Because no two persons are alike, there are broad differences in how people adapt to maturity. Everyone has known those who seem old at 40 and others who are young at 80. It is individual adaptation that makes growing old perplexing to some people. Why some people begin to decline in the middle forties and others seem to grow in judgment, friendliness, generosity, and other personal qualities has no ready answer. There are those who think that genetic inheritance predetermines the general pattern of life. Others believe that how one grows old is a matter of mental health and is based on many complex, interacting factors that include heredity, physical health, experience, interpersonal relationships, attitudes of self-esteem, and future goals in life.

Generally speaking, the early adult years are the period of greatest physical activity. During middle adulthood, people are concerned with establishing a career, rearing a family, and planning and working for financial security. By the time that most adults have reached their personal goals and their children are living their own lives, they are facing old age.

Americans tend to attach much importance to the value of keeping young. The idea that youth is the best time of life is widely prevalent. The philosophy of modern thought on aging was expressed by the French writer Victor Hugo when he said: "Forty is the old age of youth and fifty is the youth of old age." It is, therefore, not surprising to find people of middle age lamenting their youth as gone and attempting to create the impression that they are younger than their years. Dissatisfaction and dislike of oneself arising from the awareness of increasing age are mental health problems tied to the idea that youth is superior to age. The "youth of old age" can be a beginning. As involvement with one's family decreases, there is more time for friendships and leisure-time activities, both important values of middle age.

Aging is a continuous process that begins when life begins. Every cell of the body has its own life span in the normal maintenance of the body. The human body has been compared to a machine in that it requires food for energy, but, unlike a machine, the body has the ability to repair itself. How efficiently the repairs are made varies from person to person because of many individual differences. No two persons age in the same way at the same time, and emotional and physical stress take their tolls in different ways in persons. Just as the impact of day-to-day living affects length of life, so too do accidents, disease, and emotional stress. This is not to say that the aging person inevitably becomes a sick old person. He does not. Many old people are affected very little by the chronic illnesses that are associated with aging. Most individuals proceed confidently into old age, maintaining their health, alertness, and interest to life's end. A happy and healthy old age can more likely be achieved if one starts early in life to bring it about. Healthful living during the first 40 years of life is a priceless contribution to the second 40.

Because no two persons do things in the same way, people will adjust to change with the same individuality. Everyone's experiences are different, and everyone reacts in relation to his past experience. The cantankerous old person was very likely a hard-to-get-along-with young person. He did not become that way overnight, and as he grew older he became more like his real self. The reactions he displays need not be the result of aging but instead may very well reflect his true personality. The adjustments of youth and of middle age are no less demanding; they only differ in kind and time. The ability to cope with stress in a mature manner is evidence of sound mental health. The world of the space age is fast moving and rapidly changing and requires great adaptability on the part of all men and women. Those who are prepared can meet the problems of today's living with wisdom and flexibility.

HOW PEOPLE AGE

People age in different and interrelated ways. Chronological age is measured in years. Biological age indicates where one is physically in the total life span. Psychological age is the result of inherited characteristics and adaptive effort in meeting change brought about by chronological age. Social age is measured by a person's ability to perform the various roles expected of him in his community. While there is a degree of sameness in the way individuals age, there are also wide differences. Changes do not occur at the same rate nor with the same degree of intensity. Also, the effects of aging are not the same. Some older people have great physical strength and endurance. Others have great intellectual power. Some are emotionally strong in the face of fear or of disappointment, while others cannot tolerate stress without breaking. Some have great resistance to disease, and others are frequently ill.

The physical or biological changes in aging are the most evident. Graying hair, wrinkled skin, and bowed shoulders are common aging signs that occur at different times in different people. Because there is interest in knowing what physical changes to expect, what the possible effects are, and what can be done about the effects, a brief description of the aging process is presented here.

The Aging Process

Areas and Types of Expected Changes	Possible Effects of Physical Changes	Examples of What To Do
1. *Body tissue and bony structure* Mineral salts, particularly calcium, shift from bone to tissues and blood vessels.	Bones are more brittle and more easily broken.	Obtain periodic physical examination. Guard against tripping and falling. Wear well-constructed shoes with a broad medium-high heel and wear an ankle support too if needed. Keep stairways and ramps uncluttered, well lighted, in good repair, and equipped with handrails.

Areas and Types of Expected Changes	Possible Effects of Physical Changes	Examples of What To Do
Cell division and capacity for cell growth and tissue repair is retarded.	Blood vessels are less elastic. Heart must work harder to supply needed blood to internal organs.	Use aids for circulation and muscle relaxation, such as rocking chairs and footrests. When lying down to rest, elevate the legs and feet to the level of the heart.
2. Dentition Lost dental enamel is not replaced.	There is a tendency for teeth to deteriorate and for gums to change, with possible infection when decay occurs.	Obtain regular dental care. Keep mouth clean and free from infection. Eat a well-balanced diet.
Teeth may be lost.	Diet habits may change. There may be some change in facial appearance.	Obtain dental care, including properly fitted dentures. Keep dentures in the mouth. Keep mouth and dentures clean.
3. Hearing Hearing is progressively lost in one or both ears.	Person may be unaware of his handicap or may refuse to acknowledge it, and frequently misunderstands when he is spoken to. He may withdraw from group activities with resultant loneliness.	Accept help in adjusting to and accepting handicap. Obtain necessary medical care and treatment. Learn to use a hearing aid if it is recommended.
	Accidents may occur because of inability to hear.	Remind family, friends, and others of the need to face the person and to speak slowly and distinctly when talking to the hard of hearing.
4. Circulation Blood vessels become narrowed and obstructed, slowing the flow of blood.	There is a tendency for clots to form. If varicose veins exist, they may break down, forming ulcers.	Keep as active as possible to promote circulation. Obtain medical care for ulcer infection or open skin lesions. Keep skin dry.
Adjustment to temperature and to activity is slower and circulation is poorer in the extremities, especially in the legs.	A person is more sensitive to cold, and body temperature usually remains low.	Prevent loss of body heat with additional warm clothing. Keep floors and house comfortably warm.

Areas and Types of Expected Changes	Possible Effects of Physical Changes	Examples of What To Do
5. *Nervous system* Sensory perception and motor strength are reduced.	Sensory and motor impulses and reactions to external stimuli are retarded, and the person is slower to react to danger.	Use caution when applying heat or cold to the body. Regard pain as a danger signal. Write things down to compensate for memory loss. Use caution so that accident hazards are not overlooked or forgotten. Obtain prompt medical care and treatment as needed.
6. *Vision* Changes may occur in the lens and in the blood vessels of the eyes. Near vision may be impaired.	If vision changes interfere with occupational or recreational activities, the person may have an emotional reaction. Accidents are more apt to occur because of poor vision. Person may have blurred or restricted field of vision. Cataracts and glaucoma may develop.	Provide increased lighting for close work and for reading. Rest the eyes frequently. Eat an adequate diet. Avoid cluttered floors or having any objects about that may be a hazard. Have regular eye examinations.
7. *Skin* Aging of other organs affects the skin. Circulation changes reduce the blood supply and retard the transfer of sensory and motor impulses.	Extremities, especially the feet, may be swollen, cold, burning, or otherwise uncomfortable. The skin bruises easily and is prone to infection, especially in the legs and feet. The skin may become uncomfortably dry and wrinkled.	Keep the feet clean and dry and elevate them when resting. Report any rash or open sore to the doctor. Lubricate the skin with mild cream or lotion to keep it soft, pliable, and in good condition. Use soap sparingly. Use caution when applying external heat because of danger of burning.
Decreased gland activity and other aging factors may influence the color, amount, and texture of the hair.	Hair may become gray, dry, and thinner.	Keep the hair clean and brush it gently at least once a day to stimulate circulation of the scalp and to keep well groomed.

Areas and Types of Expected Changes	Possible Effects of Physical Changes	Examples of What To Do
8. *Sleep* Sleep patterns change. Lessened activity decreases the need for long periods of sleep, and there is a tendency to nap during the day.	Increased leisure encourages more frequent rest and sleep periods. Sleeping at night may become briefer.	Resist inactivity. Do not become overtired, but keep activities within limits of tolerance.
9. *Nutrition* Less food is required because of lessened activity.		Try to stay at or less than the average weight for your height and age.
Taste buds become less sensitive.	A reduced appetite may occur, and indifference to food may develop. Eating may become too much trouble for the person and, therefore, his nutrition may suffer.	Eat a balanced diet. Eat smaller and more frequent meals. Avoid foods that experience has shown to be hard to digest.
10. *Sexual* The cessation of menstruation and menopause occur in women.	Usual menopausal symptoms are hot flashes, excessive sweating, and irritability.	Develop understanding of this phase of the life cycle.
There is a diminution of sexual activity in men.	Men and women may have periods of anxiety and worry and may become despondent.	Plan interesting activities to keep occupied.

The aging process cannot be reversed, but some of the changes that occur can be retarded by the observance of sound personal health practices. The following are important rules for keeping healthy as long as possible:

- Eat adequate daily meals.
- Use good posture.
- Take suitable exercise and alternate it with appropriate rest.
- Pay attention to personal safety.
- Obtain periodic physical examinations.
- Develop good mental and emotional attitudes.

Diet

All through life the foods that make up the daily meals help in keeping the body strong and in protecting it against weakness and infection. A well-nourished body has greater recuperative power when illness does occur.

The need for good nutrition does not end when one stops growing. When many older people of today were growing up, some of the important foods were scarce and expensive and little was known about their special value in the diet. The citrus fruits were regarded as a luxury, and their vitamin C content, with its important function of helping the body to resist infection, had not yet been discovered. The importance of milk throughout life to preserve the characteristics of youth and to increase the years of usefulness also was not then known. Today these foods are plentiful and within the reach of most pocketbooks. However inexpensive they may be, many older people still neither understand their nutritive value nor have they learned to eat them. Now they must be encouraged to follow good eating habits—and it is never too late to learn.

As one grows older, certain physiological changes occur that may decrease the amount of food needed or wanted. A person becomes less active physically, the digestive juices decrease and food is digested more slowly, and the ability of the body to absorb and utilize some food essentials is lessened. Another difficulty for many older people is the loss of some or all of their teeth, which may affect their ability to chew.

The physiological changes that occur with aging may result in failure to eat the very foods that in later life the body needs in larger amounts. Meat, fruits, and vegetables, which are rich in protein, calcium, iron, and vitamins, are the protective foods needed in abundance. Because older people are less active and their digestive processes tend to slow down, they require fewer high calorie foods, such as fats and oils, starchy foods, and sweets. The intake of these foods should be limited so that the body can keep a desired weight level while still maintaining adequate nutrition.

Very often some of the complaints of older people, such as tiredness, inability to sleep, anxiety, and depression, have their origin in poor eating habits and undernutrition. Eating should be a source of both health and pleasure. Appetite and digestion are influenced by the appearance, smell, and taste of food as well as by the emotional climate in which food is eaten. Fatigue, worry, or anger at mealtimes can destroy appetite and upset digestion and assimilation of food. Meals that are well prepared, served attractively at regular hours, and eaten in pleasant surroundings with congenial companions tempt the appetite and, more important, aid the body in making better use of food.

Posture

Posture is the way one holds his body. It is the relationship that one part of the body has to the other parts when a person sits, stands, lies down, or walks about. Maintaining good posture makes one feel better because it lessens strain on the muscles and joints and prevents fatigue. Good posture also conserves energy and promotes better functioning of all parts of the body. Generally speaking, the muscles of the body act in groups and in opposition to each other. When one muscle group contracts or shortens, its opposite extends or lengthens. It is this action that makes movement possible and that achieves body balance through coordinated action. Walking is an example of the alternate lengthening and shortening of the muscles attached to the joints at hips, knees, and ankles and of balance achieved by muscle coordination.

The tiring that results from most activity is normal and to be expected. When activity is accompanied by alternate periods of rest, the body systems are able to rid themselves of accumulated waste materials and to replenish their energy-giving supplies and there is no ill effect on muscle tone, strength, or one's health. It therefore follows that adequate nutrition together with alternate periods of rest and activity greatly influence body posture.

The emotions and mental attitudes have an influence on body posture. Depression, happiness, grief, pain, and even one's attitude toward life are reflected in body position. Bearing changes as the emotions vary, and judgments of the emotional and the physical health of people are often made from observations of their posture.

Good posture is important both in activity and in rest. Holding the head up and the shoulders back and pushing the chest forward makes the space in the chest cavity larger and breathing more efficient. Many tasks can be performed while the individual is sitting down, thereby saving the energy required to stand and do the same amount of work. A kitchen table and a sink at convenient heights eliminate stooping and stretching that tire the back and the shoulder muscles. Learning how to lift and move heavy objects prevents muscle strain and fatigue. Frequent changes of a person's position when sleeping are unconscious reflex actions taken to relieve fatigue.

Exercise

Exercise should be a daily activity to prevent extreme fatigue and undue strain on muscles and joints. Limiting athletic exercise to the week-end is an example of what not to do. Regular physical exercise has many benefits. It stimulates respiration, improves the appetite, relieves nervous tension, provides relaxation, helps to control the weight, and aids the circulation. Exercise should be selected on an individual basis according to age, ability, tolerance, and personal preference and, in some cases, on the advice of the doctor. Walking is an excellent form of exercise for most people, and even such simple exercising as rocking in a rocking chair has great value.

If the older person is not used to exercising, the activity should be started slowly and increased gradually. A person is never too old to participate in recreational exercise that is within the limits of his endurance, nor is there a set age at which he should stop accustomed activities. True, not every older person should, for example, play tennis, but if it is a game that he has played since youth, perhaps he needs only to decrease the time spent in this activity.

A well-known heart specialist has made the following observations:

"To be sure, no hard and fast rules about exercise can be laid down for everyone of a certain age, in the first place, because no two persons have exactly the same physical needs or psychological preferences and, secondly, because chronological age is not the same as physiological age. Also it is true that some individuals live to be old and free from disease despite the fact that the only exercise they get is in breathing, eating, talking, and in tending to the minimal physiological processes of mother nature; what percentage of healthy older persons belong in this category has not been determined, but it appears to be considerably in the minority.

"Naturally, in extreme old age, when physical strength and mental ability steadily decline, there comes a time when exercise beyond that of the simplest acts of living is no longer possible, but in the early and middle years of old age exercise can be very beneficial. It is important to recognize that here is a difference between positive health and the mere absence of disease." *

Personal Safety

The physical condition of an elderly person seems to correspond to his susceptibility to accident. Quite often, however, accident prevention is within the control of the individual himself. Many accidents are the result of long-standing habits of which the individual is no longer aware. Others are the result of physical changes, such as changes in vision, hearing, and reaction time. Most accidents happen in the home, and falling is the most common accident that happens to older people.

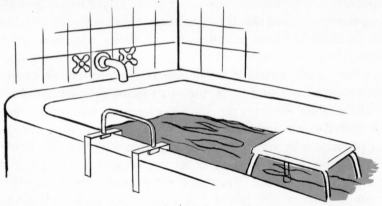

Many of the accidents that occur in getting in and out of the bathtub can be prevented by the use of grab bars, a rubber suction mat, and a stool or tub seat.

Much has been said and written about the influence of attitudes in the prevention of accidents. Actually, an attitude is not in itself a response but a gradually developed pattern of action, a habit, or a way in which a person acts under certain circumstances. Daydreaming, inattention, aggression, or frustration may be the trigger that sets off the train of events that culminate in an accident. Personal problems are factors too, because they create stress and tension.

* Paul D. White, "The Role of Exercise in the Aging," *Journal of the American Medical Association*, 165, No. 1 (September 7, 1957), 70.

There is also a close relationship between accidents and house-keeping. As safety precautions, homes in which older people live must be well lighted and the floors should be kept uncluttered. There should be no highly polished floors or slippery scatter rugs. Conveniently placed handrails are recommended for stairs and hallways. If accidents are to be prevented, people must acquire habits of caution and alertness, become aware of places and situations where accidents are most likely to occur, and work toward the elimination of these hazards.

Medical Supervision

The periodic physical examination is an inventory of the person's current health status and therefore is an essential health practice. The examination is a preventive measure for the early detection of progressive and disabling conditions and will many times avert or delay serious illness. The fact that most of the long-term illnesses the aged are likely to have can be controlled or their severity lessened if they are discovered and treated early is a compelling reason for continuous medical supervision. Early detection of disease is more important than the most skillful treatment after disease has become advanced.

Every family should have a family physician. Not only is he the doctor when someone is ill, but he becomes a friend and coun-selor. The family physician should be selected before illness oc-curs so that he can get to know the individual when he is ap-parently well, when circumstances are not influenced by stress and anxiety, and when the patient's behavior is less likely to be altered by emotion. To recognize significant change, the doctor must know how the patient behaves under average conditions.

The doctor needs to know the medical history of the patient. Information about a person's past illnesses and injuries, his reaction to certain drugs, and his general health in terms of nutrition, sleep patterns, rest and relaxation, stressful situations, and personality characteristics all become a part of the patient's medical record. This information is necessary for the doctor to be able to appraise the patient's general health.

What the older person probably wants most when he talks about himself to the family physician is interest and attention. What the older person can do to help his doctor most is to report to him any noticeable changes such as pain or persistent discomfort, bleeding or spotting from any body opening, and the appearance of a growth or mass of any kind, particularly if it tends to become larger. Any

125

noticeable change in function of any part or organ of the body are danger signals that demand immediate attention.

The physical examination provides an opportunity to find out whether the older person requires immunization or vaccination against certain communicable diseases to which he may be susceptible. It is essential and practical to utilize these safeguards. Also, a routine physical examination will show the doctor any changes in the patient's elimination, circulation, digestion, skin condition, and body weight. Sometimes sleep patterns have changed. Sleeping less or more, difficulty in getting to sleep, restlessness, and periods of wakefulness are all matters of concern to the doctor. Changes in vision, hearing, taste, smell, or sensitivity to heat or cold are symptoms that should be reported to the doctor to help him appraise the patient's general health.

Another aspect of illness is its cost. Many families have insurance to cover both hospital and medical care, and some insurance contracts provide payment or part-payment for drugs, laboratory examinations, and loss of income during illness. It is wise for the individual to tell the doctor the amount and kind of insurance coverage carried and to discuss with him fees for office visits and for home calls. The patient should also find out in advance what preference about local hospitals his doctor has and where he usually sends his patients when they are ill.

Mental and Emotional Attitudes

Personality is the sum total of one's physical and mental activities and attitudes. As one ages, personality characteristics are intensified and one becomes more and more like oneself. Illness is one of the stress situations in which changes in personality and attitudes are intensified and become more marked, because sickness is often a threat to the individual, and his own estimation of himself may be lowered. When illness occurs to the well-adjusted person, he uses his personality and emotional strengths as defenses against the increased stresses and thereby makes sickness and disability less overwhelming and less apt to disturb his image of himself as a whole person. One of the main needs of everyone is to learn to understand and to accept himself. As a person must learn to live with a physical handicap, so must he learn to live in harmony with his personality. His own insight into why he reacts and behaves in certain ways is essential to his mental health. When a person has learned to understand himself he can more easily

126

make the effort to be friendly and outgoing, and then life becomes richer and more satisfying.

Mental attitudes play an important part in how people adjust to life physically, for physical and mental health go hand in hand. Good mental health has its own distinguishing aspects that are easy for anyone to recognize. The ability to get along with oneself, the ability to get along with others, and the ability to adjust to changing situations are the identifying characteristics of the mentally well person. Although everyone may have times when one or more of these factors is temporarily upset or out of balance, his ability to make adjustments in his daily living is basic to his mental well-being. People everywhere want about the same things from life: something to do, someone to love, a place to live, health, and

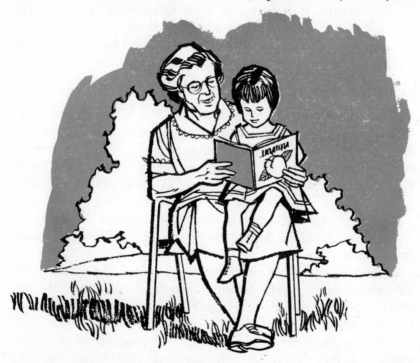

A strong attachment between children and older people contributes to the emotional health of both.

security. Their greatest problems are likely to be loneliness and a deep sense of not being wanted, needed, or noticed, all of which are stressful situations. No one can escape stress in some degree, for it is a part of living. But how one reacts to love, hate, pleasure, injury, or illness is the result of past experience, training, inherited tendencies, and habit.

Although there are no hard and fast rules for solving life's problems, the worry and tension they bring can be lessened. Many people have found the following guides to be helpful:

- Take time for play. There are many inexpensive hobbies that provide relaxation.
- Share your troubles with someone. A good friend or a pastor or a priest can often help to put the problems into proper perspective and to find a solution.
- Do not bottle up anger. Relieve it by physical activity. Take a long walk, go swimming, dig in the garden, do something that brings on healthy fatigue.
- Accept what cannot be changed. It is futile to fight against circumstances over which one has no control. Also, for one's own mental health it is better to learn to understand and accept people as they are than to try to change them.
- Keep physically fit. Mental health and physical health are closely related, and physical conditions affect one's outlook on life.

SUGGESTED STUDENT ACTIVITIES

1. Get a copy of the report on *The 1961 White House Conference on Aging* and discuss some of the recommendations presented there. (Reports on the various sections of the conference may be obtained for a small fee from the U.S. Government Printing Office, Washington, D.C., and are probably available at your public library.)

2. Discuss "ageless" persons whom you know or about whom you have read. What do you think are the qualities that make them "ageless"?

3. Dramatize a home situation in which an older person takes his rightful place in the family, makes his contribution to the group, and is treated by each family member with consideration and affection.

4. Plan a party for residents of an old people's home. Make suggestions for games and activities that both young and old people could participate in together.

5. If there are Golden Age clubs or similar recreation centers in your community, arrange with the instructor to invite one of the club leaders to speak to the class about the program. What suggestions do you have for youth participation in the activities of the center?

6. Make a list of desirable health practices for yourself. Do they differ from those recommended for the aged person? In what way?

9

THE PATIENT WITH A LONG-TERM ILLNESS

Long-term illness can occur at any time of life. Although this kind of illness is primarily associated with the older person, heart disease, arthritis, rheumatism, disabling accidents, and chronic illness as an aftermath of acute communicable disease make the very young as vulnerable as the aged. A characteristic of much long-term illness is its insidious course. Usually the onset of disability is slow. The symptoms may develop so gradually that the individual, particularly an aged person, may overlook or may minimize them. The disease can be well advanced before it causes sufficient discomfort or restricts activity enough for the sufferer to seek medical attention. A regular physical examination is a safeguard for everyone so that illness can be recognized early and treatment started.

Today people are living longer, and the number of people who live to old age increases every year. There are several reasons for this. Increased medical knowledge has resulted in the control of acute communicable disease and in better infant and maternal health. In the past, infants, children, and mothers were especially vulnerable to infection, and their death rate was high. Modern drug therapy has dramatically reduced the acute infectious illnesses that affect all age groups, and better nutrition has improved their health.

Despite scientific advances, as people live longer, their bodies tend to slow down and wear out. The older they become, the more likely they are to be affected by some chronic disability or illness and, with added years, the more certain they are to need medical and nursing care. The trend in the United States is toward caring for the sick at home. It is estimated that in this country eight out of ten patients with a long-term illness are being cared for at home. There is an advantage to this, for in many instances the patient does better in the warm, loving atmosphere of his home than in a hospital or a nursing home.

Many medical, nursing, and other health-related groups in the community have joined with social agencies to serve families in caring for the sick at home. This plan makes it possible for some patients to remain at home and for many who are hospitalized to go home earlier. More and more hospitals are providing progressive care. The seriously ill patient requires and receives the greatest amount of nursing care. As he improves and can do more for himself, he receives less nursing service. This plan prepares convalescent patients to take care of some of their own nursing needs both while they are hospitalized and when they return home. In some communities, housekeeping services are provided for convalescents who need this assistance. Although these forward-looking services are not available in all parts of the country, interest in them is growing. It is likely, however, that for some time to come, perhaps always, most of the responsibility of caring for persons who have a long-term illness will rest with the family. Certainly this will be true in the event of a national disaster of any kind, when a shortage of medical, nursing, and institutional personnel and facilities could be expected.

WHEN ILLNESS OCCURS

The patient with a long-term illness needs essentially the same kind of nursing care as does any other sick person: to be kept clean, well nourished and as comfortable as possible, and to have his disabilities treated. He needs emotional support, encouragement, tolerant understanding, and acceptance of him as a person to aid him in recovery and a return to optimum health.

The illness of an elderly person is likely to be progressive, with symptoms increasing so slowly in number and in intensity that there may be delay in recognizing them. In contrast, the illness of a young person tends to have an acute, almost explosive onset that is so conspicuous that it cannot be overlooked.

The patient who has an acute illness usually goes to bed until he has been seen by the doctor and a diagnosis has been made. Bedrest has positive advantages for him. Keeping warm, quiet, relaxed, and comfortable provides rest, builds resistance, and helps repair damage caused by the illness. Going to bed at the first appearance of illness may prevent the spread of a communicable disease. To be on the safe side, the person with a fever, headache, nausea, sore throat, or running nose—all symptoms of many of the communicable diseases—should go to bed in a room by himself or at least isolate himself from other family members until the doctor sees him or until he feels better.

Bedrest for the patient with a long-term illness is a different matter. When the doctor tells such a patient to stay in bed, he is prescribing a form of treatment that is often as important as medicine and without which sometimes medicine can do little good. However, because of the rapidity with which physical changes may occur, complete bedrest has dangers and is prescribed only when it is absolutely necessary. Whether bedrest is to be partial or complete and for how long it should continue are matters for the doctor to determine. There are times when there is no substitute for enforced immobility, and at these times the nursing care that the patient receives is vital in the prevention of complications. It is more difficult for the aged to recover from enforced bedrest than it is for the average young adult.

During bedrest muscles lose tone and develop weakness and changes occur so rapidly in the joints, tendons, and muscles that in about 3 weeks contractures can occur that are very difficult to overcome. The muscles lose their power, and the patient may be unable to stand or to maintain balance when he is allowed to get up. It is only by active exercise that muscles maintain their strength and tone, and motion is the only way to maintain mobility of the joints.

Circulatory changes also occur with prolonged bedrest. These changes are demonstrated by swelling of the feet and the legs, by dizziness, and even by fainting when the patient gets out of bed. They can occur after only a few days of inactivity. In general, heart action is slower when a person is at rest, as shown by a slower pulse and a decrease in blood pressure.

In addition, studies have established that prolonged bedrest upsets metabolic balance. This imbalance results in rapid excretion of both nitrogen and calcium, which in turn causes a change in the patient's muscle tissue and bone composition. The excretion of calcium through the urinary system may result in the formation of mineral deposits in the kidney and in the bladder.

Pressure sores, or decubiti, are another complication of prolonged bedrest. They usually occur at the bony prominences of the body, such as the shoulder blades, the elbows, the heels, and the lower end of the spine, where the weight is borne. Their primary cause is that the patient has remained in one position so long that circulation in the skin is impaired. The withdrawal of nitrogen from body tissues during illness results in loss of weight, accelerates the breakdown of the skin, and slows healing. Pressure sores can be more easily prevented than cured. The best precaution against them is to keep the patient's skin clean and dry and to change his position frequently.

UNDERSTANDING THE SICK

Sick people of any age react emotionally to illness. To understand why they behave as they do, one must be aware that everyone has certain innate needs. He wants recognition, love, security, success, and, above all, self-esteem. One of the fears of the sick, especially of the older person, is that he will become helpless and unable to care for himself and thus will lose his independence. Long-term illness and permanent disability are threatening situations that bring anxiety to the individual and threaten his image of his personal worth. The ill person should be allowed to do everything he can for himself even if it is no more than to wash his face. Self-help has emotional significance that should not be underestimated.

As a rule, the older person should not be hurried. His reaction time has slowed, and he does not coordinate physically as efficiently as he once did. These reactions are intensified for the elderly sick. To show them impatience and to do things for them that they can do for themselves if given enough time are threats to their dignity. The danger of doing too much for the patient is that he may cease to do for himself and may become totally dependent on others. People who are ill for a long time have a common pattern of behavior: the longer they are ill, the more dependent they become and the more they feel that they are unable to do for themselves. In time they may even come to think that their situation is hopeless and may refuse to do anything for themselves unless aided and encouraged.

The effect on children of chronic illness or a handicapping condition is largely determined by the feelings and attitudes of their parents and those about them. There is no doubt that an ill child experiences insecurity and that illness has permanent psychological effects. Helping the child to accept his handicaps and to use his remaining abilities, both physical and emotional, makes it more likely that he will develop desirable attitudes as he matures.

Elderly people are often as troubled by the evidences of the

132

slowing down of their mental processes as they are by the physical changes that occur. They find it impossible to keep as many things in mind as once they could and may forget something that has real importance for them. This lapse of memory sometimes causes a person to feel inadequate. Failure to remember names, dates, and, especially, recent occurrences is annoying to anyone and is particularly troubling to the aged.

The job of the home nurse and of the other family members in caring for someone with a long-term illness is often a hard one that may require adjustments in living habits and even in attitudes. To maintain a balance between being over-protective and being callous to the suffering of the patient requires maturity, endurance, and a sense of humor. The family should appear cheerful in the patient's presence because cheerfulness has an encouraging effect on the sick. Flexibility in the management of the patient when it does no harm and firmness when it is necessary are advisable. Kindness toward him is always essential. It is particularly important for family members to understand the behavior of the older person, who sometimes appears not to appreciate the care and attention given him. His irritation and resentment probably arise from frustration at being unable to care for himself.

The key to successful handling of the tense and anxious sick person is to help him to learn how to live with his handicap, particularly when his convalescence is prolonged. He must learn to accept what cannot be helped and to make the best of the abilities and faculties that remain. How he does this is largely determined by his personality and mental health and by the effort he puts into making a new life for himself. There must be a compelling desire to learn new skills, new ways of doing things, and new patterns of living. Without this drive to succeed he will fail. To learn to do for oneself is indeed the primary component of rehabilitation. Rehabilitation of the long-term ill, either young or old, should begin when illness begins and should continue until the patient is restored to an optimum of his pre-illness abilities. However, no one can retain his mental health without the stimulation of friends and loved ones. Because this support becomes even more necessary when illness occurs, the role of friends and family in the care and rehabilitation of the sick is an important one. At all ages love and security are fundamental to emotional and physical health. Respect for the person as an individual who has the same desires and needs as others, tolerance for his foibles, and kindness aid in his adjustment to illness and disability.

THE SICKROOM

The room selected for the patient confined to bed for some time should meet both his needs and those of the person who will be giving the nursing care. The sickroom should be sunny and airy. It should provide quiet and privacy, be near the bathroom, and offer a convenient and uncluttered arrangement of personal belongings and furniture.

For the convenience of the home nurse in caring for the patient, a hospital bed is recommended. Many times a hospital bed can be borrowed from the local visiting nurse association, the health department, or other health or welfare agencies in the community. A hospital bed can be rented or bought from any hospital supply company. One of the advantages of using a hospital bed is that it is high enough to allow the home nurse to give care to the patient without strain to her back and shoulder muscles. In addition, it can be operated mechanically to provide a backrest and other supports and has side rails to keep the patient from falling out of bed. The side rails are also an aid to the patient in turning or in changing his position in bed. If a hospital bed is not available, an ordinary bed elevated on blocks to make it the proper height for the home nurse is entirely satisfactory, and equipment for the comfort and the safety of the patient can be improvised. However, when the patient is to be in and out of bed daily, an elevated bed should not be used because it creates a hazard for him. As a further precaution, the casters should be removed to make the bed stable.

A good firm mattress is essential to the comfort of the patient with a long-term illness. The mattress should be enclosed in a washable cover for protection and cleanliness. If a waterproof cover is needed, it should be thin and should fit the mattress snugly to prevent wrinkles. For added comfort a cotton mattress pad can be placed over the waterproof cover. A sponge rubber mattress is excellent for the patient who must spend most of the time in bed. A special air mattress, called the alternating pressure mattress, is recommended for the patient who is likely to develop bed sores or who may already have them. Turning the mattress regularly from end to end and from side to side will distribute pressure and wear as evenly as possible, although modern mattresses are built to give extra support at the heaviest parts of the body. It may be necessary to use bedboards to make the mattress firm and level. Masonite or ¾ inch plywood is good material to use for this purpose. The board should be cut large enough to cover the bed springs to prevent the mattress from sagging. Exposure to sun and air for a few hours once a week if possible and regular thorough brushing with a vacuum cleaner appliance will keep the mattress clean and sweet smelling.

Large sheets are necessary for both comfort and cleanliness. The 108-inch length provides an ample amount to anchor the bottom sheet well under the conventional size mattress and to fold the top sheet over the blanket to keep the blanket clean. The bottom sheet must provide a tight smooth surface. Contour bottom sheets are convenient, and their snug fit makes them wrinkle free. Nylon contour sheets wash more easily and dry more rapidly than cotton sheets and require no ironing. A draw sheet placed across the center of the bed may offer additional protection to the bottom bedding and is an aid in moving the patient in bed.

Blankets should be clean, soft, light in weight, and sufficiently warm for the patient's comfort. An extra long blanket has the advantage of reaching high enough to keep the patient's shoulders warm and still provide enough length to anchor under the lower end of the mattress to assure that his feet will stay covered. The fabric is a matter of personal choice. Cotton blankets wash well and are suitable for use in mild weather. Woolen blankets and those made from synthetic fibers are warmer than cotton blankets but need special care in washing if they are not to be dry cleaned. If an electrically heated blanket is used, precautions should be taken to follow carefully the directions for use. If a bedspread is used, a lightweight cotton one that can be laundered easily is preferable.

The temperature of the sickroom should be warm enough to keep the patient comfortable and to prevent chilling when he is bathed or is uncovered for any reason. Adequate ventilation should be provided at all times, and the room should be aired daily.

Light should not shine directly in the patient's eyes. Preferably, the bed should be placed so that light from a window comes from the side or the back of the bed; if neither is possible, the shades should be lowered or a screen placed to avoid glare. Light from a bedside lamp should come over the patient's shoulder to prevent strain and tiring of the eyes. When a night light is needed, a small light plugged into the wall outlet or a flashlight is usually sufficient.

A comfortable chair in the room will encourage family members and guests to sit down and talk with the patient and help him keep in touch with family activities and feel that he has a part in them. Plants, an aquarium, or a household pet, if they are permitted, can be a source of great pleasure to the patient whether he is young or old. A radio, a record player, or a television set can provide recreation for the patient who has to be alone much of the time.

Cleanliness and order in the sickroom are important to the welfare and comfort of the patient and they are a real timesaver for the home nurse. Cleanliness involves keeping the patient and his bedding free from perspiration and body discharges, promptly removing all soiled articles from the room, and keeping down dust that might carry disease germs to or from the room. Careful washing of the hands before and after giving nursing care is a basic precaution against spread of infection.

Noise is upsetting to the ill person, and small noises are often more disturbing than loud, unaccustomed sounds. Recurring sounds such as those made by creaking doors, rattling windows, flapping shades, and dripping faucets are the chief offenders. Talking or whispering outside the room of a patient, particularly one with an acute illness, may also be disturbing. Conversations that the sick person should not hear should take place completely out of his hearing.

PLANNING THE PATIENT'S CARE

Any illness of a family member has a disrupting effect on the family, but when the patient has a long-term illness and is to be cared for at home, the impact is apt to be more severe. This situation affects the division of work, the recreation, perhaps the living arrangements, and more often than not the money available for daily living expenses. Often many adjustments will have to be made, but, if the attitudes and relationships of family members toward one another are good, there will be a sharing of responsibility and work even though one person may be designated as the home nurse. The home nurse and the other members of the family can do their best for the patient only when they themselves get sufficient rest, food, and recreation to keep fit.

Obviously, the routine of the patient's day will vary according to the nature and severity of the illness, but the nursing care will always include providing meals, medicines, and treatments. Help with personal grooming and with dressing may be needed if the patient is allowed up. The patient may need assistance in getting necessary exercise and rest periods. The important thing in planning the nursing care is to work out a schedule that will permit the patient to get the care he needs at the time he needs it. The schedule should take into consideration among other things the usual habits of the sick person. Many older people have formed habits that are harmless although sometimes annoying to others. As long as these habits do not endanger the patient or anyone else, he should be allowed to continue them. If the sick person has been accustomed to taking a bath at night before going to sleep, this practice should probably be continued. Then washing his hands and face and rubbing his back in the morning substitutes for a bath in the morning. Many people eat a light meal at lunch time and have the main meal of the day in the evening. Reversing this practice may be upsetting to the sick. Certainly during illness is not the time to make an issue of a habit that is harmless and needs only an adjustment of the nursing care schedule.

PREVENTING PHYSICAL DEFORMITIES

The posture of the patient has a direct relationship to the prevention of body deformities, particularly those known as contracture deformities. A contracture or shortening of the muscle produces a deformity if it is allowed to continue. Because a strong muscle tends to pull a weaker one, strict attention must be paid to the body position of the ill patient. For example, the patient may find that he is more comfortable if the knees are bent and supported, but if this position is constantly maintained, the knees may become stiffened and permanently fixed so that the legs cannot be straightened. The patient who has paralysis must have the affected part of the body supported so that contractures will not occur. (See "Positioning the Patient in Bed," chapter 13, pages 201-211.) A paralyzed leg tends to turn either inward or outward, allowing the foot to drop to the side. A rolled blanket or a sandbag can be placed alongside the leg to hold it in proper position, and the feet should be placed against a support that holds them and the ankles in good alignment with the body. When a patient is to lie on his side for some time, the uppermost arm and leg must be supported. Pillows or other supports should be properly placed to maintain body position and to relieve strain on hip and shoulder joints. Sometimes holding a firmly rolled cloth in the palm of the hand when the hand is at rest helps to prevent a contracture of the fingers. A hand towel or heavy washcloth rolled to a diameter of at least 3 inches serves very well.

In the prevention of contracture deformities, exercise is as important as the maintenance of correct body posture. Muscle tone is lost rapidly when the patient is in bed, and the joints become less flexible so that, unless they are exercised, contractures may

137

develop fairly quickly. The patient can aid in preventing contracture deformities by doing as much as he can for himself and by moving about in bed. The doctor may prescribe range of motion exercises, and if the patient cannot perform these exercises unassisted, someone in the family will have to help with them. A doctor, a nurse, or a physical therapist can teach the home nurse and the patient, by explanation and by demonstration, how the exercises have to be done. Prescribed exercise for the handicapped patient is a form of treatment and should be followed as ordered by the attending physician. The doctor will determine how often and for how many times the exercises are to be done.

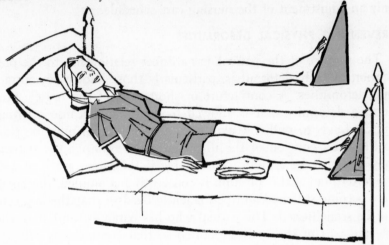

Keep the patient's head in line with the trunk of the body and supported comfortably for proper body positioning. A firm, flat support, such as a folded bath towel, may be placed under the slightly flexed knees. Place a slanted foot support so that the feet are firmly braced against it.

Every joint in the human body has a normal range of motion, but the range will differ from one person to another according to what the joint has been accustomed to do. For example, athletes and dancers have greater range of joint motion than has the average person because they exercise and use their joints more. People suffering from certain diseases, for example arthritis, have a restricted range of motion because the affected joints have become tight and stiff. Regular range of motion exercises are especially important for patients with a handicap or a long-term illness. The exercises are intended to be restorative, to help the patient to return to a maximum of activity, and to prevent crippling, but the rehabilitation of the patient is a long slow process that takes practice and the will to do it. Any sick person needs encouragement, but the patient with a long-term illness needs praise for even small accomplishments to help him to achieve greater goals. The activities of daily living, those things which all of us do automatically for ourselves from hour to hour, become complex tasks to the weak and handicapped individual. For him, it takes perseverance and effort repeated many times to do such apparently simple things as eating, dressing, and getting out of bed. Once the patient realizes he can do much to help himself, his will is strengthened and his morale is improved.

ELIMINATION

Elimination usually presents no problems for the well person, but long-term illness, inactivity, drugs, or changes in the amount and kind of food eaten sometimes cause a change in normal bowel activity. It is not unusual for the patient in bed to become constipated because of the slowing down of all body processes. If he has difficulty in using a bedpan, he may aggravate and increase the tendency to constipation by delaying when he feels the impulse for a bowel movement.

Under normal conditions the lower bowel is emptied at regular intervals, which vary from one person to another. Fecal material passes through the intestines by muscular contractions that are set in motion by the intake of food. When the waste material reaches the rectum, the nerve endings are stimulated and a feeling of needing to have a bowel movement is created. If the stool is soft and formed, it can usually be assumed that elimination is normal. A hard dry stool indicates constipation. Older people are more likely than young to have fecal impactions, a condition in which the dry hardened stool packs in the lower bowel and cannot be expelled. Advanced age is an important factor in that the senile patient is unreliable and may not remember when he last had a bowel movement. An aged person may be constipated or he may have diarrhea, with the frequent passage of small amounts of fluid stool that by-pass the impaction. If the patient is incontinent, one should suspect a fecal impaction. An enema may be all that is required to empty the lower bowel, but this treatment should not be attempted until recommended by the doctor. If an enema is not successful, further relief measures will be carried out by the doctor.

CARING FOR THE INCONTINENT PATIENT

Incontinence is the inability to control the escape of urine from the bladder or of stool from the rectum. When incontinence occurs, voiding and defecation are involuntary. This condition may be only temporary, but with some types of disability or injury and often in senility it is chronic and more or less permanent. For example, the patient who has suffered a back injury that has caused paralysis of the lower part of the body usually is incontinent, while the patient who has had a stroke may have temporary incontinence. The acutely ill or the unconscious patient is usually incontinent for a short time, and the long-term ill person may be incontinent only at times.

Neither the patient nor his family should accept incontinence as a problem that has no solution. Incontinence is a medical problem, and the physician must give guidance to the home nurse in its solution. Each patient must be evaluated and the training program planned to meet his individual needs and abilities. The home nurse and other members of the family will have to accept the problems that arise with caring for an incontinent patient. Every effort must be made to keep him clean, dry, and free from odor. In addition to his daily bath, the patient needs to have his bed linen changed and his back, buttocks, and genitalia bathed and carefully dried each time he becomes wet to keep him comfortable and to prevent the formation of decubiti or pressure sores. The skin must receive extra attention because chemical changes in the urine form ammonia which is very irritating. Wearing a urinal to keep dry is usually more successful for male patients than for females. Sometimes a retention catheter is inserted into the patient's urinary bladder to allow the urine to drain into a bottle. Using disposable absorbent pads and adult-size diapers saves nursing care time and cuts down on the laundry. In some communities adult diapers can be rented from a regular diaper service.

Although diapering of incontinent patients is practiced in most hospitals, nursing homes, and in the home, discretion should be used because of the psychological effect it has on the patient. He may regress to infantile patterns of behavior and actually impede a program of bladder and bowel training. Judgment must be used by the home nurse in gearing the care of the patient to what is best for him psychologically as well as physically.

If there is no physical impairment or other apparent reason for the incontinence, the patient, unless he is senile, can usually be trained to regain control. It sometimes helps to place the patient on the bedpan or to offer him the urinal at regular intervals, about every 2 hours or less, even waking the patient if he is asleep. Success with this training will vary from one person to another, and it usually takes many weeks of effort before a routine is established so that the bladder will empty automatically at a certain time. Getting the incontinent patient out of bed and on to a bedside commode or to the bathroom so that he is in a sitting position rather than having him use a bedpan or urinal while lying in bed may help him to regain muscle control. The sitting position appears to improve the general circulation, and increases his oxygen intake because he breathes deeper. The effect on his morale is favorable because incontinence is an embarrassing and distressing situation to most people, and any measure of success in its control encourages the patient and his family.

PREVENTING AND CARING FOR DECUBITI

Decubiti, or pressure sores, are the result of interference with the blood supply to some part of the body. Most commonly affected are the skin areas over the bony prominences of the body that come in contact with the bed, but a cast, a splint, a tight bandage, or even the bedding can create enough pressure to cause the skin to break down and develop sores that are difficult to heal.

A large factor in the development of decubiti is moisture, either perspiration or body discharges, such as urine or stool. Wrinkles in the bottom sheet, crumbs, or anything that causes irritation or friction contributes to the formation of these sores. In addition, care must be taken in placing and removing the bedpan so that it does not pull against the patient's skin.

In the early stages of a pressure sore, the skin is tender, warm, and slightly reddened. When the area is pressed with the fingers, the redness disappears, but the redness returns when the pressure is removed. At a later stage, the skin becomes blue or purplish red, often mottled, is no longer warm to the touch, and does not pale when pressed with the fingers. At this stage an open sore is almost inevitable because circulation has been impaired and the tisssues are dying.

The prevention of decubiti depends almost entirely on nursing care. The patient's position must be changed every 2 hours, preferably every hour, so that pressure is not maintained for long on any one body part. He should be turned from side to side and from back-lying to face-lying position. The obese patient with pendulous breasts or pendulous abdomen, where two folds of skin lie against each other, should have these areas bathed, dried, and powdered

141

frequently to prevent friction. The skin should be kept clean and dry, and if the incontinent patient can bathe in the tub, frequent baths help to keep the skin in good condition. Gentle rubbing of the pressure areas with alcohol or a lotion will help to stimulate circulation and bring needed nutrients to the skin. It is generally agreed that good nutrition contributes to the prevention of pressure sores. A firm mattress that provides an even distribution of body weight, or large pieces of covered foam rubber placed under the body at the bony prominences, will help to relieve pressure.

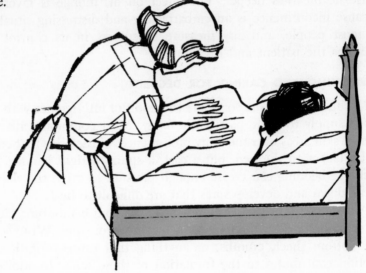

A back rub helps to stimulate circulation in the skin.

Any redness of the skin at a pressure area should be reported immediately to the doctor so that he can recommend additional measures for the care of the patient. Treatment of these areas should begin at the first sign of redness. After the skin has broken, infection nearly always follows and the treatment is much more difficult. Exposure of pressure areas to light and air is of help, and the doctor may ask that a frame to support the bedcovers be used to allow for free air circulation. He may also recommend the use of an alternating pressure mattress. This mattress has a motor that inflates and deflates alternate air spaces in the mattress so that no one part of the body receives constant pressure. Another method of prevention as well as treatment is the use of a large piece of sheepskin or of chamois skin placed under the affected part of the body, usually the buttocks, to help absorb moisture, relieve pressure, and protect the skin from irritation. If the sheepskin has fleece, the sheared wool should be placed next to the patient's body. Plain skins are effective though less resilient and absorbent than the sheep wool. A number of these pads will be needed to keep the patient dry. They may be washed and well rinsed by hand or in a washing machine, using lukewarm water and a mild soap. They must always be air dried to keep the skins soft and supple.

SUGGESTED STUDENT ACTIVITIES

1. Draw a floor plan of a bedroom to show the most satisfactory arrangement for a patient's care. Show the position of the bed in relation to the door and the windows.

2. Make and bring to class miniature flower arrangements suitable for a meal tray or a bedside table. Appoint a committee to judge the arrangements.

3. Select two or three representatives from the class to visit the nutritionist at a hospital. Have them arrange with her to observe the preparation and serving of food to the patients and give a report to the class.

4. Describe to the class how you would work out an interesting, useful project for an invalid who can do light work for a few hours a day, either in bed or sitting up in a chair.

5. Bring to class a picture of a satisfactory bed for a sick room. List your reasons for selecting the bed. What type of bedding would you choose? Why?

6. Prepare a paper on the points to be considered in selecting a nursing home for a patient with a long-term illness.

7. Arrange with other members of the class to role-play the following situation: Your mother has just returned home from the hospital. One of her friends has come to see her and has remained too long. Get the visitor to leave without giving offense or seeming inhospitable. Discuss other ways in which the desired result might have been accomplished.

HOME EMERGENCIES

There is a tendency for people to try to treat themselves when sickness occurs. Sometimes the symptoms of illness are so slight that getting medical advice seems to be unimportant. It may appear easier and more economical to use a medication already in the medicine cabinet or to stop at the drugstore and ask for a remedy or even to get a friend's advice. However, there are several excellent reasons against treating oneself unless with the advice of a doctor. There is always risk that the wrong medicine or treatment may be taken, which may make the condition worse or produce new and more serious symptoms of illness. Medication taken without advice from the doctor may mask the symptoms that make it possible for him to diagnose the illness correctly. Money may be wasted on ineffective drugs with the likelihood that medical care costs of the illness will be increased if the illness is intensified or prolonged by the lack of proper medical attention. Finally, but quite importantly, there is always delay in obtaining the correct treatment.

When a person is injured, the idea that someone other than a physician can tell what is wrong may prove to be a costly mistake. Obviously, the doctor cannot be called to treat every little ache or injury. This is why it is important for one or more members of the family to be able to recognize symptoms of illness, especially those that recur and those that are characteristic of the common communicable diseases, and to know how to give first aid.

THE VALUE OF FIRST AID TRAINING

First aid is the immediate and temporary care given a sick or an injured person until the services of a physician can be obtained.

The person who has been properly trained to give this care is able to assist people when they need help the most. The purposes of first aid training are to prevent accidents, to train people to do the right thing at the right time, to prevent additional injury, and to provide safe and proper transportation for the injured.

The American Red Cross has developed a practical course in first aid that is offered by its chapters throughout the country and has published a textbook that covers in detail the treatment of common emergencies that are likely to occur in the home. Emergencies occur in every household. The information in this chapter is not intended as a substitute for a first aid course, but as a review and an aid to the home nurse in meeting and preventing common home emergencies. Information on home nursing and first aid is available through many community agencies. There are many corporations and industrial companies that not only provide safety training for their personnel but also offer to the public free materials on accident prevention and emergency first aid.

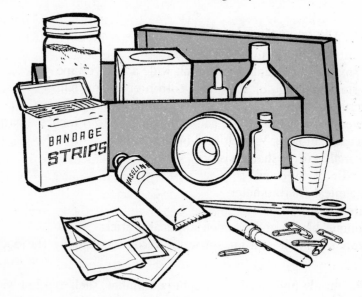

Keep first aid supplies assembled in a container. Store in a safe, easily accessible place.

EMERGENCY AND FIRST AID SUPPLIES

Every family should have on hand a small supply of medicines and first aid supplies. A list of the preferred drugs and supplies should be obtained from the family physician. He will suggest specific medications, such as an antiseptic, a laxative for occasional use, a headache remedy, a lotion for the treatment of poison ivy or insect bites, and an ointment to be applied to superficial skin burns. Since some drugs deteriorate with age and become either ineffective or unsafe to use, he will indicate which medicines should be purchased in small amounts and replenished regularly. (For more about this, see "Medications," chapter 16, pages 282-290.)

Perhaps the most convenient and safest way to store emergency supplies is in a covered box that can be placed where it is readily accessible to adults and out of the way of children. A metal or plastic box makes a good container, but a covered cardboard box will do as well. The important thing is for the container to be large enough to hold the supplies and to keep them arranged so that a desired article can be found quickly without unpacking the entire contents of the box. Usually the bathroom medicine cabinet is unsuitable for this storage because it is often within the reach of children and too small to accommodate the needed supplies.

Supplies to be kept on hand are:

- A tube of lubricant or petrolatum
- A small roll of ½-inch or 1-inch wide adhesive tape
- A small package of absorbent cotton or cotton balls
- Sterile adhesive dressings in assorted sizes and shapes
- Several packets of sterile gauze dressings 2 to 4 inches square
- Gauze bandages ½-inch to 2-inches wide
- A small pair of sharp scissors
- A pair of tweezers
- A clinical thermometer
- Safety pins
- Tongue blades and wooden applicator sticks
- Burn ointment and an antiseptic recommended by the doctor

The family may need additional equipment, such as a hot water bottle, an ice cap, an enema outfit, an electric pad, a steam vaporizer, a bedpan, and a waterproof rubber or plastic sheet. All of these articles are found in many homes. It is not recommended that they be purchased unless there is an actual need for them, as many times they can be borrowed for short-time use. Any electrical device should be inspected to make sure that it is safe and in good condition, and it should be stored and used according to the manufacturer's directions.

146

GENERAL PROCEDURE AT AN ACCIDENT

Many injuries are minor in nature and the first aid needed is obvious to the trained person. If the injury is serious, the following steps generally apply:

Determine whether the injured person requires speedy care. Act quickly if there is severe bleeding, stoppage of breathing, or poisoning. In these cases, seconds count. Have someone call a doctor immediately. Give the indicated first aid at once. In the majority of accidents, however, great speed is not essential and often may be harmful. There is usually time to study the situation, to plan carefully, and to give first aid deliberately. A quick glance at the patient and a moment's survey of how the accident happened generally tells whether or not one is dealing with an emergency.

Keep the patient lying down, comfortably warm, and do not move him unless necessary. Use judgment in applying external heat or in placing blankets over the patient, particularly if he is unconscious. A coat or a blanket placed under the patient may conserve body heat more effectively than covering placed over him.

Examine the patient carefully for injuries. Clues to the nature and extent of the injury are furnished by the story of what occurred as told by the patient or an observer, the reactions of the patient to the injury, and the findings disclosed by examination.

Plan what to do. Get a physician or ambulance or obtain medical advice by telephone. Discuss with relatives or friends at the accident scene what is to be done, or with the patient if he is conscious. Give helpers careful instructions in what they are to do.

Carry out the necessary first aid.

SHOCK

Shock is a term used to describe disturbed body function resulting from circulatory failure and is commonly associated with injury. Because the patient in shock has very unstable circulation he should be handled gently and moved no more than absolutely necessary. Evidence of shock may be delayed, and every injured patient should be treated as a potential shock victim and observed carefully. However, his injuries should receive immediate attention, and fractures should be splinted and any bleeding controlled. Shock is more apt to develop in the very old, the very young, and the weak and undernourished.

The symptoms of shock are quite evident. The skin is pale, moist, and cool. If shock is caused by bleeding, the skin, lips, and fingernails take on a blue tinge. Usually the patient perspires around the

147

mouth, on the forehead, and in the palms of the hands. His pulse becomes rapid and may be so weak that it is imperceptible. He is weak, dizzy, apprehensive, excessively thirsty, and nauseated, and frequently he vomits. His respirations may be rapid and shallow or they may be deep.

If the patient has no difficulty in breathing, he should be kept lying down to provide a greater flow of blood to the head and chest where it is needed most. If he has been severely injured or has lost a great amount of blood, his feet usually should be elevated from 8 to 12 inches. This procedure should not be followed, however, if the patient has a head injury or if elevation of the feet increases difficulty in breathing or causes pain. In any of these circumstances, the patient's head and shoulders should be elevated.

Adequate but not excessive covering both under and over the patient should be provided to maintain normal body heat. External heat from hot water bottles, electric pads, or an electric blanket should not be used except in extremely cold weather. Heat in excess of that needed to maintain normal body temperature tends to increase the state of shock through loss of body heat and body fluids from perspiration. Also, there is danger of burning the patient because he is more susceptible to and less aware of heat.

Fluids are valuable in the treatment of shock *but only if they cause no additional harm to the patient.* When the victim is placed under medical care shortly after injury, the doctor decides what and how much fluid he may have. If medical care is not available or will be delayed for a considerable length of time, the patient may be given small sips of water. If no nausea or vomiting develops, the amount of fluid given may be increased, and about every 15 minutes the patient may have a half glass of a solution of ½ level teaspoon each of table salt and baking soda to a quart of water. In general, stimulants, such as coffee or ammonia, have no value for the patient who is in shock.

If the patient has an abdominal injury, if he is vomiting, or if it appears that he will need immediate surgery, he should not be given fluids by mouth. Instead, if he is able to follow directions, he may *rinse* his mouth with water to help satisfy thirst.

TYPES OF WOUNDS

A wound is a break in the skin or in the mucous membrane lining the body cavities. A great many wounds are the result of minor accidents and are neither serious nor in need of much attention. The basic function of a dressing, the material placed directly over the wound, is to protect the wound and keep out infection. Because some wounds heal just as well or better when left uncovered, the doctor will decide whether a dressing or a bandage should be used. He will also determine whether other treatment should be given.

Wounds are of four general types:

Abrasions: caused by rubbing or scraping the skin against a hard or rough surface. The skinned knee that a child sustains in a fall on the sidewalk or the playground is an example. This type of wound may or may not bleed, depending on the depth of the injury to the skin.

Incisions (cuts): caused by sharp objects, such as knives, glass, or razor blades. This type of wound generally bleeds freely.

Lacerations (tears): usually jagged and irregular and often caused by objects such as handtools, saws, or machinery. People who are struck by flying wood, stone, or metal in a tornado incur this type of wound. There is often considerable damage to the tissues and profuse bleeding.

Punctures (piercing wounds): commonly caused by nails, needles, ice picks, bullets, and knives. The size of the wound will depend on the object that caused it and the force of the penetration into the tissues. Often the wound is deep and has a small skin opening. There may be very little external bleeding but severe internal hemorrhage as, for example, after a gunshot or a stab wound.

There are two common dangers with any wound, bleeding and infection. In a sense, moderate bleeding is an advantage in that it washes the wound and helps take away any dirt and bacteria. Puncture wounds are hazardous and require special attention to prevent infection. Bacteria are introduced deep into the tissues in this type of wound, which closes quickly and is hard to clean. A doctor should always be consulted about the treatment of a puncture wound because of the danger of tetanus or lockjaw.

Bleeding Wounds

The first objective in treating a bleeding wound is to stop the hemorrhage as quickly as possible by applying pressure directly over the wound. A life may be saved by rapid action. If a large blood vessel is cut, death may occur in less than a minute from loss of blood. Pressure should be applied at once to the wound with a thick pad of clean cloth. In an emergency, a piece of clothing or even the bare hand will do, but the cleaner the object used, the less the danger of infection later.

After the bleeding is controlled, additional padding of folded cloth should be applied and bandaged firmly in place over the dressing. If the padding becomes saturated, apply another dressing and additional pressure directly over the wound. The patient should be placed under medical care as soon as possible.

If the bleeding from a wound is not severe, the proper procedure is to apply a dressing and get the patient to a doctor for further treatment. Whenever possible, dressings should be sterile. Touching the wound, especially with the fingers, should be avoided and no medication should be put on it. Adhesive and absorbent cotton are never to be applied directly to the wound because both will adhere and may cause additional bleeding when removed.

Home treatment even of minor wounds carries some hazard. The family physician should advise what to do. He may suggest that small wounds be cleansed with soap and running water or that an antiseptic be used before a dressing is applied. (For more information on care of wounds, see chapter 17, pages 291-293.)

Puncture Wounds

Common puncture wounds are those caused by nails, pins, knives, splinters of wood, missiles, and other sharp objects. A puncture wound is always hard to clean and because it is caused by a foreign body it is apt to become infected. The wound closes easily, sealing out oxygen and providing a perfect place for the growth of lockjaw or tetanus bacteria. If bleeding occurs, infection is less likely because blood washes out the dirt and bacteria or disease-producing germs. A doctor should be consulted and he will decide whether or not the patient should receive tetanus antitoxin and/or tetanus toxoid.

If the skin around the wound is dirty it should be washed with soap and running water or with boiled water that has cooled. An antiseptic should be applied and the wound should be covered with a sterile dressing.

Infected Wounds

The patient with an infected wound should always be under the care of a physician. If the wound is in an arm or a leg, the injured part of the body should be elevated and supported on a pillow and kept at rest. Constant motion is harmful and favors the spread of infection. If it is not possible to obtain the advice of a doctor or to have him see the patient for an extended period of time, it is safe to apply hot moist dressings to the wound. A hand or a foot can be soaked in a solution of 2 level tablespoons of table salt, or of

6 level tablespoons of Epsom salts (magnesium sulphate) to a quart of water, for 15 or 20 minutes every 1 or 2 hours to help localize the infection. (See "The Effects of Heat," pages 258-259 and "Hot Moist Compresses," pages 274-276.)

INTERNAL BLEEDING

Bleeding from any body opening requires the immediate services of a doctor. The patient will exhibit signs of shock in greater or less degree, and treatment should be started at once, even before the doctor comes. The patient should be put to bed and kept quiet.

Blood may come from the stomach or the lungs through the mouth or the nose. Blood from the stomach is usually dark red, while that from the lungs is usually frothy and bright red. If bleeding is from the stomach or the lungs, an icecap placed on the chest or over the stomach may reduce the internal bleeding. The conscious patient may be given crushed ice for thirst. If he becomes unconscious, he must be turned on his side, with his head and chest lowered to prevent aspiration of fluid into the lungs.

If the bleeding is from the rectum, vagina, or bladder, the patient must be kept lying flat, with the foot of the bed elevated from 12 to 18 inches. It is especially urgent that the patient receive prompt medical attention if bleeding occurs during pregnancy.

NOSEBLEED

The person having a nosebleed should remain quiet, either sitting with his head held back or lying down with his head and shoulders raised. Usually the bleeding is near the tip of the nose, and pressure may be applied by pinching the nostrils together. It may be necessary to pack the nostrils with gauze to stop the bleeding, but this should be done by a doctor. Sometimes cold wet towels applied to the face will aid in stopping the bleeding.

Nosebleeds may be the result of injury or of disease or they may occur spontaneously. Such diseases as high blood pressure and rheumatic fever may be the cause. Nosebleeds sometimes occur at high altitude, following athletic activity, or as the result of a cold. Ordinarily they are not serious. However, if the bleeding persists more than 10 or 15 minutes, the doctor should be called. Recurrent nosebleeds should be investigated to determine the cause.

BURNS

There are three general causes of burns: heat, light, and chemicals. Although burns are classified according to the depth or degree of tissue destroyed and the amount or extent of the body surface involved, it is not always possible to determine the degree of a burn at first. Also, the degree frequently differs in different parts of the burned area. A first degree burn is superficial and involves only the upper layer of the skin. There are no blisters, but the skin is reddened, swollen, and painful. In a second degree burn the top layers of the skin are destroyed, blisters occur, and, although the tissue regenerates and heals, there may be some scarring. A third degree burn destroys the skin, the hair follicles, and the sweat glands, and the surrounding surface may appear charred. Third degree burns are slow to heal and may have to be skin-grafted.

Application of an anesthetic burn ointment usually relieves the pain of a first degree burn of relatively small area. If the burn is more severe, a dry sterile pressure dressing is applied to keep out infection, relieve the pain, and prevent loss of body fluids. If clothing adheres to the burned area, any portion not adhering should be carefully cut away. Severely burned patients develop shock and should be placed under medical care as quickly as possible. (See "Care of Burns," chapter 11, pages 172-173.)

Chemical Burns

In a chemical burn, the chemical should be quickly washed off with copious amounts of cold water. Immersion of the burned part of the body in ice water relieves the pain and is believed to facilitate recovery. If the chemical that caused the burn is identified, the label of the container may recommend specific treatment. In the absence of such specific information, no additional chemicals should be applied in an attempt to neutralize the harmful agent.

Chemical burns of the eye are extremely serious. Irrigation with tap water should be started at once and continued for a minimum of 5 minutes. The patient's head should be held under the tap or water poured over the eye from a bottle, a cup, or whatever is at hand. Immediate medical attention should be procured. When the patient's eyes have been irrigated thoroughly, a pad or a piece of cotton should be placed over his closed eyes and bandaged in place before he is taken to the doctor.

Sunburn

Sunburn is caused by the action of ultra-violet rays. Slight overexposure to the sun's rays reddens the skin, but as overexposure increases, the tissues are injured, swelling occurs, and blisters appear, accompanied by pain, fever, and headache. A severe sunburn may be acquired on a cloudy day, particularly at the shore or on the water.

The most effective way to prevent sunburn is to time the exposure. The first exposure should be no more than 15 minutes. The length of subsequent exposures should be gradually increased. On sea and lake shores and at high altitude, the initial exposure time should be limited to 10 minutes and increased gradually.

As with thermal or heat burns, the treatment of sunburn depends on the degree of the burn, and the burned area should not be exposed to the sun again until complete healing has taken place. A dressing should be applied if blistering occurs. Medical care is needed for severe cases.

Numerous preparations for the prevention of sunburn, both lotions and ointments, are available. They vary in their effectiveness, and some people may have an allergic reaction to them.

Snowburn

Snowburn, a deep burn caused by reflection of the sun on snow, may be painful, especially to the eyes. It sometimes causes temporary blindness. Long exposure should be avoided. The eyes should be protected with sunglasses and if affected by the sun, they should be treated by the application of cold compresses. A doctor should be consulted. The skin can be protected against snowburn by wearing gloves and a face covering. First aid to the skin is the same as for any other burn.

SIMPLE FAINTING

Fainting is caused by a diminished blood supply to the brain. It may be precipitated by fatigue, hunger, the viewing of an injury, or some powerful emotion, such as fear or joy. Usually the person knows that he is going to faint. He becomes dizzy and weak, his skin is cold, moist and pale, and he loses consciousness. The person who feels faint should lean forward, with his head between his knees, or better yet, he should lie down. Rapid and spontaneous recovery occurs as soon as gravity brings an increased blood supply to the head. However, the patient should remain at rest for at least 10 minutes, or fainting may recur. If he has not recovered consciousness within 10 minutes, a doctor must be called. If fainting occurs during an illness, or when a person who has been ill is thought to be convalescent, the doctor should be informed at once.

CONVULSIONS

A convulsion is a violent, involuntary contraction or spasm of the muscles. It is a symptom of illness, not a disease. Generally, the onset of a convulsion is sudden, its duration brief, and the seizure subsides of itself, regardless of any treatment given. There is nothing that anyone other than a physician can do to stop a convulsion. Protection of the patient from injury is of primary importance. If he is in bed, he should be protected against falling out of bed. If the patient is a small child in a crib, it may be necessary to pad the crib bars. A padded spoon or piece of wood should be placed between the teeth at the side of the mouth to prevent the patient from biting his tongue.

Some infants and young children up to the age of 4 or 5 are likely to have convulsions when their temperatures begin to rise during acute illnesses. This reaction can be compared to the chill that an adult may have at the onset of illness and that is followed by a rise in body temperature. Infection and injury may also be the cause of convulsions in the young child. Though alarming to the parent, when these episodes are brief and occur only occasionally during early childhood, they probably have no lasting or ill effect.

Following a convulsion a child usually falls into a deep sleep. He should be kept quiet and permitted to rest.

In adults convulsions are usually caused by a head injury, an internal disturbance, or an infection such as tetanus, meningitis, or the eclamptic seizures that sometimes occur as a disease complication of pregnancy. Convulsions during pregnancy or during delivery are considered to be especially serious.

HEATSTROKE

Heatstroke or sunstroke is caused by exposure to too much heat, usually from the rays of direct sunlight. It generally occurs outdoors but may occur indoors, and it is likely to happen in climates where there is no relief from the heat at night. The cause is somewhat obscure but appears to be a breakdown in the functioning of the sweat glands that results in extremely high and sometimes fatal body temperature. Old people are particularly susceptible to heatstroke, and most deaths in this age group occur with the first hot spell of the summer season.

The symptoms of heatstroke are a rapid, pounding pulse, dry skin, and, in many instances, unconsciousness. Medical care is needed at once, and the patient should be taken to a hospital as soon as possible. In the meantime, the patient should be kept quiet and sponged freely with alcohol or with cool water to reduce his fever. (See "Sponge Baths," chapter 15, pages 280-281.) Stimulants are not to be given. Fluids by mouth are not urgently needed because the patient does not perspire. If he is conscious, he may be permitted to have small amounts of water or of salt water made by adding ½ teaspoonful of salt to a half glass of water.

HEAT EXHAUSTION

Heat exhaustion is the result of salt depletion in the body; it is fairly common and may be mild or severe. In mild cases the patient feels unusually tired and frequently has dizziness, a headache, and nausea. In severe cases weakness is pronounced, the skin is pale and moist, and perspiration is profuse. Usually there is no elevation of body temperature, and unconsciousness is rare.

Heat exhaustion usually can be prevented by taking large amounts of fluids and salt, both of which are lost through excessive perspiration. If the patient is conscious, fluids may be given by mouth. If there is nausea, it usually subsides after a period of bedrest. Fluids can then be tolerated without vomiting. Medical care is needed if heat exhaustion is severe.

HEAT CRAMPS

Heat cramps are commonly associated with severe heat exhaustion. The condition usually affects the abdominal and the leg muscles. It is the result of a decrease in the salt content of the blood, which is excreted mainly through excessive perspiration. Drinking water that has had salt added usually affords relief, and the application of moist heat to the cramping muscles may be of some benefit.

FROSTBITE

Frostbite is caused by prolonged exposure to extreme cold. It usually affects the extremities because the blood becomes chilled as it flows away from the trunk of the body, where the blood is kept warm. The nose, ears, and cheeks are also susceptible to frostbite because they are less well protected from cold than the trunk.

Before frostbite occurs, the skin is usually flushed because the blood vessels dilate as a first response to cold. Soon the affected parts become painful, and a tingling sensation is followed by numbness. When sensation is lost and pain has ceased, the tissues have been seriously injured by the formation of ice crystals in the tissues. At this stage the skin appears white or greyish-yellow, and blisters may appear. The result is serious inflammation and sometimes gangrene or decay of the affected area.

The objective of treatment of frostbite is to reestablish circulation in the affected part. The patient should be sheltered from the cold, usually taken indoors, as soon as possible and should be given warm fluids to drink. The frosted area of the body should be handled with great care and rewarmed by immersion in water of body temperature. *Hot water should never be used* because it causes sudden dilation of the blood vessels and may cause them to rupture. If lukewarm water or the means to immerse the frosted part is not available, the patient should be wrapped in wool blankets or in woolen clothing so that his body heat will accomplish the thawing process. Neither hot water bottles nor heat lamps should be used, and the patient should not be placed near any kind of radiant heat because it may increase the damage to the tissues. Firm pressure against the frozen part with the warm hand is of some help in relieving discomfort, but rubbing with the hand or with snow should never be done because it increases the risk of further tissue damage. Once circulation is reestablished, the patient should be encouraged to exercise his fingers and toes. If blisters are present, care should be taken to prevent breaks in the skin. Any broken places in the skin should be protected by applying a sterile dressing to avoid possible infection.

HEART ATTACK

An acute heart attack has two principal symptoms, dyspnea or difficult or labored breathing and severe pain. Pain, which is usually acute and frightening, appears most often in the chest under the sternum or breastbone. In some cases severe pain appears in the left arm and shoulder. Nausea and vomiting frequently accompany a heart attack and may lead the person to think that he has indigestion.

If the patient has difficulty in breathing, his head and shoulders should be elevated. He should be persuaded to lie down and remain quiet to lessen strain on the heart muscles. *A doctor must be called at once.* If the patient has been under medical supervision for a known heart condition, he may have medicine prescribed for such an emergency. If he is conscious, the person helping him should inquire about prescribed medicines and assist him to take any that may have been ordered.

Generally it is necessary to hospitalize the patient, but, because any activity causes additional exertion, moving him should not be attempted until medical advice can be obtained. In an emergency, if a doctor cannot see the patient where he is within a reasonable length of time, he should be taken to the hospital. While he is being moved he should be kept lying down and disturbed as little as possible.

APPENDICITIS

Appendicitis may occur at any age but is most common between the ages of 15 and 30. The characteristic site of pain is in the right lower quarter of the abdomen. However, pain may be felt in the upper part or generalized throughout the abdomen. Often the patient is constipated, and, while it is not usually the case, he may have diarrhea. Fever may or may not be present. Usually the patient has nausea and vomiting.

When these symptoms occur, the doctor should be called at once. An icecap placed over the lower right side of the abdomen may give some relief from pain. Small amounts of cracked ice or of water may be given to relieve thirst. No medicines, treatments, or food should be given, and the patient should be kept in bed. Heat should never be applied to the abdomen because it may increase the inflammatory process.

CROUP

Croup is the term used to describe an inflammation of the larynx or voice box. The patient has a characteristic hard, barking cough of spasmodic nature that causes difficulty in breathing. Usually there is an accompanying hoarseness and sometimes loss of voice. Croup occurs chiefly in children under 5 years of age. Attacks nearly always come at night and may last from 30 minutes to 2 or 3 hours. During the attack, the inspirations are difficult and there is a stridor or a harsh, high-pitched whistling sound, with a retraction or pulling in of the soft tissues above the clavicle or collar bone, between the ribs, and at the base of the sternum. Expiration is quieter and less difficult.

When croup occurs, the throat should always be examined carefully. If it is red or has greyish-white spots anywhere on it, the doctor should be notified at once. Although immunization against diphtheria is commonly carried out during infancy, there is always the possibility that the child has not been sufficiently protected and may have diphtheria. Laboratory examination of discharges from the throat may be necessary before the doctor can confirm the diagnosis.

A steam inhalation is recommended to relieve the spasmodic coughing. Various drugs that quickly evaporate may be ordered by the doctor to use with the steam, but the essential relief agent is the warm moist air. Hot compresses or an icebag applied to the throat may relieve the spasms. A mucous plug in the throat may be dislodged by getting the child to vomit.

The child who has repeated attacks of croup should be under the doctor's care so that the condition causing the attacks may be corrected. Building up the child's general health and protecting him from extremes of weather may help to overcome the condition.

FOREIGN BODY IN THE EYE

Any foreign body in the eye requires prompt treatment. Because of the danger of infection and injury to the eye, the object should be removed by a doctor immediately whenever possible. A soft pad should be placed over both eyes and bandaged loosely in place before taking the individual to the doctor. The most common place for a foreign body to lodge is on the inner surface of the upper eyelid. If, for any reason, he cannot be seen promptly by a doctor, the following procedure is recommended: Have the patient sit with his head back, facing a good light, or have him lie down. Ask the patient to look down so that the edge of the upper lid may be grasped with the fingers. Place a matchstick or a pencil across the lid and turn the lid inside out so that the inner surface may be seen. Remove any object on the lid by touching it gently with a moistened cotton applicator or the corner of a clean folded cloth.

If the object is not on the lid but can be seen on the surface of the eye, ask the patient to wink several times in an effort to dislodge it. Sometimes tears will wash it away. If the object is embedded in the eye, do not attempt to remove it. Get the patient to a doctor as soon as possible. Caution the patient against rubbing the eye, because rubbing may cause more serious damage. If the patient is a child, observe him carefully to prevent him from rubbing his eyes. Adequate medical followup after the removal of a foreign body that has penetrated the eye is extremely important because of the danger of infection.

FOREIGN BODY IN THE EAR

Foreign bodies in the ear, such as a seed, a bead, a pebble, or an insect, require the attention of a doctor. The efforts of an untrained person may push the object farther into the ear canal, perhaps cause injury to the ear drum, and make the object more difficult to remove. A sharp instrument of any sort should never be used in an attempt to remove the object because of the danger of further injury. Medical attention should not be delayed, particularly if the foreign body is a dried seed, such as a pea or a bean, that may absorb moisture and swell, making it harder to remove.

If the foreign body is an insect, the patient should be turned on his side and warm oil dropped into the affected ear canal. This will stop the buzzing because the insect usually drowns in the oil, and it may float the insect to the top of the oil where it can be removed. The oil may be drained from the ear canal by tilting the head to one side. If this treatment is not effective, the doctor should be consulted.

FOREIGN BODY IN THE NOSE

When an insect, a grain of corn, or any other small object becomes lodged in the nose, a few drops of oil may be put into the obstructed nostril to relieve irritation and discomfort. There is usually no immediate danger from such an accident, but the person should be taken to a doctor as soon as possible to have the object removed.

FOREIGN BODY IN THE THROAT OR IN THE AIR PASSAGE

A foreign body in the throat or in the air passage may cause a serious, even fatal accident. The most common offender is a particle of food. Small children should never be given peanuts, popcorn, or foods containing nuts until they have their first teeth and have learned to chew their food before swallowing. Meat should be finely cut for the same reason.

When a foreign body lodges in the throat or in the air passage, it usually causes violent coughing, which sometimes causes the object to be expelled. If it passes into the lung, it will cause an infection unless it is removed. Removal is a procedure that can be performed only by a doctor. No attempt should be made to remove such an obstruction from the throat with the fingers, because doing so may push the object down and make it harder to remove. There should be no interference with the attempt of the patient to cough it out. If the person is a small child, he should be turned upside down and slapped sharply on the back between the shoulder blades. Persons other than small children should be placed across a bed or a table, with head and shoulders hanging over the side. They too should be slapped sharply between the shoulder blades in an effort to dislodge the object from the air passage. The patient should always be taken to a doctor or to the emergency room of the nearest hospital unless the object is expelled, even though the choking and coughing subsides. Cessation of choking and coughing may mean only that the object has passed into one of the lungs.

If breathing stops, artificial respiration must be started immediately and an attempt made to clear the airway by pulling the tongue forward with the fingers. These actions are urgent lifesaving measures. (See "Artificial Respiration," chapter 17, pages 294-297.)

FOREIGN BODY IN THE FOOD PASSAGES

Children frequently swallow such objects as coins, pins, tacks, buttons, and safety pins. These objects may or may not do harm, depending upon their nature and their size. Treatment should not be attempted by the home nurse. A doctor should be called for advice or the child taken to him at once.

Solid objects that are swallowed are not apt to cause trouble; and, if they are opaque, their progression through the stomach and intestines may be observed with X rays. A *long* solid object, however, may cause some trouble in passing through the curves of the bowel, and sharp solid objects may cause a perforation. A bobby pin or an open safety pin may pass safely through the digestive tract, but there is a definite danger that it may become lodged or may instead have passed into the air passage. The doctor must *always* be consulted when it is known that a foreign body has been accidentally swallowed. If it is necessary to provide food to the patient because of delay in receiving medical attention, he should be given liquids or soft foods. *The patient should never be given a cathartic.*

INSECT BITES AND STINGS

The toxic secretion of the insect is an acid that causes local inflammation and itching. The application of an alkali, such as baking soda, household ammonia, or soap, helps to neutralize the acid and to give relief from the pain of the sting. In addition to the acid component, the poison of bees, wasps, yellow jackets, and ants contains an alkaline and a histamine-like fraction to which some people have violent allergic reactions. When people known to be allergic to specific insects receive a sting on an extremity, the use of a constricting band applied above the bite is advised to slow absorption. Ice applied to the sting probably has the same effect and gives some relief from pain.

160

FOOD POISONING

Food poisoning is an acute inflammation of the intestines usually caused by any of the salmonella germs or organisms and is induced by eating contaminated food. Common offenders are meat, milk, puddings, salad dressings, custards, whipped cream, and other foods that are usually prepared some time in advance of eating and have not then been properly refrigerated. Despite the fact that refrigeration inhibits the growth of harmful bacteria, many foods may be safely refrigerated for a limited time only.

The symptoms of food poisoning include nausea and vomiting, diarrhea, and severe griping abdominal pain. Usually the onset is sudden and occurs within a few hours after eating the contaminated foods, but illness may occur as much as 72 hours later. Generally the illness lasts 1 or 2 days, and treatment is dictated by the severity of the symptoms. In severe cases there may be prostration and collapse, but the patient usually recovers rapidly as the symptoms abate and the toxins are excreted.

ANIMAL BITES

Animals may inflict any type of wound. Because the bites carry into the wound germs from the animal's mouth and from the skin and clothing of the person, a variety of infections are possible. The greatest danger is that of rabies. Warm-blooded animals are susceptible to rabies, and it has been found that many species of wild game are infected, as well as the common source of infection, cats and dogs. Healthy pets may be vaccinated against rabies, and in many communities the vaccination of pets is mandatory. One injection is believed to give immunity for 4 years or more and to prevent the animal's transmitting rabies to human beings or to other animals.

In case of an animal bite, the wound should be washed thoroughly with soap and water to remove the saliva and then rinsed with clean running water and a sterile dressing applied. A physician should be consulted at once. If at all possible, the animal should be caught and confined so that it may be observed for symptoms of rabies. If it is necessary to kill the animal in order to protect people, shooting in the head should be avoided, because the brain tissue will have to be examined to determine whether the animal was rabid. The dead body should be kept refrigerated until it can be sent to the laboratory for examination. The doctor will decide whether it is safe to postpone rabies treatment of the patient while the animal is under study and will treat the wound to guard against infection. If the animal is found to be rabid, everyone who has had any close contact with it should be given rabies vaccine at once.

POISONING BY MOUTH

The primary objective in the treatment of poisoning by mouth is to dilute the poison as quickly as possible. The patient should be placed under medical care at once. If the poison is known and if the antidote is specified on the label of the container, the antidote should be given as directed.

First aid should be given immediately to all poison victims. In most cases, large amounts of fluid, either water or milk or both, should be given to dilute the poison. Milk protects the lining of the digestive tract to some degree and slows the absorption of the poison.

The symptoms of poisoning vary greatly. The fatal dose of any poison is the smallest amount known to have caused death, but there are several conditions that modify a poison's action: the amount taken, the age of the person, individual tolerance of and reaction to certain drugs such as narcotics, health status, the condition of the stomach, that is, whether empty or full, and how the poison is taken. A poison that is given hypodermically is more powerful than one taken by mouth. A poison that is inhaled as a gas or vapor is fast and potent, while those absorbed through the skin are slower.

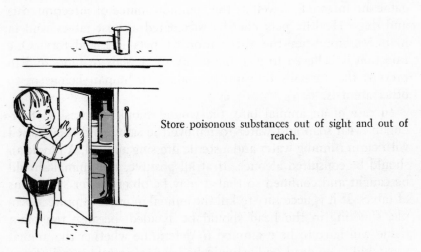

Store poisonous substances out of sight and out of reach.

Most poisons taken by mouth are swallowed either accidentally or with intent to commit suicide. Most victims of accidental poison-

162

ing are small children who have not been adequately protected. Bleaches, detergents, soaps, water softeners, waxes, polishes, lighter fluid, cosmetics, kerosene, insecticides, and all types of drugs and medicines are offenders. Nearly all cases of accidental poisoning could be prevented if parents of preschool age children would observe proper precautions by keeping medicines and all other poisonous substances under lock and key or out of reaching and climbing distance of children.

POISON CONTROL CENTERS

In 1961, there were more than 700 poison control centers in all of the 50 states, the District of Columbia, and Puerto Rico. Some of the centers are located in health departments, but most of them are in hospitals, frequently in children's hospitals because many of the poisoning accidents happen to children. When the centers are in hospitals, both information and treatment are available at all times.

In some cities, the telephone number of the poison control center is listed with the fire, police, and other emergency numbers. If the center is not listed in one's telephone directory, he should learn from his doctor or from the local health department where the nearest center is and what the telephone number is and should record this information where it will be quickly available. In an emergency, if a nonmedical person calls a poison control center, he will usually be given first aid instructions and advised to call his doctor.

Although some poison control centers give emergency treatment, their chief function is to furnish to doctors information about the ingredients in trade-name poisonous products, the antidotes for them, and other treatments. There is no legal requirement that the ingredients of some of these products be printed on their labels. However, through a voluntary arrangement more than 200 major producers of products containing potentially poisonous substances inform the national clearinghouse for poison control centers about the ingredients in the drugs and household preparations they manufacture as well as their antidotes. In turn, the clearinghouse transmits to the local poison control centers the data received from the cooperating producers.

SUGGESTED STUDENT ACTIVITIES

1. Ask to be permitted to examine the school first aid cabinet or chest. Compare it with the medicine chest suggested in the home

nursing textbook. Suggest reasons for any differences you note.

2. As a class project, equip a medicine chest and a first aid kit. Select a class representative to demonstrate to another class or to a school assembly the proper use of the items they contain.

3. If your school has no safety committee, how could your class assist in organizing one?

4. Discuss the advantages and disadvantages of keeping the school first aid cabinet locked.

5. Make a report to the class on school safety programs.

6. Keep a scrapbook of reports of accidents to children. Suggest ways in which each of the accidents could have been prevented.

7. Make a list of hazards present in homes and schools. Inspect your school and your home to determine what hazards are present. What can you do to remove those you discovered?

8. Using the telephone directory, make a list of the name, address, and telephone number of the following: family physician, dentist, hospital, pharmacy, poison control center(s), ambulance, police department, and fire department.

9. Suggest several ways that you could identify or mark a bottle containing poison so that anyone could recognize it in the dark. Prepare an example and bring to class.

10. Discuss the advisability of keeping the home medicine cabinet locked to prevent accidents, especially to children.

11

DISASTER-CAUSED EMERGENCIES

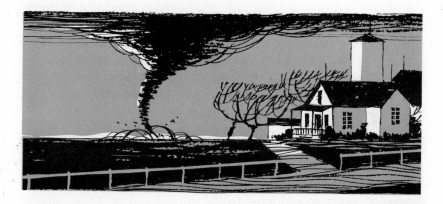

Disaster-caused emergencies may be classified as natural or enemy caused. Natural disasters result from tornadoes, floods, fires, explosions, hurricanes, transportation accidents, and epidemics. Enemy-caused disasters result from various weapons systems, such as chemical, biological, thermonuclear, and conventional methods of warfare.

In either a natural or an enemy-caused disaster numbers of people are plunged into helplessness and suffering and, as a result, may be in need of food, clothing, shelter, and medical and nursing care. In addition to causing illnesses and injuries, both types of disaster can result in the separation of family members, damage to or destruction of homes, and loss of possessions that may represent the savings of a lifetime. Experiences of this kind affect families deeply and often result in emotional shock to individual members, anxiety, confusion, hardship, and discouragement.

RESPONSIBILITY FOR CARE OF DISASTER VICTIMS

The U.S. government and the American Red Cross have plans that help communities meet their disaster-caused needs.

When a natural disaster occurs, the Red Cross is responsible for providing food, clothing, shelter, and medical, nursing, and hospital care as determined by the needs of the victims. In addition to this emergency aid, the organization assists in the rehabilitation of families unable to meet their continuing needs. The government is responsible for the protection of life and property, for the maintenance of public health and welfare, and for repair and maintenance of public property.

In the event of an enemy-caused disaster, the government, through its civil defense authorities, assumes the additional responsibility of providing food, shelter, clothing, and medical, nursing, and hospital care for the victims. In such a disaster, the Red Cross would assist to the extent of its ability by making available its trained personnel and any of its resources that might be needed. To make the plans of their government and the Red Cross effective, responsible people throughout the nation must be informed about the plans and be prepared to do their part.

PREPARATION FOR DISASTER

Self-help is fundamental in time of disaster. Immediately following a natural disaster, professional medical and nursing care is necessarily centered on the critically injured and ill. Home nurses are needed to care for patients at home and to help nurses in mass care shelters and hospitals.

In the event of an enemy-caused disaster, national in scope, survival would become a strictly personal affair, since it is probable that there would not be enough doctors and nurses to care for the ill and injured during the emergency period. The outcome would depend in part upon what each individual could do for himself, his family, and his neighbor after such a catastrophe and in part on how well individuals and families prepare for emergencies. The magnitude of the problem would be such that people with only minimum training would be called upon to perform nursing duties they would not be expected or permitted to perform in a natural disaster situation. People outside the affected area would have to be prepared to care for the sick in their communities without aid from the outside and in addition to provide food, clothing, shelter, and medical and nursing care for refugees evacuated to their communities.

Survival items for each family should include a battery-powered radio, a flashlight or a lantern or candles and matches, food, fuel, first aid supplies, medication, bedding, and clothing. Strict conservation must be practiced to insure that these essentials are not wasted or used too rapidly.

Enough food and water to last a minimum of 2 weeks should be stockpiled and stored in the family shelter area because regular sources of supply may be cut off. Eight gallons is the recommended water supply for each child up to 3 years of age, and 7 gallons for every other person. Foods should be stockpiled in sealed packages, jars, or cans to maintain their quality and to protect them from radioactive dust.* To provide a balanced diet, they should include fruit, vegetables, juices and beverages, milk, stews, soups, cheese, meat, fish, infant foods, bread, and crackers. Food supplements, such as jellies, jams, sugar, salt, seasoning, chewing gum, and hard candy, make meals more appetizing.

Salty foods should be avoided because they cause an increase in the consumption of drinking water. Dried and canned foods are preferable to frozen foods, which will spoil when defrosted. Much of the food should be edible without heating. Small-size cans of food, preferably for one meal only, are recommended because of the difficulty of preserving leftovers safely. As familiar foods are likely to be more acceptable in times of stress, instant coffee and tea, dried milk, and chocolate drinks should be included. If a family member (for example, someone with diabetes) requires daily medication and special foods, provision must be made to keep on hand adequate amounts of essential drugs and equipment and the necessary foods.

It would be advisable to consult the family physician about the drugs or medications that should be stocked for first aid or preventive treatment.

DISASTER INJURIES AND ILLNESSES

In either natural or enemy-caused disasters a variety of injuries and illnesses may be anticipated. The most common of these are:

- Open cuts and wounds from glass, metal, and other debris
- Fractures
- Bruises
- Pressure or crushing injuries
- Concussion and other head injuries
- Hemorrhage, both internal and external
- Burns from heat, fire, steam, chemicals, or hot water
- Illnesses resulting from fatigue, exposure, and overcrowding

---

* *Family Food Stockpile for Survival,* Home and Garden Bulletin No. 77, U. S. Department of Agriculture, 1961.

With any of these injuries the victim may sustain some degree of shock and should receive supportive treatment. (See "Home Emergencies," chapter 10.) Also, he may have more than one illness or injury at the same time (for example, the individual may be suffering from hemorrhage, broken bones, and a head injury), and his need for nursing care is therefore multiplied. Childbirth, premature and at term, may be anticipated during or following a disaster.

Immediately following a disaster, when people are living in crowded shelters or have taken other families into their home, the risk of contracting a communicable disease is multiplied. The common cold and influenza frequently follow exposure to the inclement weather of a tornado or a hurricane when the individual's resistance is lowered through fatigue, insufficient rest and sleep, or improper eating. Carriers of infectious or communicable disease, who may have no outward evidence of illness, can be a source of great danger to others. The importance of keeping up protection against communicable disease by periodic immunization and vaccination cannot be overemphasized. Health authorities occasionally carry out immunization programs for the entire population, as, for example, typhoid inoculations following a flood or hurricane when the water supply has become unsafe.

In an enemy-caused disaster, in addition to the usual injuries and illnesses, radiation sickness could occur as a result of a thermonuclear explosion. The symptoms of radiation sickness may occur the first day but often are delayed for a week or more. Among the factors to be considered in making the diagnosis are the protection that the victim had at the time of the bomb burst and his distance from the explosion. Radio instructions from government authorities would keep the people informed concerning the areas in danger from fallout. Local civil defense authorities will provide the public with information on the effects of radioactive fallout or on any illness resulting from chemical or biological warfare.

CARE OF DISASTER PATIENTS

The first concern in the emergency care of disaster patients is to maintain breathing by keeping the air passages open, to stop bleeding, and to treat for shock. The need for nursing care may extend over a period of time. The amount and the kind of care to be given depend upon the needs of each patient, the doctor's orders, and the people available to provide the nursing care.

Patients should be kept quiet, made as comfortable as possible, provided with warmth and shelter, and given whatever foods and liquids are permitted and available. Reassurance not only to the ill and injured but to other survivors as well is especially important at this time. Cleanliness in the care of patients must be observed to the fullest possible extent. Persons with colds or other suspected communicable disease or infections should be kept apart from apparently well persons.

Much ingenuity will be needed in feeding the ill. Food supplies may be limited both in variety and quantity, and eating utensils and cooking equipment may have to be improvised. Modification in feeding may be made in accordance with the number of people to be fed, their individual needs, and the food available. For example, if milk is in scarce supply it would be given first to babies, children, and pregnant women. Attention would have to be given to the food for those with diabetes to try to provide the essentials of a balanced diet and prevent diabetic shock or coma. Many patients will need assistance with eating, and the individual helping them should observe their needs and give help accordingly. Because illness and anxiety interfere with normal eating patterns, some people may have to be urged to take both food and fluids.

WHAT THE HOME NURSE MAY DO IN DISASTER

People with nursing skill and knowledge are an invaluable resource to professional medical and nursing personnel in the care of victims following a natural disaster. These volunteers work in Red Cross mass care shelters under the supervision of a registered professional nurse and may perform the following duties:

- Accompany patients to hospitals, homes, and doctors' and dentists' offices
- Help prepare children, the aged, and the chronically ill for meals and assist in feeding them
- Help prepare patients for treatments and examinations
- Help bathe patients
- Assist in teaching the shelter inhabitants to make up cots and keep their personal belongings in order
- Keep linens in order
- Help improvise equipment for the use of the nursing staff in caring for patients
- Report any unusual signs or symptoms immediately to the nurse in charge
- Assist in the taking and recording of temperatures

169

When patients are in temporary quarters they should be protected against hazards such as loose plaster, shattered glass, gas leaks, leaking roofs, wet floors, and fires. The home nurse should be alert to such conditions and should report them immediately to the person in charge. Sometimes it is necessary to set up temporary infirmaries to care for the injured and professional personnel are not available in sufficient numbers to staff the facilities adequately. This situation provides a real opportunity for community service by those people who have had training and experience in giving general nursing care. Occasionally the services of trained volunteers are used to supplement the nursing care of patients in hospitals and in nursing homes.

In an enemy-caused disaster, it is anticipated that home nurses would be needed to assist with additional nursing care duties. They may be assigned to:

- Observe patients receiving intravenous fluids
- Care for patients coming out of anesthesia
- Assist with special treatments
- Admit patients to a facility for care
- Prepare patients for transfer to another facility

Care of Patients Receiving Intravenous Fluids

An intravenous injection is the introduction of a fluid directly into a vein to replace or maintain body fluids, as in giving blood or plasma to a patient who has hemorrhaged. The fluid is given slowly, and the process may take several hours. The container holding the blood or other solution is suspended from 18 to 24 inches above the vein in which the solution is entering, and the rate of flow is controlled by a device on the tubing. The equipment (container, tubing, and needle) used for an intravenous injection must be sterile.

The procedure must be started by a doctor or by a professional nurse. However, after the needle is in place in the vein and the rate of flow established, someone other than a nurse or a doctor may stay with the patient. This safeguard for the patient is frequently provided by a responsible member of the family, who is asked to remain with him until the procedure is completed. Usually the solution is introduced into a vein in the arm, ordinarily at the inner aspect of the elbow, and preferably in the left arm if the patient is right handed. The arm is immobilized by fastening it to a board or a splint so that the patient has some freedom of movement of other parts of his body in order to relieve muscle fatigue and strain. Immobilizing the arm also helps to prevent the needle from coming out of the vein.

It is important for the person staying with a patient who is receiving an intravenous injection to observe carefully the following instructions:

• Keep the patient quiet, especially the part of the body where the insertion has been made so that needle stays in place.
• Report to the nurse in charge if the fluid stops flowing from the container.
• Watch for and report any swelling around the needle, an indication that the needle is not in the vein and that fluid is entering the tissues around the point of the insertion.
• Watch for and report immedaitely any signs that the patient is chilly, shivering, or faint. These usually indicate an adverse reaction to the solution he is receiving. Remain with the patient until the doctor or the nurse arrives.

Care of Patients Under Anesthesia

Keeping the air passage free is a lifesaving measure. (See "Artificial Respiration," chapter 17, pages 294-297.) A patient coming out of an anesthetic may have difficulty in breathing because the relaxed tongue has dropped back in the throat and closed off the airway or because vomitus, mucus, or fluid has collected in the throat. To keep the air passage free, the patient should be placed on his side. If the patient stops breathing he will show a marked change in color (cyanosis or blueness). *Help should be sent for at once.*

Because the patient has a tendency to perspire when under anesthesia he must be protected against chilling. Minor movements of arms and legs are permitted, as restraint causes him to become more restless. Frequently the patient is nauseated. Necessary equipment such as a basin and wipes should be kept at hand. The patient will be able to hear and comprehend spoken instructions before he can talk; therefore care should be taken to avoid any conversation that he might misunderstand or that would cause him to worry. The patient should not be left alone until he is completely conscious. After surgery and anesthesia the patient usually complains of dry mouth and thirst. His lips may be moistened for comfort. Fluids should be given only as ordered and never to an unconscious patient.

The person assigned to stay with a patient under anesthesia should observe the following instructions:

- Observe at all times any evidence of difficulty in breathing. To help the patient to breathe, push the lower jaw forward by pressing on the angle of the jaw just below the tip of the ear. If breathing is not resumed, grasp the tongue with a piece of gauze or a wipe to prevent the fingers from slipping and pull the tongue forward, turn the head to one side, and cleanse the mouth.
- Note the color of the skin. Pallor or blueness may indicate shock and should be reported to the doctor or the nurse.
- Keep the patient quiet, comfortably warm, and dry and lying on his side.
- Watch for vomiting; provide a basin and assist the patient. Keep his head turned to the side so that the fluid will run out of his mouth easily.
- Take and record the pulse rate frequently; report any marked change in rate, rhythm, or volume to the doctor or the nurse.
- Watch for and report any signs of bleeding on dressings.

Care of Burns

Under ordinary circumstances there will be a doctor or a professional nurse in charge at the shelter or the emergency hospital to give instructions and to provide over-all supervision of the care of the injured. The care of patients who have received extensive burns may have to begin before the patient can be brought to a physician. It is essential to keep burns covered for cleanliness, to prevent infection, and to give some relief from pain. Closely woven gauze or other soft material should be used next to the skin. These materials are not likely to adhere to the burned area. Absorbent cotton should never be placed on a burn, because it is difficult to remove. Only large, easily separated foreign particles, such as pieces of clothing, should be removed before applying the dressing. Care should be taken to avoid breaking blisters if any are present on the burned surface of the body, because every break in the skin is a potential source of entry for infection.

Unless specific orders have been given for caring for the burn, the following method may be safely used:

- Dressings should be large enough to cover the burned area completely.
- Apply the dressing and hold in place with a bandage, using firm, but gentle, even pressure in applying the bandage.
- Fasten the bandage with a knot or a safety pin.

- In some instances bleeding will occur from wounds already dressed and the fluid will saturate the dressing. Do not remove the original dressing, but apply another over it for reinforcement.
- Bandage snugly to provide for control of bleeding; use a tensile (stretch) type bandage to allow for swelling.

Admitting Patients to a Facility

A home nurse may be requested to assist with the admission of patients to mass shelters, hospitals, or other medical care stations. Among other duties, she may be assigned to:

- Prepare identification records
- Care for valuables
- Observe signs and symptoms of illness and injury
- Reassure patients and their families

Transferring to Another Facility

Patients may have to be transferred from emergency centers to hospitals or to other centers for further care. It may be the responsibility of a home nurse to help prepare these patients for the transfer. She will be expected to:

- Reassure the patient
- Make the patient comfortable on the carrying vehicle, with the body in proper position, and provide support for any injured part
- Make sure that the litter bearer or accompanying person has orders about the position of injured parts, and, if necessary, show him how to place and maintain the needed support
- Make sure that any extensive wounds are securely bandaged and labeled if bleeding has required a second pressure bandage
- Make sure that the patient's medical record accompanies him and that the last medication or nursing care given is recorded
- Give a drink or nourishment, if permitted. Offer the bedpan or urinal if trip is to be time consuming

RESUME OF DISASTER INJURIES AND ILLNESSES AND RECOMMENDED ACTION

The ability to recognize the nursing needs of the patient and to aid others in carrying out the doctor's orders safely, swiftly, and effectively, may save a life in a disaster. The conditions that nursing personnel and their assistants encounter most frequently in emergency situations and suggestions for the home nurse on what to observe, what to do, and what to report to the person in charge are presented in chart form at the end of this chapter.

173

DISASTER INJURIES AND ILLNESSES AND RECOMMENDED ACTION

Condition	What To Observe	What To Do	What To Report
Cuts and Wounds	Bleeding	Stop bleeding and apply sterile dressing. Keep wound clean and covered. Apply more dressing over original one if it becomes saturated, using firm pressure directly over wound.	Symptoms of shock or bleeding
	Symptoms of shock	Treat for shock.	
	Glass or other debris in wound		Evidence of foreign object in wound
	Evidence of pain	Support the affected part. On doctor's orders, move joints to help prevent stiffening and prevent decubiti.	Location, type, and intensity of pain
	Discharge (amount and odor)		Changes in color, odor, or consistency of discharge from wound
	Swelling or discoloration—Red streaks leading from wound		Swelling about the wound and discoloration—Red streaks leading from wound
Hemorrhage (internal)	Air hunger (gasping for breath or deep sighing)	Notify doctor or nurse *at once.*	
	Rapid pulse that is growing weaker	Reassure patient and keep quiet.	Any symptoms of internal hemorrhaging
	Sense of smothering	Keep patient comfortably warm.	
	Excessive thirst, with dry mouth	Supply fluids *if ordered.* Begin with about 1 cupful every hour if tolerated.	
	Restlessness	Give no stimulants.	
	Skin that is cold, clammy, pale, or bluish		
	Apparent source, such as lung, rectum, or other		

Condition	What To Observe	What To Do	What To Report
Burns	Symptoms of shock	Treat for shock.	Symptoms of shock
	Reddened skin, accompanied by pain; blisters; cooking or charring of the skin	Apply thick, firm, dry sterile dressing; bandage without wrinkling and overlapping; separate the fingers and toes when applying the dressing.	Any sudden rise in temperature
	Extent of the burn		Changes in amount, color, or odor of urine
	Evidence of infection		
	Pain	Keep patient comfortably warm.	
		Give medication as ordered by doctor.	
		Take temperature.	
		Measure and record fluid intake and urine output.	
Severe Bruises and Crushing Injuries	Symptoms of shock	Treat for shock.	Symptoms of shock
	Difficulty in breathing	Elevate and support injured part in correct position.	Change or difficulty in breathing
	Flattened or crushed extremities, with or without accompanying bleeding; discolored skin areas (black, blue, or red)	Elevate the head and shoulders if there is breathing difficulty or tilt up the chin.	Unconsciousness Discharges from or change in color and texture of injured part
	Breaks in the skin	Treat any break in the skin as a wound.	
	Bloody or serous drainage	Apply heat or cold only when instructed to do so.	
	Evidence of pain	Measure and record fluid intake.	Change in color or amount of urine
		Take temperature.	Rise in temperature
		Turn on side with the head and chest lowered to prevent aspiration of fluid into the lungs, if unconscious.	

175

Condition	What To Observe	What To Do	What To Report
Fractures	Evidence of pain when trying to move the injured part Inability to move an extremity or other injured part Wrong shape or out of line Swelling and blueness of skin Lack of feeling when touched	Keep broken part quiet. If an extremity, keep joint above and below the break immobilized with firm splint, using a rolled magazine or piece of board. Secure the splint above and below the fracture and above and below the adjacent joint. Apply clean dressing and bandage before splinting if bone protrudes through the skin. Do not turn the victim if back or neck is injured. *Move only if necessary* and keep victim in the position in which he was found.	Deformity of injured extremity Breaks in skin Bleeding Pain or swelling Blueness of skin
Concussion and Other Head Injuries	Complaint of headache Period of unconsciousness Unusual behavior (excitable, stuporous, or confused) Change in rate, rhythm, or volume of pulse Heavy or irregular breathing Bleeding or discharge from nose, ears, mouth, or a wound Vomiting, especially if forceful	Keep patient lying down. If breathing is difficult, keep air passages open by turning head to one side to allow fluid to run out. If necessary, push lower jaw forward by pressing on the angle of the jaw just below tip of ear. Keep patient comfortably warm. Apply sterile dressing to any wound.	Source of bleeding (ears, nose, mouth, or open scalp wound) Symptoms of shock Unconsciousness Sudden change in pulse or respiration Forceful or projectile vomiting Rise in temperature

Condition	What To Observe	What To Do	What To Report
Concussion and Other Head Injuries (cont.)	Swelling or lump on the head Face pale or flushed Evidence of dizziness, pain, or convulsions	Give fluids only when ordered by the doctor. Do not give alcoholic beverage or stimulants, such as coffee, tea, or cocoa. Do not swab inside ears or nose. Count the pulse frequently during the 24 hours following injury to note any change in rate, rhythm, or volume. Measure fluids given and the urine output. Take temperature.	
Reaction from intravenous injections of plasma, whole blood, or other fluids	Swelling around point of injection Chilling, shivering, or faintness Stoppage in the flow of fluid	Stop the flow of fluid. Obtain help from doctor or nurse immediately. Reassure the patient.	Swelling around point of injection Complaint of chilliness, or noticeable shivering Cessation of the flow of fluid—displacement of the needle
Radiation Sickness	Nausea and vomiting Bleeding from gums and other mucous membrane Evidence of sore throat Tiny hemorrhages (discolorations) in the skin, which gradually become larger and break open Weakness and headache Diarrhea; blood in stool	Keep patient away from others who have a cold or other communicable disease. Keep all wounds clean and covered with sterile dressings. Keep patient as quiet as possible. Take temperature.	Signs of shock Nausea and vomiting Bleeding from gums or other mucous membrane Enlarging, bruise-like areas on skin Bloody diarrhea Evidence of sore throat Rise in temperature

SUGGESTED STUDENT ACTIVITIES

1. Prepare a brief report of the natural disasters that have occurred in the last 10 years in your city or county. What is the present potential for natural disasters in your community, such as those caused by weather, fire, explosions, or transportation hazards?

2. Help the instructor to procure and show one of the Red Cross films about disaster. Discuss the implications of the film as it relates to your community.

3. Collect newspaper articles describing natural disasters that occurred in this country during a 2-week period. Tabulate the disasters in order of kind and frequency. How do they differ in number of people injured and made homeless and the total destruction caused?

4. Arrange with the instructor to invite a representative of your Red Cross chapter disaster committee to talk with the class about the rehabilitation phase of a disaster operation.

5. Take a poll in your apartment house, block, or neighborhood to find out in how many families there is at least one member trained in home nursing or in first aid. What do the results of your poll indicate?

6. Using your family as the example, prepare a list of the foods and the amounts of each you would stockpile for 2-week survival needs.

7. Read one of the studies that have been made about changes in behavior under stress or anxiety. Describe your own feelings at a time when you were badly frightened. Were they like or different from those described in the study? Discuss how you can improve your reaction to stress.

8. Arrange with the instructor to invite your school doctor or nurse to explain to the class how different anesthetics are administered. Why are different methods and anesthetics used? Report on the discovery and first use of anesthesia.

9. If there is a branch of the weather bureau in your community, try to arrange with the instructor for the class to make a field trip to see the instruments used in collecting and interpreting weather information.

SECTION II

Home Nursing Procedures

12

PATIENT CARE SKILLS

GENERAL INTRODUCTION

The simple home nursing procedures presented in Section II can be carried out in the home. Each skill is clearly explained step by step, and line drawings provide visual aids to assist with the explanations. Because it may be more difficult to learn the skills without help, it is recommended that at least one person in every family become prepared to care for the sick at home by taking a Red Cross home nursing course. In class the skills are demonstrated and opportunity provided for guided practice. This section of the book will serve as a ready reference for those who have had this preparation.

Care of the patient at home is often more desirable than care in a hospital or a nursing home because at home the patient is in familiar surroundings, has fewer financial worries, and receives affection and emotional support from the family. The home nurse and other members of the family who are concerned with giving care to the sick at home need to remember that competent physical care must be accompanied by an understanding of the emotional needs of the patient as expressed by his behavior. These reactions will vary from person to person.

It is taken for granted that the doctor has confidence in the ability of the home nurse to give competent care to the sick person and that home conditions are such that necessary treatment can be given as ordered.

Comfort, safety, economy, effectiveness, and appearance are the components of nursing care, and they are related to manual skills, whether used in caring for a patient or in performing household tasks. An understanding of these components and their application to specific skills are important to both the home nurse and the patient. Some helpful points to remember are:

- It is easier to care for the patient and to do the necessary daily tasks if there is a flexible plan or schedule to follow.
- It will save time to assemble all the necessary equipment before starting a task and to put everything away as soon as it is finished.
- One's health is safeguarded by practicing correct body mechanics, by having adequate nutrition, and by getting sufficient rest, recreation, and sleep.
- Recovery will be hastened by guarding the patient against infection, by providing proper body support whether the patient is in bed or out of bed, by encouraging him to do as much for himself as possible, and by providing emotional and spiritual encouragement.

HAND WASHING

The home nurse should always wash her hands thoroughly before and after caring for a patient to help protect the patient, herself, and others from infection. Running water should be used for hand washing. If tap water is not available, water for both soaping and rinsing may be poured over the hands from a pitcher. Grasping the pitcher by its handle with a piece of clean paper or a towel will keep it from slipping. Towels of paper or cloth may be used to dry the hands, but if towels are not available, the hands may be dried by shaking them.

In some situations, such as disaster, water for hand washing may be limited or not available. An acceptable method of cleansing is to rub the hands and the wrists with a liquid detergent, hand or baby skin lotion, cold cream, or witch hazel solution. Alcohol can be used, but because of its drying action precautions should be taken to prevent breaks in the skin. The small foil-wrapped packets of paper impregnated with moist soap or lotion that are sold in drug and department stores can be used to cleanse the face and the hands satisfactorily.

Equipment

Running water
Soap
Clean towels
Container for soiled towels

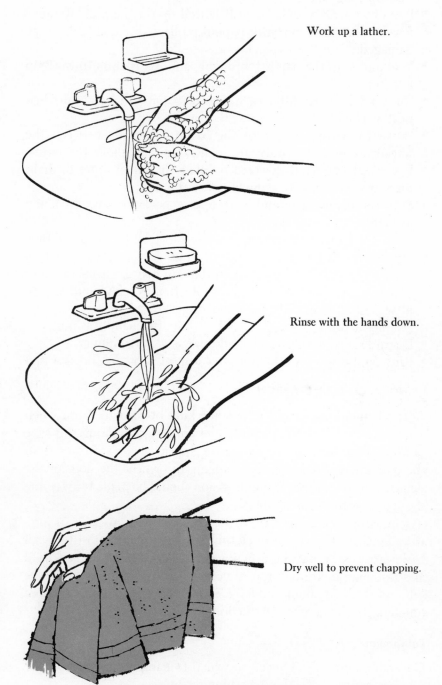

Work up a lather.

Rinse with the hands down.

Dry well to prevent chapping.

For protection, wash the hands thoroughly.

Procedure

- Roll up long sleeves.
- Remove a wrist watch or push it well up on the arm. Remove jewelry that may hurt the patient, collect dirt and soil, or be damaged.
- Wet and soap the hands thoroughly and use friction to work up a lather.
- Rinse off bar soap after each use so that it will be clean when next needed.
- Wash the entire surface of the hands, especially between the fingers, around and under the nails, and well above the wrists.
- Rinse with the hands lowered to allow the soiled water to drain directly off the hands, removing dirt and oil.
- Soap the hands again and work up a good lather, using friction as before.
- Rinse the hands well, taking care to remove all the soap and dirt.
- Dry the hands for comfort and to avoid chapping, using a clean towel. Wet skin or dried soap on the skin may cause chapping or breaks in the skin that may admit infection. Rough hands are unattractive and uncomfortable, but the skin can be kept soft and pliable by using lotion or a hand cream after hand washing.
- Discard soiled towels in the laundry or a waste container.
- Rinse and dry the washbasin after disposing of the soiled water.

USING A COVERALL APRON

The home nurse should wear some kind of coverall apron when giving direct care to the patient. The purpose of wearing this type of apron is to help in preventing the spread of disease to or from the patient. It should be kept hanging in or near the door of the sickroom ready for use. Some provision should be made for washing the hands before it is removed.

A pinafore apron similar to the one pictured on page 61 provides excellent protection to clothing. An acceptable substitute can be improvised by putting a man's short-sleeved shirt on backward and fastening it. If an apron is worn in caring for the patient, the bib and the skirt should be large enough to keep one's dress from touching the patient or the bedding.

Equipment

Coverall apron	Object on which to hang the clothes hanger
Clothes hanger	Hand washing facilities

Procedure

- Wash the hands.
- Slip the arms into the sleeves of the apron without touching the outside of the garment, which will be next to the patient.
- Fasten the apron at the neck and the waist for security and ease in working.
- Wash the hands after caring for the patient and before removing the apron.
- Unfasten the apron at the neck and the waist to remove the garment. Slip the arms out of the sleeves and place the apron on a clothes hanger with the inside in to keep it clean.
- Hang up the apron with the opening facing outward so that it can be put on easily.

THROAT INSPECTION

The throat is one of the first areas of the body to signal illness. There are many kinds and degrees of intensity of throat infections. Many times a sore throat is an early symptom of a cold, but it may also be a symptom of an acute communicable disease. Early recognition and treatment of a sore throat are particularly important when the patient is among a large number of people, for example, in school or in a shelter.

Sore throats may cause some difficulty in swallowing, although in general small children do not complain of this difficulty. Because infection is present, the lymph glands in the neck may become enlarged and tender. Another accompanying discomfort is earache, caused by inflammation and infection traveling through the Eustachian tube, which connects the throat to the ear.

It is wise to practice inspecting a child's throat while he is well. If he has had previous inspections, he is likely to be cooperative when he is not feeling well. If the home nurse is unable to see the back of the throat on the first attempt, she should let the patient rest and try again.

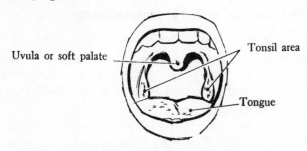

Diagram of opening to the throat

The purpose of throat inspection is to see if there is marked redness or swelling or any other unusual condition in the throat and to be able to describe the observed condition to the doctor.

Equipment

Wooden tongue depressor or clean teaspoon
Handkerchief, preferably paper
Flashlight, if extra light is needed

Procedure

- Explain to the patient what is to be done.
- Place the patient facing a good light, near a window or a lamp, or use a flashlight.
- Give the patient a handkerchief and instruct him to cover his mouth if he should have to cough suddenly.
- Support the patient's chin with one hand and, to help open the throat, ask him to say "Ah." Stand to one side to avoid being in direct line of possible cough spray.
- Depress the tongue by placing on it a wooden tongue depressor or a spoon handle about two-thirds back, using pressure as necessary so that the back of the throat is in clear view. Ask the patient to say "Ah" again.
- Inspect the back and the sides of the throat for redness, swelling, spots, or patches, noting also the condition of the tongue, the gums and teeth, and the odor of the breath.
- Discard the wooden tongue depressor. If a spoon has been used, take care not to touch the part that has been in contact with the mouth until the spoon has been washed with hot, soapy water and rinsed with boiling water.

If white, gray, or yellowish patches are observed or if the throat is unusually red and swollen, put the patient to bed and keep others away from him. Take his temperature and report the condition to the doctor.

CARE AND USE OF THE CLINICAL THERMOMETER

A clinical, or fever, thermometer is one used to take body temperature. Because it is made of glass, it is fragile and must be handled with care. When not in use, the thermometer should be kept in a safe place and protected from heat. The bulb end must be kept clean at all times.

The clinical thermometer differs in its construction from most other thermometers. The glass tube narrows at the mercury-filled bulb end to prevent the mercury from returning to the bulb until it is shaken down. The thermometer operates on the principle that mercury expands when exposed to heat. When subjected to body heat, the mercury rises in the glass tube and remains at the highest point registered until it is shaken down.

There are two kinds of clinical thermometers: oral and rectal. Oral thermometers usually have a long, slender bulb, while rectal thermometers have a short, stubby bulb, either round or pear-shaped. Most clinical thermometers have the shape shown in the cross-section drawing below, but some have a thin, flat tube. If only one thermometer can be purchased, it should be the one with the stubby bulb, because it can be used to take the temperature by mouth, by rectum, or at the axilla, or armpit.

Curvature of glass magnifies the mercury in the tube; white coating makes a background for the mercury.

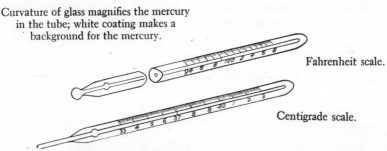

Fahrenheit scale.

Centigrade scale.

Diagrammatic drawing of a clinical thermometer.

Clinical thermometers use either the centigrade or the Fahrenheit scale. The centigrade thermometer is marked from 34.5° C. to 43.4° C., while the Fahrenheit thermometer is usually marked from 94° F. to 110° F. To convert a centigrade reading to a Fahrenheit reading, multiply the centigrade reading by 9, divide by 5, and add 32. To convert a Fahrenheit reading to a centigrade reading, subtract 32 from the Fahrenheit reading, multiply by 5, and divide by 9.

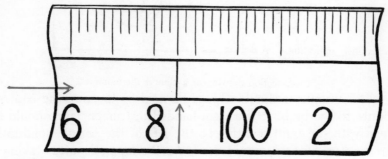

Detail of the thermometer. Arrow indicates average normal temperature.

The scale markings are the same on all clinical thermometers: the long lines designate degrees and short lines designate two-tenths (⅕) of a degree. These lines appear above the numbers. The average mouth temperature, which is 98.6° F. or 37° C., is indicated on the tube by a small arrow. The front of the thermometer is ridged to magnify the mercury column in the glass tube. The back of the thermometer is made of opaque glass so that the mercury will be easier to see. For an accurate reading the bulb end of the thermometer must be kept in the mouth or the rectum for at least 3 minutes. When the temperature is taken in the axilla the thermometer must be held in place for 5 minutes. Mouth temperature should not be taken immediately after the patient has been smoking or has had a hot or a cold bath, or hot or cold food or drink. Rectal temperature should not be taken immediately after the patient has had an enema. The temperature registered under such circumstances may not be the true body temperature.

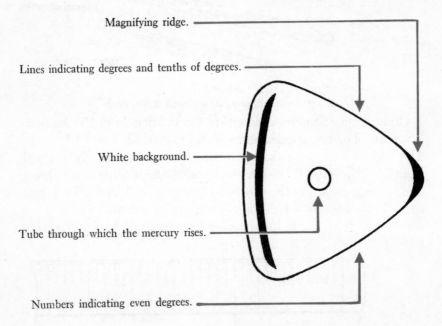

Magnifying ridge.

Lines indicating degrees and tenths of degrees.

White background.

Tube through which the mercury rises.

Numbers indicating even degrees.

Cross section drawing of a clinical thermometer.

A thermometer should always be held by the top, the end opposite to the bulb. It is a right-handed instrument and should be read with the bulb pointing to the left of the person holding it. If the home nurse cannot read the thermometer after taking a temperature, she should cleanse it and put it away until someone else can read and record the temperature.

POINTS TO REMEMBER ABOUT USING THE CLINICAL THERMOMETER

When shaking down the mercury:

- Stand away from the furniture to avoid striking the thermometer against an object and breaking it.
- Hold the thermometer firmly by the top between the thumb and first two fingers.
- Shake with a loose wrist movement, as though shaking water off the hand, to bring the mercury to 95° F. (35° C.) or below.

To insure correct registration:

- Make sure that the mercury is shaken down to 95° F. (35° C.) or below before taking the temperature.
- Allow sufficient time for accurate registration of the temperature.
- Verify any marked rise or fall in the temperature by taking it again, if necessary with another thermometer.

When reading the thermometer:

- Make sure the light is adequate for accurate reading of the thermometer.
- Hold the thermometer by the top.
- Locate the clear bubble just above the bulb at the constriction in the thermometer. Rotate the thermometer slowly until the bubble can be seen at its widest point. To the right of the bubble the mercury will be seen as a silver ribbon in the glass tube.
- Read the scale to include the degree and nearest two-tenths of a degree.

For the safety of the patient:

- Have the patient sit or lie down when taking the temperature.
- Take the temperature in the rectum or the axilla when it cannot be taken safely or accurately in the mouth.
- Cleanse the thermometer immediately after use, return it to its case, and put it in a safe place.

TAKING THE MOUTH TEMPERATURE

Equipment

Clinical thermometer
Container of wipes: absorbent cotton, paper tissues, toilet paper, or pieces of clean gauze or cloth
Container of cool, clean water
Soap
Waste container

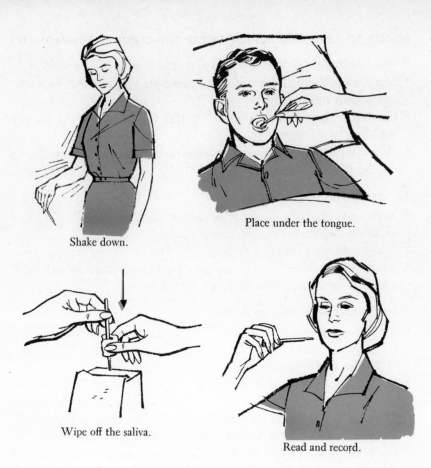

Shake down.

Place under the tongue.

Wipe off the saliva.

Read and record.

Taking the mouth temperature.

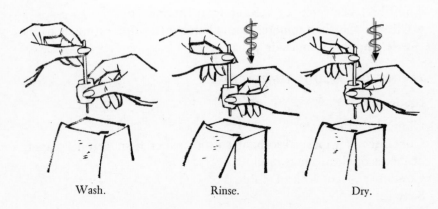

Wash.

Rinse.

Dry.

Cleansing the thermometer.

Procedure

- Have the patient sit or lie down.
- Hold the thermometer firmly by the top.
- Shake the mercury down to 95° F. (35° C.) or below to insure accurate registration.
- Moisten the thermometer with clear, cool water to make the instrument easier and more pleasant for the patient to hold in his mouth.
- Place the bulb in the patient's mouth, well under the tongue and a little to one side.
- Tell the patient to keep his lips closed, to breathe through his nose, and not to bite down on the thermometer or to talk.
- Leave the thermometer in place for 3 minutes to insure accurate registration.
- Remove the thermometer, holding it securely at the top.
- Remove saliva from the thermometer with a wipe, using a firm, rotary motion from the top downward over the bulb for cleanliness and to make reading the thermometer easier. Discard the wipe in a waste container.
- Take the thermometer to a good light, still holding it by the top, and read and record the temperature.
- Cleanse the thermometer immediately:
    Moisten a wipe with cool water and soap it well. Hold the instrument by the top, with the bulb down, over a waste container. Beginning at the top, wipe down with a firm, rotary motion, using friction and getting well into the grooves of the tube and over the bulb. Discard the wipe.
    Moisten a fresh wipe with clear, cool water and rinse the thermometer, using the same downward, rotary motion.
    Soap and rinse the thermometer again.
    Dry it with a fresh wipe, using the same motion.
- Put the thermometer away in its case, bulb end first, for safety and cleanliness.

If there is a marked rise or fall in the patient's temperature, check the reading by taking the temperature again. Report the results to the doctor at once if the second reading confirms the first.

TAKING THE RECTAL TEMPERATURE

Because of large blood vessels in the walls of the rectum that bring warm blood to that area, the temperature is usually approximately 1 degree higher in that part of the body than in the mouth. Therefore, the average normal rectal temperature is 99.6° F. (37.5° C.). For the information of the doctor, the daily record should always indicate that the temperature has been taken rectally.

Equipment

The same equipment will be needed as for taking the temperature by mouth, except that a thermometer with a stubby bulb should be used and a lubricant such as petrolatum will be needed.

Procedures

For an adult:
- Explain to the patient what is going to be done and tell him to lie on his side.
- Shake the mercury down to 95° F. (35° C.) or below to insure accurate registration.
- Lubricate the bulb end of the thermometer with petrolatum, oil, or cold cream so that it will slide easily into the rectum.
- Slip the bulb end of the thermometer about 1 inch into the anus, or opening of the rectum. Hold it in place for 3 minutes to make sure that the thermometer registers the actual temperature. Let the patient insert the thermometer and hold it in place if he is able to do so.
- Remove the thermometer and read and record the temperature registered.
- Cleanse the instrument in the manner described on page 191.

For a child or an infant:
- Explain to an older child what is going to be done.
- Shake the mercury down to 95° F. (35° C.) or below to insure accurate registration.
- Lubricate the thermometer in the same way as when taking the rectal temperature of an adult.
- Place the child on a bed or a table, lying on his side or his abdomen so that the anus is visible.
- Place an infant on his back on your lap or put him on a bed, a bathinette, or a table. Grasp his ankles with one hand and gently bend his knees so that the anus is visible.
- Insert the bulb of the thermometer gently about 1 inch into the anus and hold it for 3 minutes. *It must be held in place at all times.* Help may be needed to hold a restless child.
- Remove the thermometer and take and record the reading.
- Cleanse the thermometer in the manner described on page 191.

TAKING THE AXILLARY TEMPERATURE

Temperature taken in the axilla may be called skin temperature. It is about 1 degree lower than the mouth temperature. Therefore, the average normal axillary temperature is 97.6° F. (36.5°). For this reason the daily record should show that an axillary temperature has been taken. The axillary method may be ordered for infants or when other methods are difficult to follow. In order for the axillary method to be reliable, the procedure given below must be followed carefully.

Equipment

The same equipment will be needed as for taking a mouth temperature.

Procedure

- Shake the mercury down to 95° F. (35° C.) or below. Do not moisten or lubricate the thermometer.
- Dry the area under the arm.
- Place the dry bulb end of the thermometer in the axilla and have the patient press his arm firmly against his body, putting his hand on his opposite shoulder and holding the thermometer in this position for 5 minutes. It will be necessary to stay with a child and hold the thermometer in place until the temperature registers.
- Remove the thermometer and take the readings.
- Cleanse the thermometer in the manner described on page 191.
- Write the temperature and the manner of taking it on the daily record.

COUNTING PULSE AND RESPIRATION

The pulse is the throbbing caused in the blood vessels by contractions of the heart muscles as they force blood through the vessels. Respiration is the act of breathing, or the twofold process of inspiration, by which the body takes in oxygen from the air, and expiration, by which the body gives off waste products, chiefly carbon dioxide, from the lungs. The rate, volume, and rhythm of both pulse and respiration vary with age, sex, size, and physical and emotional activity. In general, as the temperature rises, both pulse and respiration increase. Therefore, the count of the pulse and of respirations is an index of the patient's condition.

Watch or clock with a clear dial and a second hand.

Procedure

- Have the patient lie or sit down, with his arm and hand in a relaxed position, thumb up, supported on a chair arm, a table, or a bed.

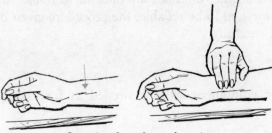

Counting the pulse at the wrist.

- Locate the pulse by placing the fingers, not the thumb, on the thumb side of the patient's wrist between the tendons and the wristbone.
- Count the pulse beats for one-half minute and multiply the number counted by 2 to get the rate per minute. If there is any doubt as to accuracy, count the beats again.
- Count respirations while the fingers are still on the wrist. The patient is less likely to change his rate of breathing if he is unaware that it is being counted. Count the rise and fall of his chest for one-half minute and multiply the number counted by 2 to get the rate per minute.
- Write on the patient's daily record the time, date, and rate per minute of the pulse and of respirations.

USING THE BEDPAN AND THE URINAL

If the patient is to remain in bed, the home nurse will need to provide a bedpan and a urinal. They should be placed on a protected area for cleanliness and be out of sight when not in use.

Equipment

Bedpan, warmed if necessary
Bedpan cover
Bell or other call system
Bed protector: a covered rubber, plastic, or oilcloth sheet or a cloth-covered newspaper bed pad
Urinal and cover

Newspapers to protect the furniture and the floor
Basin of warm water, soap, washcloth, and towel
Toilet paper

Procedures

For using the bedpan:

- Bring the covered bedpan, the bed protector, and the toilet paper to the bedside. Make sure that a bell is within the patient's reach.

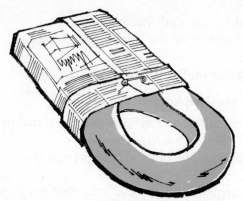

Bedpan with cover made of newspapers.

- Fold back the top covers at the side of the bed to prevent their becoming soiled. Keep the patient covered.
- Have the patient flex his knees.
- Place the bed protector under the patient's hips.
- Place the bedpan on the bed beside the patient with the open end toward the foot of the bed. Hold the pan at the side or the back to avoid handling the open end.
- Place one hand under the small of the patient's back; on signal, help the patient lift his hips. With the other hand, slip the pan under the patient's hips and adjust it for comfort.
- Raise the patient to a sitting position if the doctor permits, placing supports at his back.
- Put the toilet paper where the patient can reach it; leave the room to give him privacy unless he is too ill to remain alone.
- Cleanse him if necessary, putting the soiled tissue in the pan. Avoid soiling the bed covers.
- Remove the pan promptly when the patient has finished, helping him to lift his hips so that the pan does not rub the skin.
- Remove the bed protector.
- Cover the pan and take it to the bathroom.
- Allow the patient to wash his hands and make him comfortable.

- Observe the contents of the pan and, if unusual, save for the doctor to see.
- Note observations on the patient's daily record.

For using the urinal:

- Help the patient place the urinal if help is needed. Avoid exposing the patient.
- Remove the urinal promptly after use, cover it, and take it to the bathroom.
- Allow the patient to wash his hands.
- Observe the contents of the urinal and, if unusual, save for the doctor to see.
- Note observations on the patient's daily record.

For caring for the bedpan and the urinal:

- Empty the contents of the bedpan and the urinal into the toilet unless the doctor has ordered otherwise.
- Rinse the bedpan with cold water to prevent stool from sticking to the sides.
- Cleanse the utensils thoroughly, using hot soapy water and a commode brush.
- Rinse them well and dry the outside.
- Put them away covered and keep them out of sight when not in use.

PLACING THE HELPLESS PATIENT ON THE BEDPAN

Ordinarily one person should not attempt to place a helpless patient on the bedpan. A patient able to use his arms can lift himself by using a trapeze bar above the bed. For example, a patient in a body cast or with a paralysis of one or both legs might have no loss of strength in his arms and could assist greatly in lifting himself for the placement and the removal of the bedpan. The completely helpless patient, however, is not able to assist, and the home nurse will need a helper to work opposite her at the bed.

Equipment

In addition to the equipment listed on pages 194-195, several protected pillows or folded blankets will be needed to make a body-length platform to support the helpless patient while he is on the bedpan.

Procedure

- Turn the patient on his side and steady him in that position.

196

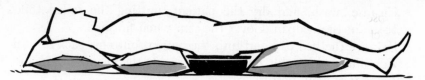

Note position of pillows and bedpan after it has been placed under the helpless patient.

- Place a large pillow or two small ones lengthwise against the patient's back from his shoulders to the upper buttocks. Place a large pillow or two small ones lengthwise against the patient from his thighs to his feet, building a platform on which he can be placed.
- Protect the ends of the pillows and the bed between them with a waterproof bed pad or a protective sheet.

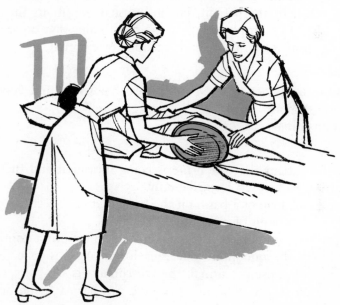

The home nurse will need a helper to assist in putting a helpless patient on the bedpan.

- Place the pan on edge against the patient's buttocks, as precisely in the desired position as possible, hold it in place, and roll the patient back onto the pan and the platform of pillows.
- Allow the patient time to use the bedpan.
- Hold the bedpan flat on the bed while the helper rolls the patient toward her, onto his side, off the platform.
- Remove the bedpan and set it aside on a protected surface.
- Remove the pillows.

- Cleanse, wash, and dry the patient, putting the soiled toilet tissue in the bedpan. Cover the pan when finished.
- Remove the bed pad and turn the patient onto his back or position him comfortably on his side. Provide the necessary supports for proper body posture.
- Observe the contents of the pan. Note on the patient's daily record the amount, appearance, and anything unusual about the stool or the urine.

MEASURING URINE OUTPUT

Measurement of urine is started at a definite time, usually the first time the patient voids in the morning, and is recorded for each 24-hour period. When urine is being measured, it is common practice to measure and record the patient's fluid intake as well. In general, the amount of urine voided will depend on the amount of fluid taken by the patient, but in unusual conditions this may not be true. Drugs or physiological malfunctioning may cause a decrease or an increase in the fluids retained or excreted.

Equipment

Measuring container, marked in ounces if possible, and kept for this purpose alone
Bedpan or urinal

Procedure

- Tell the patient that the urine is being measured and that the bedpan is to be used for urine only.
- Place the bedpan or a basin on the toilet seat or collect the urine in the catch basin of a commode chair.
- Empty the contents of the pan into the measuring container and record the amount in ounces each time urine is collected. If the patient is using a urinal, the measurements may already be marked on it. Strips of adhesive tape can be placed on an unmarked urinal to indicate measurements in ounces.
- Empty the urine into the toilet.
- Cleanse and put away the equipment.

COLLECTING URINE SPECIMENS

When the doctor requests a specimen of urine, he will state how much he needs and when he wishes it collected. It is usual to save a single specimen from the first urine voided in the morning unless a 24-hour specimen is requested; 4 to 6 ounces are usually sufficient. The patient should understand that the urine specimen must be kept separate from a bowel movement.

Because the external bladder and vaginal openings in women are so close together, the urine specimen may contain vaginal or other discharges unless special care is taken. Before the patient voids, the external genitalia should be washed with soap and water.

Equipment

Clean bedpan, urinal, or other receptacle
Clean bottle with a watertight stopper or screw top

Label for bottle.
Large, clean, covered container (when collecting a 24-hour specimen)

Procedures

When collecting a single specimen:

- Wash the genitalia before the urine is voided or have the patient wash himself if he is able. If a woman is menstruating or has a vaginal discharge, report this fact to the doctor before the specimen is collected.
- Have the patient urinate into the clean receptacle.
- Transfer the urine to the specimen bottle and close the bottle securely.
- Attach the label to the bottle and write on it the word "urine," the name of the patient, and the date and the hour that the specimen was collected.
- Send the specimen to the doctor or to a specified laboratory as promptly as possible.
- Cleanse and put away the equipment.

When collecting a 24-hour specimen:

- Wash the patient's genitalia before each voiding.
- Begin at a stated hour, usually 7:00 A.M.; discard the urine voided at this hour.
- Pour all urine voided after 7:00 A.M. into a large, clean, covered container, such as a commode or a diaper pail.
- Save all the urine up to *and* including that voided at 7:00 A.M. the following day. The urine may then be measured, if so ordered, and a sample collected from the total amount, usually 4 to 6 ounces.

Points To Remember

- Make sure that all the receptacles and the patient's genitalia are clean.
- Make sure that all measurements and labeling are accurate.

13

CARING FOR THE PATIENT IN BED

BODY MECHANICS AND POSTURE

Posture is the relationship of the various parts of the body to each other when a person is standing, sitting, lying, or moving. Body mechanics in its simplest meaning is the way the body moves and maintains balance by the most efficient use of all its parts.

It is important for both the patient and the home nurse to have alternate periods of rest and activity in order to help maintain good muscle tone and prevent undue fatigue and joint deformities. Muscles in poor tone appear flabby; muscles in good tone are firm and ready to act. To prevent patients who are confined to bed for long periods of time from developing contractures or deformity disabilities, the body parts must be kept in good alignment and the position changed frequently. Sick people have a tendency to curl up in bed with the back, hips, and knees flexed. A patient may lie in such a position to relieve pain or to keep warm, but if he remains in this position for long periods of time, it becomes more and more difficult for him to assume correct body position.

When the home nurse knows and habitually practices good body mechanics in everyday living, she saves her own energy and is better prepared to help and teach the patient.

Points to remember in developing good body mechanics and maintaining good posture are:
- Maintain a broad base of support, standing with the feet comfortably apart, one foot forward, and the toes pointed in the direction of movement.
- Maintain natural spinal curves by:
    Tightening the abdominal and buttocks muscles to stabilize the pelvis

Keeping the chest up and forward

Holding the head erect

- Stand close to the task and flex the hips and the knees when stooping or bending.
- Use the longest and strongest muscles of the arms and the legs to provide power when moving or lifting an object.
- Carry heavy objects close to the body to conserve energy and to prevent strain.
- Move a bed patient at hip level by sliding him since this method requires less effort than lifting him.
- Move the patient by rolling or turning him since this method employs leverage and momentum and therefore requires less effort than lifting.

POSITIONING THE PATIENT IN BED

Correct body position is the same whether a person is standing or lying down. The patient in bed must have proper posture and his body must be supported in good alignment. A firm but resilient mattress is needed for support. A mattress that is very soft allows the body to sag, and one that is rigid will not conform to natural body curves. The bedsprings must be strong enough to support the mattress and not allow it to sag. Although modern mattresses are built to give the greatest support at the heaviest parts of the body, it may be necessary to place a bedboard of ¾-inch plywood that fits the length and the width of the mattress on top of the springs to provide adequate support for the weight of the person in bed.

The number and type of pillows under the head and the shoulders is a matter of preference unless the doctor gives special orders. The normal curves of the spine should be maintained, with the head in line with the trunk and not pushed forward or dropped backward. The knees may be flexed slightly for muscle relaxation and comfort.

Points to remember for maintaining good posture for the bed patient are:

- Provide support for the back, maintaining the normal curves of the spine.
- Support the joints to prevent strain or deformity.
- Give attention to the positioning of the extremities to prevent contractures.
- Change the body position from time to time to promote circulation of the blood and to prevent pressure sores.

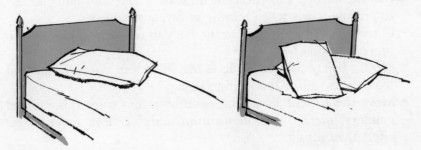

Place two pillows lengthwise, crossed at the top and with bottom corners together.

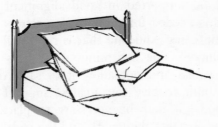

Place the third pillow crosswise at the top under the head and reaching to the shoulders.

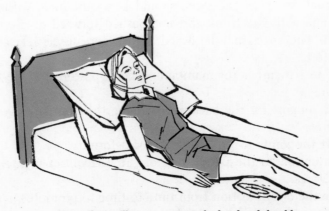

Using three pillows to support the head and shoulders.

- Encourage movement to maintain range of joint motion and to promote good muscle tone.

SUPPORT FOR THE PATIENT LYING IN BED

Equipment

Firm mattress and springs
Several pillows or substitutes, such as folded blankets or bath towels

Bedboard if needed for firmer support
Foot support

Procedures for the Patient Lying on His Back

Using one pillow:
- Place the pillow, reaching to the shoulders, under the patient's head.
- Place a vertical foot support so that the patient may brace his upright feet against it. The support should extend about 2 inches above the toes to protect them from the weight of the bedding.

Using three pillows:
- Place two pillows lengthwise, crossed at the top, with the bottom corners together and extending under the patient's shoulders.
- Place one pillow crosswise at the top, under the head and reaching to the shoulders.
- Place a small pillow at the lower back if necessary for support.
- Place a flat, firm pad or a folded bath towel under the patient's knees if necessary for support and for comfort.
- Place a foot support. (See picture page 204.)

Procedure for the Patient Lying on His Side

- Place one pillow under the patient's head.
- Place a pillow at the patient's back lengthwise and anchor it by pushing the edge of the pillowcase under his back. Fold the outer side of the pillow under and tuck it in snugly against the patient to give support.
- Place a small support, such as a folded or rolled bath towel, under his abdomen.
- Flex the hip and the knee of his uppermost leg, bringing the leg forward so that it does not rest on the lower one. Extend the lower leg comfortably.
- Place a pillow lengthwise under his uppermost leg to provide correct support and position of the knee and the foot. The pillow should extend well under the foot so that the ankle and the foot do not drop and are kept on the same plane.

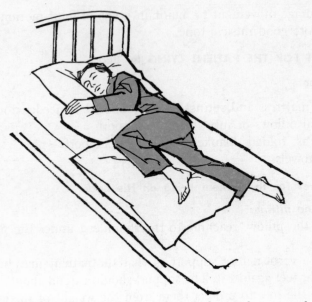

To achieve proper posture in bed, the body must be supported
in good alignment.

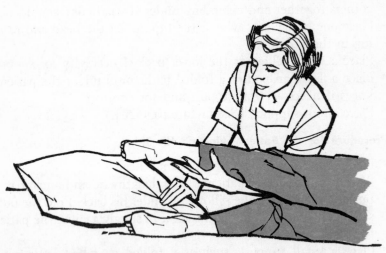

Support the knee and ankle on the forearm and hand when lifting the leg to
place a pillow support.

- Fold and place one pillow on a level with his shoulder for support of the uppermost arm and hand so that there will be no strain on the shoulder joint.
- Have the patient place his hand and his arm on the pillow in a position that is comfortable for him and correct in relation to the position of the rest of his body.

SUPPORT FOR THE PATIENT SITTING UP IN BED

Equipment

Back rest   Small pillow
2 to 5 large pillows   Slanted foot support

Procedure

- Help the patient to sit up in bed and brace himself with his arms. Remove the pillows.
- Place the back rest so that its slanted side is toward the patient.
- Place three pillows on the back rest as described in the procedure for lying in bed using three pillows.
- Help the patient to lie back on the pillows.
- Place a slanted foot support so that he may brace his feet against it.
- Place pillows at both sides to support his arms and shoulders.

MOVING THE PATIENT IN BED

The purpose of changing the position of the bed patient is to relax him, to improve circulation, to prevent continued pressure on any part of his body over too long a time, to avoid strain on his joints, to prevent deformities, and to change his position for comfort or for giving treatments.

Whenever the home nurse cares for a patient who is in bed, she should both allow and urge him to do as much for himself as possible. Helping himself provides exercise for the patient, is a positive rehabilitation measure, and gives him the mental and moral support that is necessary for his ultimate recovery. However, when assistance is needed, it should be provided.

In order to let the patient cooperate to the greatest extent of his strength, the home nurse should always tell him what is going to be done and should arrange with him a signal so that both the patient's and the home nurse's efforts are coordinated. For example, the home nurse may count "One, two, three," or say, "Ready." Any simple cue will do that enables the patient to understand when to do his part.

Procedures When the Patient Can Help

Moving to the side of the bed:
- Place the hands, palms up, under the pillow, supporting the patient's head and shoulders. On signal, pull toward the near side of the bed.

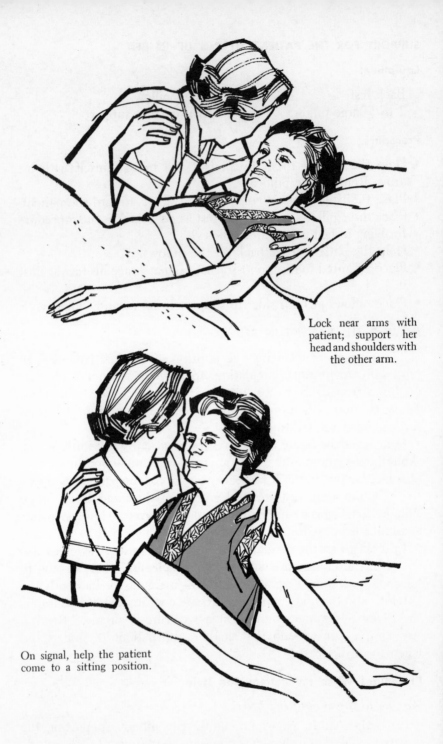

Lock near arms with patient; support her head and shoulders with the other arm.

On signal, help the patient come to a sitting position.

Helping the patient to sit up.

- Place the hands, palms up, all the way under his hips and, on signal, pull.
- Place the hands under his knees and his ankles and, on signal, pull.
- Adjust his body for correct alignment and for comfort.

Sitting up and lying down:
- Help the patient to flex his knees.
- Face the head of the bed, with the outer leg forward.
- Lock near arms with the patient by putting the arm under the patient's arm with the hand at his shoulder. The patient braces his arm with his hand at the home nurse's shoulder.
- Avoid directly facing the patient to prevent the exchange of nose and mouth secretions.
- Support the patient with the other arm, making a cradle for his head and his shoulders, and adjust posture for leverage.
- On signal, help the patient to sit up. Pause and provide support if he feels dizzy.
- Have the patient support himself by bracing his hands behind him on the bed. Give assistance as needed.
- To help the patient lie down, reverse the procedure.

Moving up and down in bed:
- Assist or have the patient come to a sitting position.
- Have him support himself by placing his hands behind him on the bed, keeping his arms as straight as is comfortable.
- Move toward the head of the bed and face the bed. Place one hand low on the patient's back; place the other hand, palm up, well under his thighs. On signal, help the patient to move backward as he digs in and pushes with his heels.
- To move toward the foot of the bed, the procedure described above is repeated, except that the patient digs in with his heels and pushes with his hands as he moves forward.

Procedures When the Patient Is Helpless

A drawsheet can be used to move a helpless or an aged patient from side to side or up and down in bed. The drawsheet should extend above the top of the patient's head and below his hips. Except in the case where the patient is being turned, the procedures described below should not be attempted without assistance. The number of people needed to assist will depend on the size and the condition of the patient, but they should work in pairs on either side of the patient.

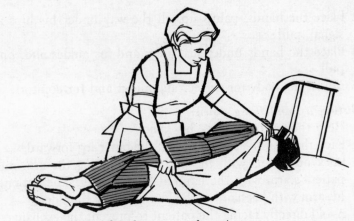
Using a drawsheet to turn the patient.

Moving up and down in bed:
- Have the patient on his back on the drawsheet.
- Gather the drawsheet into a loose roll on either side of the patient so that it can be grasped easily.
- Face the foot of the bed with one foot forward, if moving the patient up in bed.
- Grasp the rolled sheet firmly at the patient's head and hips.
- Pull toward the head of the bed on signal.
- To move the patient toward the foot of the bed, stand facing the head of the bed. Grasp the rolled sheet firmly near the patient's feet and thighs and pull toward the foot of the bed.

Turning onto the side:
- Move the patient to the near side of the bed.
- Free the covers; have or help the patient flex his knees for ease in turning.
- Place the patient's near arm across his chest. Flex his far arm at the elbow, placing his hand near his head so that it is out of the way.
- Face the side of the bed with the knees bent and one foot forward for balance.
- Place one hand on the patient's shoulder, heel of the hand down, with fingers flat. Place the other hand in the same position on his hip.
- Roll him away on signal, maintaining the grasp on his hip and his shoulder for security.
- Bring the hand from his hip to his shoulder to maintain support, slipping the free hand under his lower shoulder to adjust his position for comfort and for security.

- Shift hands again and pull his underneath hip into position for comfort, good body alignment, and security.
- Support his ankle and his knee joints from beneath and lift his uppermost leg forward so that it does not rest on his lower leg.
- Straighten his lower leg in a comfortable position.
- Support the patient with pillows or a folded blanket as necessary to maintain his position. Adjust the covers.

Turning onto the back from a side-lying position:
- Free the covers and remove any pillows or other support.
- Place the patient's knees and ankles together in a flexed position, supporting the joints from beneath.
- Stand at the patient's back, facing the side of the bed, with one foot forward.
- Place one hand on his near hip and the other hand on his shoulder, palms down, and roll him onto his back.
- Adjust his position for proper bed posture and straighten the covers.

Turning from one side to the other:
- Free the covers and remove any pillows or other support.
- Stand at the patient's back, facing the side of the bed, with one foot forward.
- Adjust his arms, flexing both elbows and folding his arms across his chest.
- Support the patient's ankles and knee joints from beneath and place them together in a flexed position.
- Place one hand on the patient's hip and the other on his shoulder and, on signal, quickly but gently roll him onto his back. Shift hands quickly to the patient's other hip and shoulder to maintain support and continue rolling him toward the near side of the bed.
- Place the patient in the correct side-lying position.
- Provide supports as necessary and straighten the covers.

Turning from the back to the face-lying position:
- Remove all pillows or supports.
- Have the patient on a drawsheet, arms at sides, with a flat support (a small pillow or a folded bath towel) placed on his abdomen.
- Have the helper at the same side of the bed.
- Gather the drawsheet into a loose roll at the patient's side.
- Grasp the rolled drawsheet and pull the patient close to the edge of the bed.

- Supporting the patient's body while the helper goes quickly to the opposite side of the bed and, reaching over the patient, grasps the rolled sheet at the patient's shoulders and hips.
- Have the helper pull the drawsheet, rolling the patient over while the home nurse supports his head. Release the drawsheet.
- Have the helper protect the patient while the home nurse pulls the patient to the center of the bed on the drawsheet.
- Position the patient for comfort and for good body alignment. Keep his head flat, his face turned to one side.
- Tighten the drawsheet and tuck the ends under the mattress at both sides for comfort and for neat appearance.
- Place small pads or pieces of foam rubber under each shoulder to keep the shoulders from dropping and to facilitate breathing.

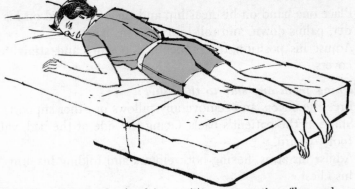

With the patient in the face-lying position, remove the pillow and turn the patient's face to one side. Pull her down in bed, with her feet over the end of the mattress.

- Pull the patient down in bed, if the knees are not to be flexed, until his heels and toes are beyond the end of the mattress to prevent pressure on the toes. Or flex his knees and support his feet over a triangular foot support or a rolled pillow.
- Place the patient's arms in a comfortable position. They may be flexed at the elbow, with the hands placed at the side of the head, or the patient may prefer to have one arm extended along his side.

Turning from the face-lying position to the back:
- Loosen the drawsheet on both sides of the bed, remove the supports from the patient's shoulders and feet, and place his arms at his sides, palms up.
- Working with the helper at the far side of the bed, gather the drawsheet into a loose roll close to the patient, grasping it at the head, hips, and knees.

- Pull the patient close to the edge of the bed, the helper supporting the patient.
- Go quickly to the near side of the bed and tuck the patient's near hand well under the hip.
- Grasp the rolled drawsheet across the patient and, pulling the sheet, roll him gently onto his back.
- Have the helper come to the near side of the bed to assist in pulling the patient to the center of the bed on the drawsheet.
- Adjust the patient's position, place a pillow under his head, and provide additional supports as necessary.
- Tuck the ends of the drawsheet under the mattress on both sides of the bed.

Points To Remember About Moving the Patient in Bed

- Tell the patient what you are going to do to gain his cooperation and help and to lessen any apprehension he might feel.
- Have him help as much as he can. Guide his movements rather than do the lifting and moving for him unless he is helpless.
- Change his position frequently from side to side, to face-lying, and, if permitted by the doctor, to sitting up.
- Provide support to avoid strain on the joints, to prevent deformities, contractures, and bedsores, to conserve energy, and to promote comfort.
- Maintain good posture and position for both the patient and the home nurse.
- Use a helper whenever it is necessary.

THE BED BATH

The purpose of the bed bath is to cleanse, refresh, and relax the patient, to stimulate the circulation, to provide a mild form of exercise, and to aid in elimination through cleansing the skin.

For the well, active person, daily baths are necessary to keep him clean, to remove oil and dead skin cells, and to prevent body odor. As one grows older, changes occur in the skin. The glands secrete less oil and perspiration, the skin becomes drier, and there are fewer waste products to be bathed away. Many older people may refuse a daily bath. For them, daily baths are not necessary and may increase dryness of the skin. Illness, particularly if the patient has fever, may increase the need for bathing. Judgment and

211

common sense, therefore, should be used in determining how often the patient is to be bathed.

Only the acutely ill or helpless person will need to be bathed by someone else. As soon as the patient's condition permits, he should be encouraged to do as much as possible for himself. In reality it may take more time for the patient to bathe himself, but this fact is outweighed by the fact that the patient is getting exercise and is gaining self-reliance. If he can do no more than wash his face and hands, he should be allowed to do so.

Certain preparatory steps must always be made for the bed bath. The room should be comfortably warm, free from drafts, and arranged so that the patient will have privacy. All necessary equipment should be collected and made ready to use. Mouth care and treatments can be done at bath time so that the patient need not be disturbed after his bath. Also, the bedpan should be offered and used if needed.

The linen should be removed from the bed and that to be re-used should be folded and placed on a chair. Bath time is a convenient time to change soiled bed linen, including the pillowcases. A common practice is to use the top sheet as a bottom sheet and place a clean sheet over the patient when the bed is remade.

Equipment

Large basin of warm water
Container or supply of hot water
Towels: 2 bath, 1 face
Washcloth
Cotton bath blanket
Soap in a dish
Skin lotion or body powder

Tray with toilet articles: hairbrush, comb, nail file, toothbrush and mouthwash or dentifrice, and waste container
Protection for the furniture and the floor
Clean pajamas or nightgown
Clean bed linen
Wastepaper pail if not near the bathroom

Procedure

- Replace the regular blanket with the cotton bath blanket and remove unneeded pillows.
- Give help as necessary in removing the patient's nightgown or pajamas.
- Keep the water comfortably hot throughout the bath by adding hot water. Change it whenever it becomes soiled or too soapy.

212

Washing the face, neck, and ears:

- Place one bath towel on top of the bath blanket lengthwise across the patient's chest, folding one-half of it under the top of the blanket. Place the other bath towel under his head to protect the pillow.
- Wet the washcloth and wring it enough to keep it from dripping.

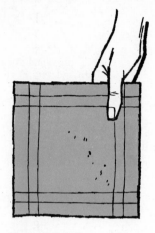

Place washcloth on palm.

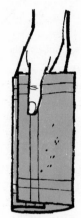

Wrap around the palm and the fingers.

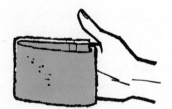

Tuck in at the top.

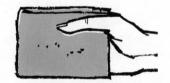

Use as a mitt.

Palming a washcloth.

- Make a bath mitt of the washcloth by wrapping it around the palm and fingers, anchoring it with the thumb, and tucking in the ends at the palm so that the corners will not drag.
- Wash the eyes gently with clear water from the nose outward toward the hairline, using a separate corner of the washcloth for each eye.
- Wash the face, forehead, nose, and cheeks, using an S-motion around the mouth and the chin. Use soap as necessary, keeping the bar out of the bath water to avoid suds. Use the flat of the hand, with long, firm strokes for effectiveness and comfort, and to stimulate the circulation.

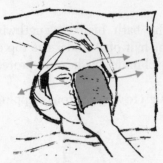

Wash, rinse, and dry the fore-head, nose, and cheeks from the center of the face toward the hairline.

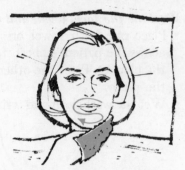

Wash, rinse, and dry around the mouth and chin in an S-motion.

- Rinse in the same order, using the same stroke. Rinse off all the soap because it has a drying effect on the skin.
- Wrap a corner of the face towel around the hand to avoid its dragging, and dry the face.
- Wash the neck and ears: first the far ear, then the front of the neck, and then the near ear. Use one continuous stroke and cleanse between the folds of the skin. Rinse and dry in the same manner.

Washing the chest and the abdomen:
- Cover the patient's chest with the towel from the pillow. Pull the blanket, still protected with the other towel, down to the abdomen.
- Soap, rinse, and dry the chest and the sides of the chest under the towel, using long, firm, but gentle strokes. Wash and dry well under the breasts. Observe the condition of the skin.
- Leave one towel over the chest. Pull the blanket down to the thighs, still keeping it protected with the other towel.
- Soap, rinse, and dry the abdomen, the sides of the trunk, and the upper surfaces of the thighs and the pubic area. Use long, smooth strokes to avoid pressure and tickling.
- Pull up the blanket and remove the towels.

Washing the arms and the hands:
- Place one towel under the patient's near arm and shoulder to protect the bedding. Place the second towel over the blanket, folding from one-third to one-half of it over the blanket edge to keep the blanket dry. Soap, rinse, and dry the arm, including the axilla, supporting the arm and using long, firm strokes.
- Place the bath basin and the soap dish on the towel at the patient's side and wash and rinse the hand in the basin.

214

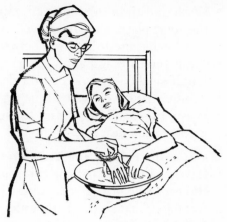

Soap, wash, and rinse the patient's
hands in a basin of water.

- Remove the basin and the soap. Dry the hand well between
the fingers, pushing back the cuticle around the nails with the
towel. Gently clean under the nails and apply hand lotion.
- Remain on the same side of the bed and repeat the procedure
with the other arm and hand.

Washing the legs and the feet:
- Help the patient to flex or bend his near knee. Fit the blanket
snugly around the thigh at the groin, keeping the far leg covered.
- Place one towel under the patient's leg and foot. Tuck the other
towel in around the edge of the blanket to keep it dry.
- Wash, rinse, and dry the leg, supporting the knee and using long,
firm strokes. Examine the skin carefully for reddened or rough-
ened areas.
- Place waterproof material under the bottom towel to protect
the bed. Place the soap dish and the bath basin on the towel and,
supporting the knee and ankle, lift the foot into the basin.

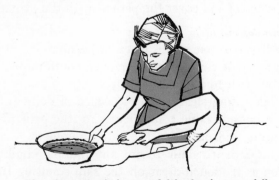

Flex the patient's knee and lift the foot carefully
into the bath basin, supporting the knee and the
ankle for safety and comfort.

215

- Wash and rinse the foot well, especially between the toes. Lift the foot, place it on the towel, and remove the basin. Dry the foot, being sure to dry well between the toes.
- Clean the nails and apply lotion to the foot and the ankle. Use lotion on the leg as needed for dryness of the skin.
- Remove the towels, extend the leg, and cover it with the blanket.
- Wash, rinse, and dry the far leg and foot in the same way, working from the near side of the bed.

Washing the back of the neck, the back, and the buttocks:
- Have or help the patient turn on his far side with his back to the near side of the bed. Adjust his position so that he is comfortable. Change the bath water so that it is clean and comfortably warm.
- Fold back the blanket to uncover the patient's back and buttocks. Place one towel over the bottom sheet and the pillow and tuck it in under the patient's shoulder and back to keep the bed dry. Place the other towel lengthwise over the patient, folding about half the width under the blanket.
- Soap, rinse, and dry the back of the patient's neck, back, and buttocks, using long, firm strokes. Examine the patient's skin carefully for reddened pressure areas or any breaks.
- Rub the patient's back, giving special attention to pressure areas.
- Have the patient turn on his back.

Washing the external genitalia:
- Place a towel under the patient's buttocks to protect the bed.
- Place the bath basin, soap, and towel within his reach if he is able to help himself.
- Allow him to cleanse and dry the genitals. If the patient is helpless or very ill, the home nurse should do this for him.
- Remove the towel and cover the patient with the blanket.

Caring for the patient after the bath:
- Help the patient to put on his gown or pajamas.
- See that the hair is combed and arranged comfortably. Women will probably wish to put on make-up.
- Make the bed, using clean linen as needed or desired.
- Arrange the bedside table conveniently for the patient.
- Remove, clean, and put away the bath equipment.
- Note on the patient's daily record any unusual conditions observed, such as reddened areas on the skin resulting from pressure; any rash, swelling, lumps, sores, and breaks in the skin; or a tendency to fatigue.

Points To Remember

- Report any unusual conditions observed to the doctor.
- Permit the patient to do as much for himself as he can.
- Avoid chilling, fatiguing, or embarrassing the patient. Place a hot water bottle at the patient's feet if needed for warmth.
- Keep the patient and the bed protected.
- Cleanse all parts of the body.
- Change the bath water whenever it is soiled or soapy. Add hot water as needed.

THE BACK RUB

The purpose of the back rub is to refresh and relax the patient, to stimulate blood circulation, and to relieve pressure.

The amount of pressure used in rubbing the back will depend on the condition of the patient and his preferences. In general, more pressure is used on the upward strokes. Warmed alcohol is refreshing and can be used for rubbing, although it has a tendency to dry the skin. Applying a skin lotion, cocoa butter, or hand cream will help to keep the skin soft and smooth. For comfort and to eliminate friction, these as well as powder are applied to the home nurse's hands and not directly to the patient's skin.

Reddened areas should be given special care for they indicate that circulation has been impaired through pressure. The area surrounding red pressure spots should be gently kneaded with the heel of the hand or the tips of the fingers to stimulate circulation. Rub *around* rather than *on* the reddened area itself to lessen the danger of causing breaks in the skin.

Equipment

Lotion or hand cream   Body powder, if desired

Procedure

- Place the patient comfortably on his side, facing away, or on his stomach.
- Bathe and dry his back.
- Lubricate the hands with an emollient, either cream or lotion, or with powder. Avoid using an excess amount of powder, which may make crumbs in the bed.
- Face the head of the bed, with the outer foot slightly forward and the knees slightly bent.

217

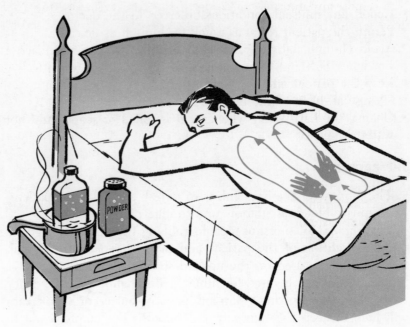

Rub the back with long firm strokes. Keep the hands flat and the fingers together.

- Apply pressure with the flat of both hands over the patient's entire back, beginning low at the back and moving upward, including his shoulders and buttocks. Use long, sweeping, firm but gentle strokes to soothe and relax the patient. As the hands move up and down the back, move forward and backward in a rocking motion, with the knees flexed. Keep the hands lubricated so that they will glide comfortably over the patient's skin.
- Observe the condition of the skin, paying special attention to bony prominences and pressure areas and giving additional rubbing around any reddened areas.
- Assist the patient into a comfortable position after the back rub.

Points To Remember

- Have the patient in a comfortable position. Do not allow him to become chilled.
- Use a stroke firm enough to relax the muscles yet gentle enough for soothing comfort.
- Continue rubbing long enough for it to be effective, from at least 3 to 5 minutes.

- Give additional rubbing around reddened areas.
- Report any unusual condition of the skin to the doctor.

MOUTH CARE

The purpose of mouth care is to cleanse and refresh the patient's mouth, teeth, and gums, to stimulate the circulation of the gums to keep them healthy, and to prevent the accumulation of sordes, the brownish material that sometimes collects in the mouths and especially on the tongues of sick people.

Equipment

Tray
Toothbrush
Toothpaste or tooth powder
Glass of warm water containing ½ teaspoon each of salt and baking soda or other mouthwash

Cotton applicators, large size (for the helpless patient)
Glass of clear, cool water
Small basin for the patient to spit into
Paper wipes
Towel or other protection
Waste container

Procedures

When the patient can help:
- Place a towel or other protection well up under the patient's chin, over the shoulders, and over the bedding.
- Have him hold the basin and clean his teeth in the usual way if he is able to sit up, rinsing his mouth well with clear water.
- Turn the patient's head to one side, if he cannot sit up, and place the waste basin near his chin.
- Pour water over the brush and apply the dentifrice, mouthwash, or salt-soda solution.
- Allow the patient to brush his own teeth.
- Provide clear, cool water so that the patient can rinse his mouth.
- Let the patient dry his mouth and chin.

When the patient is helpless:

- Place a towel or other protection over the patient's chest and shoulders, well up under the chin.
- Examine the mouth, the tongue, and the gums, carefully in a good light.
- Moisten an applicator or a swab, pressing out excess moisture against the side of the glass.

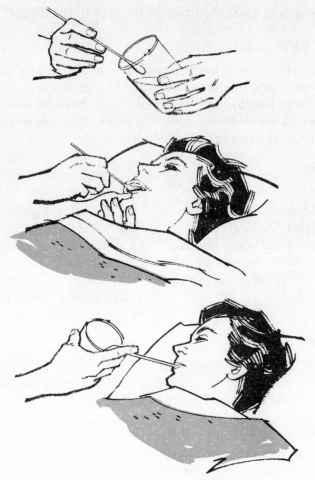

Mouth care of the helpless patient.

- Steady the patient's chin with one hand and gently cleanse the inner surfaces of the mouth, the gums, the teeth, and the tongue. Cleanse one section of the patient's mouth at a time, using a clean applicator for each section. Discard the applicators in a waste container. Repeat the process with clean applicators until the entire mouth is clean.
- Rinse, using fresh applicators dipped in clear water if the patient is unable to use the basin as he would for brushing his teeth.
- Wipe the mouth and the chin dry.
- Use an ointment or a lubricant on the lips if they are dry.
- Remove the towels and the tray and dispose of waste material.
- Note on the patient's daily record any unusual condition.

- Cleanse the patient's entire mouth and teeth as often as needed for comfort, and always after he has eaten.
- Avoid injury to the membranes in his mouth.

CARE OF DENTURES

At least once a month the patient who wears a denture should be asked whether or not it hurts him at any point. If he indicates that there is discomfort, his mouth must be inspected for signs of irritation and a report made to the doctor. When the denture is not in the patient's mouth, it should be kept in an opaque container in a safe place. The dentist who made the denture may have specified how it should be cleaned and cared for. If there are no specific instructions, the method described below is safe and generally acceptable.

Equipment

Denture brush   Cool water
Dentifrice or soap   Waste container
                       Storage receptacle

Procedures

When the patient can help:
- Place the equipment where the patient can comfortably reach and use it.
- Leave the room or move out of eyesight to assure him privacy.
- Remove, clean, and put away the equipment when the patient has finished.

When the patient is helpless:
- Ask the patient to remove his denture and to hand it to you in a paper tissue.
- Hold the denture under running water, out of sight of the patient, handling it with a tissue until one part is clean.
- Use a mild soap or the patient's dentifrice and a tooth or denture brush.
- Cleanse the denture over a basin partly filled with cold water to lessen the danger of breakage should it slip out of the hand.
- Rinse the denture in cold water.
- Rinse the patient's mouth with clear water or a mouthwash.
- Moisten the denture with cool water and return it to the patient for him to place in his mouth, or place it in an opaque container in a safe place out of sight.

BRUSHING AND COMBING THE HAIR

The hair of all patients should receive daily care and be brushed well to remove loose surface dirt and dandruff, to stimulate circulation of the blood in the scalp, and to make the patient as comfortable as possible. Cleanliness and grooming help to maintain the health of the hair, to improve the patient's appearance and morale, and to stimulate interest in personal hygiene.

Men's hair seldom requires much care beyond daily brushing and combing and regular shampooing and cutting. Regular shaving is necessary for all men to keep them well groomed. A woman's hair requires more attention. Unless cared for daily, it becomes tangled and unsightly and is uncomfortable to the patient. Usually women enjoy having their hair curled and styled, and this grooming should be encouraged.

Brushing distributes throughout the length of the hair the natural scalp oils as well as oil that may be applied to dry hair for conditioning purposes. The comb and the brush should be kept scrupulously clean and should be washed when the hair is shampooed or more often if they become soiled. The comb is used to arrange the hair and is no substitute for regular brushing. The kind of comb used depends on the personal preference of the patient. Preferably the teeth should be blunt, for sharp teeth may scratch the scalp. If any of the teeth break off, the comb should be discarded.

Equipment

Hairbrush and comb   Hair lotion or cream, if needed
Towel

Procedure

- Protect the pillow with a towel.
- Have the patient turn her head far to one side.
- Part the hair in the center from front to back.
- Begin brushing at the ends, holding the strands of hair with the fingers.
- Continue brushing until all tangles have been removed and until all portions of the scalp and the hair have been reached. Lotions and creams are available that help to loosen badly tangled hair and improve the appearance of dry hair.
- Turn the head to the other side and repeat the procedure.
- Arrange the hair in the usual manner or as the patient wishes.

222

If the patient is helpless, arrange it to give maximum comfort and to avoid tangles and inconvenience. For long hair, two braids are suggested.

- Remove the towel. Clean the equipment and put it away.
- Note on the daily record any unusual condition of the scalp or the hair.

SHAMPOOING THE HAIR

A shampoo can be given quite easily to the patient in bed, but usually it should not be given without the doctor's permission. There are many kinds of shampoo on the market: liquids, creams, soaps, detergents; shampoos for dry hair and for oily hair; and shampoos to be used with water and without water. A dry shampoo or one that cleans the hair without using water is particularly desirable for a very weak or an easily tired patient. The directions for use given on the package should be followed.

In general, liquid shampoos are more readily rinsed out of the hair. A commercial rinse can be used, but a small amount of vinegar or lemon juice added to the rinse water is quite satisfactory and is less expensive.

If the patient can be out of bed, there are few problems in giving a shampoo. In the case of an elderly patient who, because of dizziness or stiffness, finds it difficult to stoop or lean over a basin, it is often easier and safer to give the shampoo with the patient in bed.

The procedure described on page 224 can be done by one person, but it will take less time and probably be less tiring to the patient if there is another person to help. This is particularly true if the bed is low. The home nurse will need to be concerned about maintaining correct posture to avoid placing undue strain on her back muscles.

Equipment

Shampoo
Vinegar, lemon juice, or a commercial rinse
Container of warm water
Pitcher
Bath towels
Shampoo tray, if available
Waterproof protector for the bed

Protection for the floor
Chair or small, low table
Extra blanket, if needed
Heat lamp or electric hair dryer
Waterproof electric pad (for long hair)
Clean hairbrush and comb
Waste pail or small tub

Procedure

- Raise the bed to a comfortable working height.
- Protect the bed with any waterproof material available. The floor may be protected with newspapers.
- Place the waste pail or the tub on a chair or a small, low table close to the side of the bed. Place the lower end of the shampoo tray in the pail or the tub. If a waterproof sheet is used instead of a shampoo tray, drape one end of it into the pail or the tub.
- Make the patient comfortable, with the head at the edge of the bed and resting on the shampoo tray or the waterproof sheet.
- Wash and rinse the hair, working as quickly as possible to avoid tiring the patient.
- Rub the shampooed hair well with a heavy towel and dry it quickly. A heat lamp or an electric dryer may be used to complete the drying. Long hair may be spread out on a waterproof electric pad that has been covered with a dry bath towel.
- Protect the patient against chilling.
- Brush, comb, and dress the hair in the usual manner or set it in pincurls to be combed and arranged later.

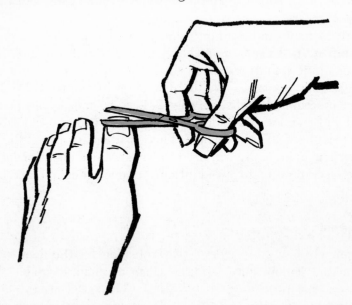

Cut the toenails straight across. Leave the corners square.

CARE OF THE FEET

The purpose of caring for the patient's feet is to provide comfort, to aid circulation, and to prevent infection.

Equipment

Warm water	Terry cloth towel
Mild soap	Lanolin, baby oil, or skin lotion
Nail clippers	Powder
Orange stick or flat toothpicks	Cotton or lamb's wool

Procedure

- Soak the feet in warm water to soften the skin and nails.
- Rub the heels and the soles of the feet to remove dead skin.
- Cut the toenails straight across, using scissors or nail clippers. If the nails are thickened and cannot be cut with scissors, do not attempt to cut them; ask the doctor what to do. If the nails tend to turn inward at the sides, use the wide, flat end of a toothpick and gently insert a very small piece of dry cotton under each turned-in nail. Remove the cotton with the fingers in 24 hours.
- Dry the feet thoroughly, especially between the toes, and powder the feet lightly. If the skin of the feet is dry, rub gently toward the body, using lanolin, baby oil, or skin lotion.
- Place a thin layer of cotton or lamb's wool between the toes if the feet perspire and remain damp between the toes.

CHANGING THE BED LINEN

The purpose of changing the patient's bed linen is to provide safety, comfort, warmth, a smooth, clean surface to lie on, and freedom of movement for the patient. The way the bed is made will vary somewhat depending on the kind of bed, the kind, amount, and size of the linens available, and the nursing needs of the patient. Contour sheets have the advantage of remaining relatively free from any wrinkles and will remain in place without adjustment. Flat sheets have to be anchored by tucking under the mattress and tend to loosen with movement of the patient.

The very ill and the incontinent patient will need to have the bottom bedding protected against moisture and soiling. A waterproof mattress cover may be used, or a rubber or plastic drawsheet covered with a cotton drawsheet can be placed across the bottom sheet to protect the center of the bed. A drawsheet may not be necessary if the patient is out of bed most of the day and is able to go to the bathroom or to use a commode. Patients frequently complain that a waterproof sheet makes them too warm. Placing this kind of drawsheet under the mattress pad provides greater comfort for the patient.

Top covers should be lightweight and warm and should be placed securely so that they will keep the patient covered. Toe space can be provided by making a pleat in the top sheet and blanket and by allowing the spread to hang loose at the bottom corners of the bed.

Equipment

Bed
Firm, smooth mattress and pad
Clean sheets and pillowcases
Blankets, suited to room temperature
Pillows

Spread, lightweight
Extra sheet for a drawsheet
A waterproof sheet or pad to protect the mattress, if necessary
Newspapers or a laundry bag for soiled linen

Procedures

When making an empty bed:

- Assemble the fresh linen, place newspapers or a laundry bag on the floor to receive the soiled linen.
- Remove the spread, blankets, pillows, mattress pad, and linen, holding the bedding away from the face and clothing to avoid contact.

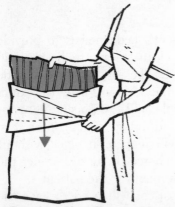

Remove the soiled pillowcase by turning it inside out.

- Remove the pillowcase by turning it inside out to avoid touching the soiled side.
- Place the soiled linen at once on the newspaper or in the bag.
- Turn the mattress and replace the pad.
- Center the bottom sheet lengthwise and place it on the bed, allowing 18 inches for tucking under the head of the mattress to hold the bottom sheet firm. (See illustration "a.")
- Make a corner at the head of the bed by grasping the sheet selvage, raising it until it forms a straight line against the mat-

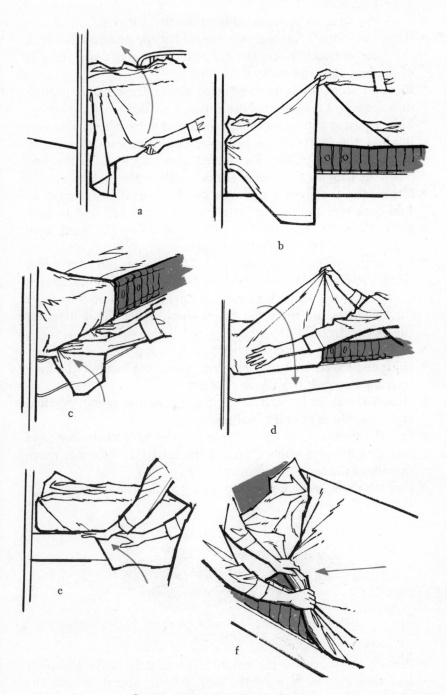

Steps in putting on the bottom sheet.

227

tress, and letting it fall back on the bed to form a right triangle. (See illustrations "b" and "c.")

- Tuck the hanging part smoothly under the mattress.
- Bring the triangle forward over the side of the mattress and tuck the sheet smoothly under the mattress all the way down the side of the bed. (See illustrations "d" and "e.")
- Place a rubber or plastic sheet across the mattress before putting on a drawsheet if additional protection is needed.
- Fold a regular sheet end to end for use as a drawsheet and place it across the center of the bed, placing it high enough for it to come under the pillow. The folded edge should be at the top. Tuck the hanging part under the near side of the mattress.
- Center the top sheet lengthwise on the bed. Allow enough to fold back over the blanket at the head of the bed and to tuck under the mattress at the foot of the bed. Leave the sheet loose at the foot until the blanket is in place.
- Center the blanket lengthwise and place the top end at shoulder height, leaving it loose at the foot of the bed. If the blanket is short, two may be used, placing one blanket as desired to cover the shoulders and the other to tuck well under the mattress at the foot of the bed.
- Go to the other side of the bed.
- Bring the lower sheet over and well under the head of the mattress and anchor it by making a corner.
- Gather the sheet in both hands, fists uppermost, close together, and above the edge of the mattress.
- Pull the sheet diagonally, beginning at the head of the bed, and tuck it tightly and smoothly under the mattress all the way down the side of the bed. (See illustration "f.")
- Pull the drawsheet smooth and tuck it under the mattress.

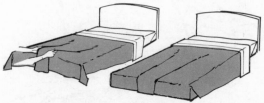

Pleats in the upper bedding provide space for the patient's feet.

- Provide toe space for the patient's comfort by making a pleat lengthwise at the foot of the bed, holding the sheet and the blanket together.

228

- Hold the pleat in place and tuck the sheet and the blanket under the mattress, making loose corners.
- Center and place the bedspread. If the patient is using the bed at once, fold the spread under the upper edge of the blanket and fold the top sheet back over the blanket and the spread. Let the spread hang loose at the bottom.
- Put on the pillowcase:

  Keep the pillow away from the face because it has been near the patient's nose and throat discharges.

  Place both hands in the clean case to free the corners. (See "a" of the following illustration.)

  Grasp the center of the end seam with one hand outside the case and turn the case back over the hand.

  Grasp the pillow through the case at the center of one end.

  Adjust the corners of the pillow into the corners of the case, maintaining grasp until corners are fitted. (See "b" of the following illustration.)

  Adjust and shape the pillow inside the case and place it on the bed.
- Arrange the bed for occupancy: fold the top sheet, the blanket, and the spread in thirds toward the foot of the bed, with the free

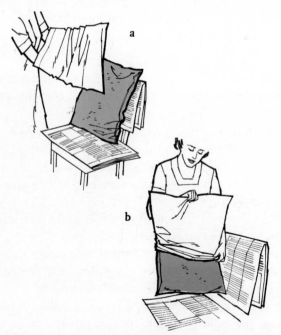

Changing the pillowcase.

229

edge toward the head of the bed so the covers may be pulled up easily.

- Remove the soiled linen.

When the patient is in bed:

- Assemble the equipment.
- For the comfort of the patient, work from the head to the foot of the bed.
- Loosen the bedding on all sides to make removal easier.
- Remove the spread, folding it lengthwise for neatness and for ease in replacement.
- Slide the top sheet down under the blanket and remove it. The patient may be asked to hold the top edge of the blanket while this is being done, or the blanket can be tucked under his shoulders to hold it in place. If the top sheet is to be used on the bottom or as a drawsheet, fold and place it over the back of a chair.
- Remove all pillows, or all but one.
- Remove the soiled pillowcases and place them with the soiled linen.
- Help or have the patient turn toward the other side of the bed in order to change the bottom sheet. Be sure to keep him covered.
- Fold the top bedding back close to the patient so that it will be out of the way.
- Gather the bottom sheet lengthwise in a flat roll and push it close to the patient. Gently pull the mattress pad smooth under the patient.
- Change flat bottom sheet:
  Center the clean sheet lengthwise, place and unfold it, allowing about 18 inches for tucking under at the head to protect the mattress, to anchor the sheet securely, and to give the bed a good appearance.
  Push the top half of the clean sheet in a flat roll under the soiled sheet against the patient's back.
  Tuck the lower half of the clean sheet well under the mattress at the head and, after making a corner, tuck the sheet well under the mattress all along the side of the bed.
  Place the drawsheet on the bed, if one is used, with the folded edge under the pillow. Tuck the drawsheet under the mattress. Lift the patient's feet onto the clean sheet.

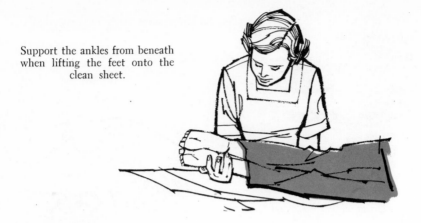

Support the ankles from beneath when lifting the feet onto the clean sheet.

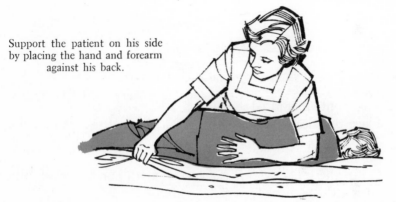

Support the patient on his side by placing the hand and forearm against his back.

On signal, roll the patient from one side to the other onto the clean sheet, giving him support while the bunched sheets are pulled out.

Roll the patient onto his back. Adjust his position and arrange the top covers.

Go to the other side of the bed.

Remove the soiled sheet, handling it as little as possible, and place it with the soiled linen.

Smooth the mattress pad and adjust the clean bottom sheet. Bring the sheet well under the mattress at the head of the bed and make a corner.

Tuck the bottom sheet securely under the mattress all the way down the side of the bed, pulling the sheet diagonally to remove any wrinkles.

Grasp and pull the drawsheet and tuck it tightly and securely under the mattress.

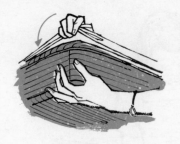

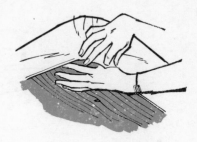

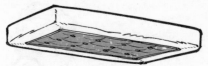

Changing a contour or fitted sheet.

- Change contour or fitted sheet:
    Place the clean sheet lengthwise on the mattress and anchor at the top and bottom corners on one side by pulling it over the mattress.
    Go to the other side of the bed, smooth out the sheet, and anchor the corners.
    Adjust the corner at the foot last since the greater weight of the patient is at the top of the bed.
- Place drawsheet as described above.
- Put on a clean pillowcase and replace the pillow. Adjust the top covers.
- Make certain that the patient is comfortable and that the call bell is within reach.
- Arrange the furniture neatly and remove the soiled linen.

Points To Remember

- Keep the bottom sheet smooth and tight.
- Use top covers that are lightweight and suited to the temperature of the room.
- Provide shoulder warmth and allow toe space.
- Handle the soiled linen with care to prevent the spread of infection.

FEEDING THE HELPLESS PATIENT

The purpose of feeding a helpless patient is to give him nourishment in a way that will be enjoyable to him, will stimulate his appetite, and will encourage his acceptance of food.

All persons whether sick or well have nutritional needs, and recovery from illness depends a great deal upon the adequacy of the diet. A well-balanced diet, with foods selected from all four of the basic food groups, is the basis of all specially prescribed diets. Modifications may be made to suit the needs of the body during illness.

Certain practices should always be observed in preparing and serving food to any sick person: season lightly, serve hot foods hot and cold foods cold, arrange food in colorful combinations and in small servings, make the tray attractive, observe the patient's food preferences as much as possible, and offer food on a regular schedule.

Before feeding a semiconscious or paralyzed patient, it is important to know that he is able to swallow. Very small amounts of water should be offered first and sufficient time allowed for swallowing before more is offered. Depending upon the patient's condition, mouth care or the use of a mouthwash before eating may improve the appetite.

Equipment

Food as ordered, arranged attractively on a tray

Napkin or other protection
Teaspoon
Drinking tube

Procedure

- Make sure that the patient is in a comfortable position at the near side of the bed with his head elevated on a pillow.
- Protect the bedding and provide a napkin.
- Sit beside the patient if the height of the bed permits easy working. Avoid hurrying.
- Test the temperature of hot foods. Liquids should sting when a drop or two touches the inner surface of the wrist.
- Fill the spoon about two-thirds full and remove any drops from the bottom of the spoon.
- Touch the lower lip with the area between the tip and the side of the spoon. Tilt the spoon toward the tip, allowing the liquid to run into the patient's mouth.
- Allow the patient time to swallow.

- When a drinking tube is used, stir the liquid to distribute the heat evenly.
- Place one end of the tube in the patient's mouth at the side, keeping the end of the tube below the level of the liquid so that no air is swallowed.

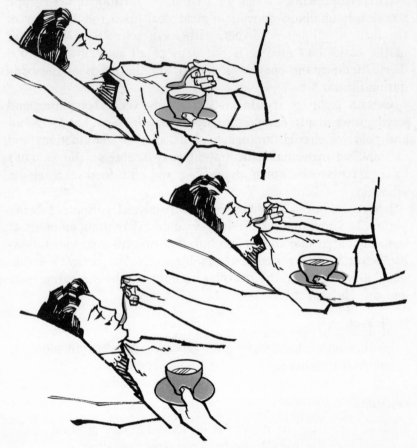

Feeding the helpless patient with a spoon.

- Support the patient's head to help him drink from a cup by placing an arm under the pillow. Hold the cup by the handle and let the patient guide the cup and control the rate of flow by placing his hand around the cup.
- Note on the daily record what the patient ate, at what time, and how much. Record appropriate comments concerning his appetite and his enjoyment of the food.
- Rinse the tube in cold water.
- Wash the patient's dishes, silver, tray, and tube in hot, soapy water and then scald and drain them dry.

- Make sure the patient can swallow.
- Give him small amounts of food to avoid choking.
- Avoid burning the patient's mouth by testing foods to be sure that they are not too hot.
- Obtain his cooperation by avoiding all evidence of haste.

CARE OF DISHES AND EATING UTENSILS

As soon as the patient has eaten, the tray should be removed from his room and the uneaten food disposed of. Solids should be placed in the garbage disposer, burned in the incinerator, or wrapped and placed in the garbage. Liquids may be poured into the sink or the bathroom commode.

Because many disease-carrying organisms are carried by the secretions from the nose and the mouth, dishes and eating utensils used by a sick person must be carefully washed with soap or detergent and hot water. Friction should be applied, especially around the rims of glasses and cups, tines of forks, and bowls of spoons where the patient's mouth has touched them. After washing the dishes and eating utensils, rinse them with scalding water and dry. In some circumstances, as an added precaution, the doctor may order that the dishes be boiled.

Because the temperature of the water used in almost all mechanical dishwashers is higher than the temperature of the water used for washing by hand, dishwashers offer certain advantages in caring for the dishes and the utensils of sick persons. To get dishes clean, the water coming into the machine should be at least 150° F., and the manufacturer's recommendations concerning soaps and detergents should be followed. Prerinse any dishes on which food has dried or been burned, or if they contain the remains of eggs, gravy, or cream sauces, before placing them in a mechanical dishwasher.

14

PATIENT ACTIVITIES

PREPARING TO GET OUT OF BED

Many patients who are unable to walk or even to stand are helped out of bed regularly because of the beneficial effects of being up and out of bed. Moving, sitting up, walking, and other physical activity improves the circulation. Better circulation increases healing and hastens general recovery from illness, improves mental alertness, induces sleep and reduces the need for sedation, improves the appetite, promotes more nearly normal bowel and urinary functioning, lessens muscle wasting and joint stiffness, and improves the patient's morale.

The ability to get in and out of bed forms the foundation of progressive, independent action if the patient is to be able to care for himself. The ability to get in and out of a wheelchair determines the scope of almost every action of the physically handicapped person. The ability to perform either of these actions unassisted depends largely on the strength of arm, back, abdominal, and shoulder muscles. Muscle tone and strength deteriorate rapidly at any age level when a person is bedfast. Early, regular, prescribed range-of-motion exercises of arms and legs are therefore essential to the maintenance or the reestablishment of muscle strength.

The physical condition of the patient determines the kind of clothing he will wear and the equipment he will need, such as a chair, a wheelchair, braces, or crutches. If the patient is going to stand or walk, he should wear Oxfords or other shoes with broad heels that will give him a feeling of security and provide support for his feet. Room temperature determines the weight and the amount of clothing he will wear. If the patient is going to be up for any appreciable time, it adds to his feeling of achievement if he can be dressed in his usual attire rather than in pajamas and a robe.

Special appliances, such as casts or braces, may mean that the clothing has to be modified. For the patient who uses the bathroom or a bedside commode, clothing should be easily adjustable to meet this need. Patients in wheelchairs who are incontinent or who void frequently especially need such clothing.

A bed that has been elevated should be lowered, and the casters should be removed to stabilize it. This important safety measure makes activity much easier for the patient. To facilitate the patient's moving back and forth from the bed to a chair, the top of the mattress should be as nearly level with the seat of the chair as possible.

SITTING UP WITHOUT HELP

The patient's ability to come to a sitting position is basic in preparing for out-of-bed activities; therefore, sitting up is the first step to be mastered in getting out of bed.

The first stage of sitting up is rolling over in bed. The second stage is sitting up in bed with support. The third stage, sitting without support on the edge of the bed with the feet and the legs over the side is such a fundamental part of the preparation to get out of bed that the patient may at first be permitted only this limited activity. Sitting balance, the ability to sit without support, must be achieved before the patient sits in a chair, dresses himself, or performs daily living activities.

The handicapped patient's ability to help himself is of primary importance. Raising himself in bed gives him exercise and develops or maintains the strength in the arm, back, shoulder, and abdominal muscles that he will need in order to get in and out of bed, to use the bathroom, to operate a wheelchair, or to walk with crutches. Probably the easiest way to come to a sitting position is to pull on a rope attached to the foot of the bed, but since this way of raising oneself does not strengthen the muscles needed to support body weight, pushing exercises must be added.

The patient may use the following procedure to sit up and lie down, using both arms:
- Have the patient lie on his back, with knees flexed, hands at his sides, palms down, and head and shoulders raised forward and up, bearing the weight of his head and trunk on his elbows.
- Have him slide both elbows back on the bed as far as possible, avoiding any outward swing of his arms or his elbows.

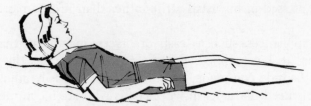

Flex the knees and bear weight on the elbows.

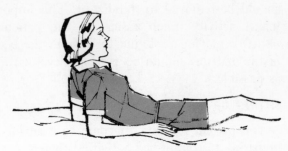

Raise the trunk from the bed by sliding the elbows back.

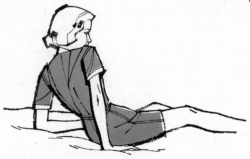

Straighten the arm and push against the mattress.

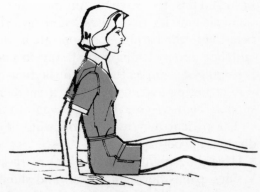

Straighten the other arm, pushing against the mattress to come to a sitting position.

Using both arms to sit up and lie down.

238

- Have him push with one hand against the mattress, extending or straightening his elbow.
- Have him push with the other hand, extending the elbow, until his body is raised to a sitting position. If the patient is not weak or dizzy, he should be able to sit up without leaning on his hands and his arms. In the beginning he should sit up for only a few minutes at a time and gradually increase the length of time he is upright.
- To lie down, reverse the procedure for sitting up. When the patient starts to lie down, have him bend his head forward to help him maintain his balance and to avoid falling backward. Have him place his hands, palms down, on the bed alongside his hips, keeping his elbows straight.
- Have him move his hands back gradually, one at a time, flexing or bending one elbow and resting the elbow and the forearm on the bed to support the body weight.
- Have him flex the other elbow, resting the elbow and the forearm on the bed, and keep his head and his shoulders forward and up until the lower back is lowered onto the bed.
- Have him bring his arms forward to his sides and lie flat on the bed.

GETTING OUT OF BED AND INTO A CHAIR

If the patient is convalescent and not handicapped by a permanent crippling condition, the objective is to get him up and walking again as soon as possible. Getting a wheelchair for this type of patient is probably a mistake, because he tends to become dependent on it for getting about instead of exercising and practicing the skills that will help him to walk.

The chair that the patient will sit in when he first gets out of bed should be comfortable, strong, and high enough to allow him to rest his feet comfortably on the floor and to rise with relative ease. If necessary, the seat may be raised by adding firm pillows or a thick foam rubber pad. The chair should have arms for comfort and for security and to aid the patient in standing and a back high enough to support the head and shoulders when the patient sits back in the chair.

There are several ways to assist a patient to get in and out of bed, and since they are equally good, the patient should use the method that he finds easiest. The weak and unsteady patient fre-

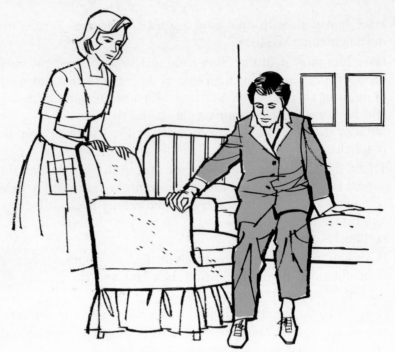

Grasp the far arm of the chair for support.

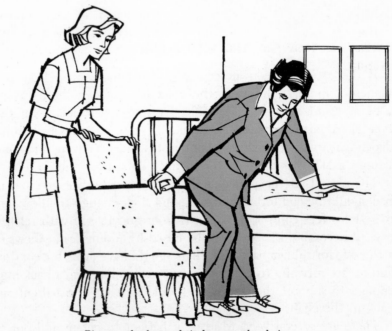

Pivot on the feet and sit down on the chair.

Getting out of bed into a chair.

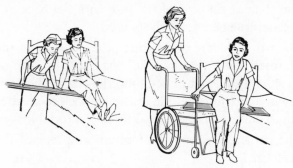

Using a board to bridge the gap from bed to chair.

quently finds that a board laid from a chair seat to the bed, when the chair seat and the mattress are the same height, provides a bridge for him to get from one to the other. Before the patient comes to a sitting position, he must raise his hips so that the board can be slipped under him, or it can be placed after he comes to a sitting position. A table leaf or a smooth board of similar size serves the purpose very well.

For the patient who lacks the strength to lift himself with his arms in order to shift to and from the chair, it may be necessary to use the following procedure:

- Place a heavy straight chair at the side and near the center of the bed with the seat facing the foot of the bed. Place an easy chair facing the bed, next to and with one corner touching the straight chair.
- Have the patient come to a sitting position with his legs over the side of the bed.
- Have him place one hand on the far side of the straight chair and the other hand, palm down, on the bed beside him.
- Stand behind the straight chair to steady it.
- Have the patient slide from the bed to the straight chair.
- Steady the easy chair.
- Have the patient grasp the far arm of the easy chair with one hand, placing his other hand behind him on the seat of the straight chair and turning so that his back is toward the easy chair.
- Have him slide into the easy chair.

GETTING INTO A WHEELCHAIR AND BACK INTO BED

The following procedures may be used to get the patient into a wheelchair.

When wheelchair has removable arms:
- Remove the chair arm next to the bed.

241

- Place the chair at the side of the bed, with the back of the chair to the head of the bed. Lock the brakes.
- Have the patient come to a sitting position, slide to the edge of the bed, reach across the chair, holding either the arm or the side of the seat, and slide out of bed onto the chair. The patient's feet may be lowered from the side of the bed before or after he is in the chair, whichever is easier and more comfortable for him.
- Place the patient's feet on the footrests and replace the arm on the wheelchair.
- Help the patient to reverse these steps when he returns to bed.

When the wheelchair has arms that are not removable:

- Place the wheelchair with its back toward the head of the bed, turning it at a slight angle to face the patient. Lock the brakes and raise the footrests out of the way.

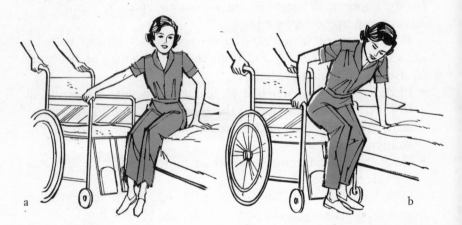

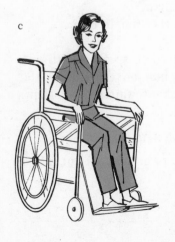

a. Place the wheelchair on an angle at the side of the bed, with wheels locked and footrests raised.

b. Patient supports body weight on hands and arms and slides from bed to the chair.

c. Patient slides back in the chair and places the feet on the footrests.

- Have the patient come to a sitting position with his legs over the side of the bed and his feet on the floor. Give him help only as needed.
- Have him place his hand nearest the wheelchair on the far arm of the chair, placing the other hand, palm down, on the bed near his hip. Have him shift his body so that the near hip is turned toward the wheelchair.
- Have the patient push with both hands to raise himself off the bed and pivot so that he can sit down in the chair.
- Place his feet on the footrests after he is seated in the wheelchair, release the brakes, and bring it away from the bed.
- Help the patient to reverse these steps when he returns to bed.
- Assist the patient as necessary in lying down, in providing proper support, and in positioning him comfortably in bed.
- Note on the patient's daily record the length of time he was up in the chair and any reactions observed.

USING A COMMODE

If the patient is allowed out of bed but cannot get to the bathroom, using a commode or a toilet chair is more satisfactory, and better for him, than using a bedpan. Getting in and out of bed to go to the toilet provides exercise for the patient, helps to improve his muscle tone, and is esthetically more satisfying to him. Also, it is an important factor in the retraining of an incontinent patient. In addition, the position on the commode is one to which the patient is accustomed and one that makes emptying the bladder and the lower bowel most effective.

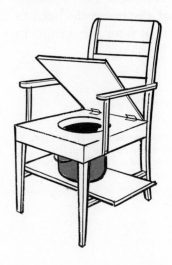

Using a chair to improvise a commode.

The top of the mattress should be level with the seat of the commode to make the patient's transfer from one to the other easy. This bed height permits the patient to rest his feet on the floor when he comes to a sitting position and lessens accident hazards when he is getting out of bed. Casters or rollers should be removed from the bed so that it will be steady.

The commode chair should be sturdy, comfortable, and of a height that makes the patient's getting on and off it easy. For comfort and for safety the commode chair should have arms. A commode with removable arms offers several obvious advantages. A commode may be easily improvised by placing a bedpan on the seat of a sturdy wooden armchair. This arrangement raises the seat level, but the few extra inches in height may be an advantage to the patient when he is getting on and off the chair. Regardless of its type, a commode chair can be made to resemble a regular chair by adding washable cushions or slip covers. It must be kept clean and free from odor at all times.

Commode chairs can be rented or purchased through dealers in invalids and hospital supplies, listed in the yellow pages of the telephone directory. Service clubs, visiting nurse associations, and Red Cross chapters may have a loan service through which such equipment may be borrowed.

The procedure for the patient's getting out of bed and onto a commode and getting back to bed is the same as that for his getting into and out of a chair.

TUB BATH FOR THE HANDICAPPED PATIENT

In the average home or apartment the bathroom door is narrow and the floor space is limited. A chair that eliminates the need to use a wheelchair to get a handicapped patient from the bedside to

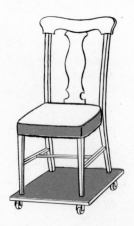

A sturdy rolling chair, narrow enough to go through the bathroom door, can be improvised. It is useful in getting into and out of the bathtub and in transferring to the toilet stool.

the bathtub may be purchased or maybe improvised by attaching wheels or casters to the legs of a kitchen or dining room chair. A chair of this type turns on its own axis and, with no arms and a seat the width of the average dining chair, it easily passes through a narrow doorway. Using a chair without arms makes the patient's transfer from the chair to the toilet seat easy and is an advantage to him in helping himself into or out of the tub. Because this chair has no braking mechanism, it should be steadied whenever the patient gets on or off it.

It is easier for the patient to get in and out of the bathtub if there is a tub seat or a stool and water in the tub.

Equipment

Rolling chair or wheelchair
Rubber bathtub mat with suction cups
Bathtub seat or stool with safety tips
Grab bar attached to side of tub

Washcloth
Towels
Soap

Procedure

- Fill the tub about one-third full with warm water.
- Have the patient undress himself and put on his bathrobe and his slippers, if he is able to do so. Help him only as needed.
- Bring the patient to the warmed bathroom in a rolling chair or a wheelchair. Place the chair so that the patient faces the side of the tub, leaving him enough room to lift his legs onto the side of the tub. Steady the rolling chair or lock the brakes on the wheelchair. Have the patient remove his bathrobe and his slippers if he can do so by himself, or help him as needed.
- Have the patient lift, or assist him in lifting, one leg at a time, so that his *feet* are over the side of the tub. Roll the chair close to the tub so that his *legs* are over the side of the tub. Again, steady the chair or lock the brakes.
- Have the patient grasp the grab bar or the side of the tub and slide forward on the chair seat to the edge of the tub, placing both feet on the mat in the tub.
- Have him maintain his hold on the tub or the bar with one hand and place the other hand on the far side of the tub.
- Give him support around the waist and help him to turn enough so that he can slide onto the bathtub seat or a stool. If there is no seat or stool, help the patient to lower himself into the tub.
- Stay with the patient while he is in the tub and give him assistance with the bath as needed.

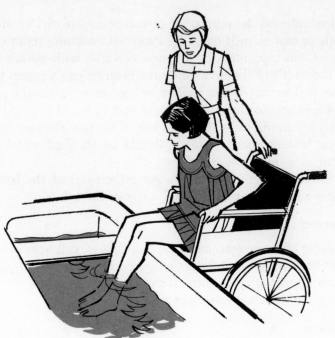

Roll the chair close to the tub, lifting the patient's feet over the side and into the tub.

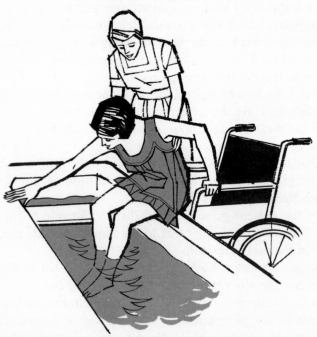

Support the patient while she slides from the chair to the edge of the tub and onto the tub seat or a stool.

Tub bath for the handicapped patient.

- To get the patient out of the tub, support him under the arms, helping him to shift to a sitting position on the side of the tub.
- After the patient's body has been dried, have him put on the bathrobe. Place the chair facing the side of the tub at the patient's back and steady the chair or lock the wheels.
- Have the patient place one hand on the rim of the tub at his side and the other hand on the side of the chair seat, and slip back onto the chair.
- Steady the chair and assist as necessary.
- If a wheelchair is being used, release the brakes after the patient is in the chair.
- Roll the chair back from the tub.
- Finish drying the patient's legs and feet and have him put on his slippers. Give no more help than is necessary for his safety.
- Take the patient back to his room.
- Give assistance as needed in dressing if he is to remain up.
- Have the patient sit in the chair while the bed is made or the linen is changed.
- Have the patient remove his robe and his slippers and get into his pajamas if he is returning to bed. Help him only as needed.
- See that he is comfortable in bed.
- Clean the tub and tidy the bathroom. Put the soiled linens in the laundry hamper.

TUB BATH FOR THE AMBULATORY PATIENT

A tub bath gives the patient an opportunity to bathe with safety, comfort, and minimum exertion.

A chair or a stool, a rubber suction mat, and handholds should be provided for safety.

If the patient prefers a shower bath, care should be taken to adjust the temperature of the water and to protect his hair before he enters the shower.

Equipment

Rubber suction mat for the tub
Bathtub seat or stool with safety tips on legs
Bathroom stool or chair covered with a pad and placed beside the tub
Bath mat

Washcloth
Towels
Soap
Blanket, if needed
Fresh clothing, warmed if necessary

Procedure

- Collect the equipment, draw the bath water, and assist the patient to the warmed bathroom. Help him undress but let him do as much as he can for himself.
- Have him grasp some secure object when he gets into the tub and give him needed support.
- Give him assistance with the bath as needed. Most people enjoy having their backs washed.
- Help the patient out of the tub to the chair or the stool only if he needs help. If he is sitting on the bottom of the tub, it will be easier for him to rise if the water is left in the tub until he is out.
- Protect him against chilling and see that he is dry.
- After the patient has dressed and has returned to his room, suggest that he rest quietly.
- Clean the tub and straighten the bathroom.

POINTS TO REMEMBER ABOUT GIVING A TUB BATH

- A low bed makes it easier and safer for the patient to help himself.
- Get a helper in advance if assistance is needed.
- Protect the patient against slipping and other accidents.
- Avoid letting the patient get chilled or fatigued.
- Note the color and condition of the patient's skin. Report any unusual condition to the doctor.

PREPARING TO WALK

After an illness, walking may have to be relearned. As with other activities, walking may be difficult and progress slow at first. However, the patient should be encouraged to cross this bridge to independence, because walking was the hoped-for outcome when he began such activities as turning over in bed, sitting up, and getting in and out of bed.

Frequently the patient is most comfortable when lying in bed, and he may wish to avoid activity designed to restore him to his pre-illness state of health, especially if movement is accompanied by discomfort. Nevertheless, it is a medically accepted fact that the patient's being up and around contributes to his own and his family's mental health as well as to his physical progress. The doctor will decide when and for how long the patient may be out of bed, and his advice should be followed to prevent the patient from overtaxing his strength and from becoming discouraged.

Just getting out of bed and walking is not a cure-all. While he is out of bed the patient needs practically as much care as when he is bedfast. Correct posture and position are still very important in the prevention of contractures and deformities. The patient still has to have an adequate diet, his personal needs must be met, and he probably requires some medicines. It is important for the patient to do as much as he can for himself. A person who finds it hard to stand by and not assist with something that the patient finds difficult to do should remember that the patient is benefited by helping himself.

In both standing and walking the patient should wear low-heeled Oxfords or other shoes that provide stability and give support to the feet. Loafers or bedroom slippers are dangerous because they slip off easily and may cause the patient to fall.

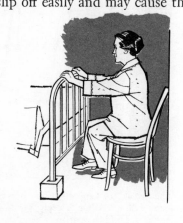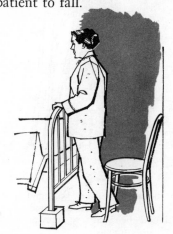

Before attempting to walk, the patient should have practice in getting up and down from chairs, in standing, and in maintaining standing balance. Low-heeled shoes or Oxfords give support to the feet.

Before attempting to walk the patient should practice standing and maintaining standing balance. Walkers are not generally recommended, except for someone with special disabilities, because a patient who uses a walker does not learn to balance himself, the gait he develops is not the normal one, and therefore he has to be weaned from it in order to learn how to walk correctly.

HELPING THE PATIENT TO WALK

To maintain good walking posture, the patient must keep his head erect, his neck, chest, and lower extremities in alignment, and his body weight evenly distributed on the joints of his feet. His

249

arms and his legs swing forward alternately in unison, right arm and left leg, left arm and right leg.

If the patient has no disability of his legs, such as paralysis, a fracture, or an amputation, but only muscle weakness as a result of

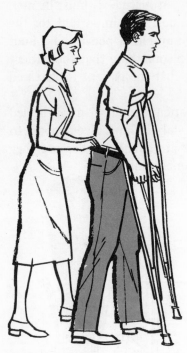

Until the patient gains skill and confidence in using crutches, some-one should be ready to provide support.

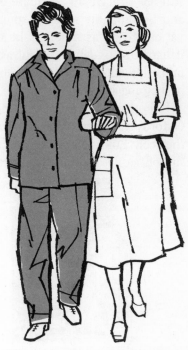

The weak or apprehensive person fears falling. Walk closely, arm-in-arm. Hold the patient's hand.

illness, it is best for him to be supported from the back at the waist, so that his normal walking position is not altered. A belt around his waist provides a good grip for the helper.

The weak or apprehensive person who fears falling may at first need additional support. The helper should walk close beside the patient, arm-in-arm, and should hold his hand. The helper's hand should be palm down on top of the patient's hand so that, if he becomes weak, she can quickly raise her upper arm into his axilla for support and, moving her outer leg sidewise to broaden her base of support, pull the patient against her hip for balance.

The procedure is somewhat different when a hemiplegic patient is being helped to walk. This kind of patient has suffered an injury, such as a stroke, to a portion of the central nervous system, and as a result one side of his body is paralyzed. The helper should stand at the patient's *affected* side, with an arm around his waist, so that the patient has both arms free. With the helper in this position, the patient has reassurance and support and his balance is not affected.

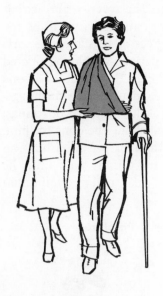

Helping the hemiplegic patient to walk.

ACTIVITIES FOR THE PARALYZED PATIENT

Sitting up and getting in and out of bed present problems of greater complexity for the hemiplegic patient than for the patient who is merely weak from illness. In addition to the limitations imposed by paralysis of one side of the body, the hemiplegic patient undergoes great mental distress, particularly if he is unable to speak distinctly. He is frightened at his inability to move an arm or a leg, especially if he cannot make himself understood. Another difficulty relates to his being right- or left-handed. The right-handed person whose right side is paralyzed must of necessity perform tasks using the unaffected left side. He finds that, to acquire a satisfactory degree of deftness, finely coordinated skills such as needlework and writing require much practice and that even to feed himself requires the relearning of what was formerly an automatic action.

An early return to activity is desirable for the patient who has had a stroke, but only the doctor can decide when activity can be started. The period of inactivity will vary with each patient, depending on the amount of damage to the vital brain centers and on the cause of the stroke. In no case is the patient gotten up until hemorrhaging has ceased, but in this interim period, posture and body positioning and exercises that prevent contractures and deformities are of great importance to insure optimum recovery. (See "Preventing Physical Deformities," chapter 9, pages 137-139.)

The problems that hemiplegic patients present differ and depend on age, previous physical condition, and the severity and extent of the physical impairment. For some patients, activity will be relatively easy. Others will need varying degrees of assistance for varying lengths of time. In any case, each patient should be offered minimum assistance and should be reminded that he still has one good side. He should be protected from accidents, given encouragement, and urged to take as much time as he needs to do things. Only those things he cannot do for himself should be done for him. Generally, there is more than one method of accomplishing an activity. Therefore, the patient should try various ways until he finds the one that is best for him and that requires minimum assistance.

Procedures for Sitting Up When One Side Is Paralyzed

Method No. 1:

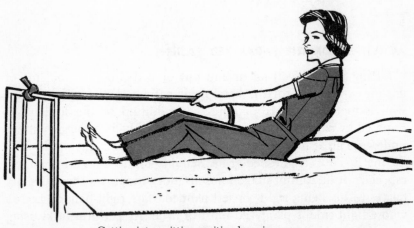

Getting into a sitting position by using a rope.

- Attach a strap or knotted rope to the bottom of the bed. A patient with one good arm will find this method the best one for sitting, lying down, or turning on his side.

Method No. 2:
- Have the patient turn on his affected side, facing the outer side of the bed, with his good knee flexed and resting on the mattress, to provide a broad base of support.

252

- Have him place his good hand, palm down, near his *affected* shoulder, with the elbow flexed.
- Have him lift his head as much as possible, push down with his good hand, straighten his elbow, and thus raise his body.
- Have the patient slide his good hand nearer his hip, swing his *unaffected* lower leg and foot over the side of the bed, and come to a sitting position. His affected arm will lie in his lap.
- With his good hand, have him shift his affected leg over the side of the bed. A sturdy straight chair at the bedside provides a hand-hold for support and a place to put his feet.

Method No. 3:
- Have the patient lie on his back.
- Have the patient slide toward the side of the bed *with the un-affected side of his body toward the outside.*
- Have him move his paralyzed leg near the side of the bed by lifting it with his unaffected foot and leg, and, with his good hand, place his paralyzed arm across his body.
- Have him lift his head and his shoulders as far as he can, grasp the edge of the mattress, and, firmly pushing and pulling against the mattress, lean on his elbow to raise his body.
- Have the patient swing his unaffected leg over the side of the bed. His paralyzed arm will lie in his lap.
- Have him place his good hand, palm down, on the bed behind him and shift his hips so that he is facing the side of the bed. When his affected leg has been lifted over the side of the bed, the patient is in position to stand.
- Place a sturdy straight chair at the side of the bed for the patient to hold onto for support. If the bed is elevated and the patient's feet do not reach the floor, place them on the chair seat or a foot-stool for additional support.

To lie down:
- Have the patient place his good hand, palm down, on the mattress and, pushing with his unaffected foot and hand, slide his hips back on the bed, turning and facing the foot of the bed.
- Have him lift his affected leg onto and toward the center of the bed.
- Have him grasp the edge of the mattress, bring his good leg onto the bed, and, supporting his body weight on his unaffected forearm and elbow, lie back on the mattress. To help maintain his balance when preparing to lie down, the patient should keep his chin forward on his chest.

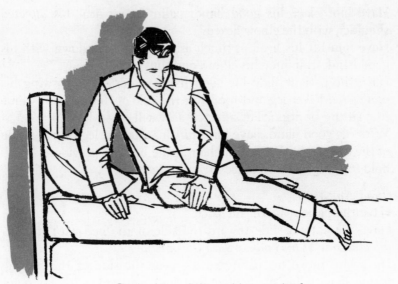

Getting into a sitting position unassisted.

Procedure for Getting Out of Bed When One Side Is Paralyzed

- Place the wheelchair or a sturdy armchair near the end of the bed at an angle, with the back of the chair toward the patient's unaffected side. If the patient is paralyzed on the left side, the back of the chair is to his right. If he is paralyzed on the right side, the back of the chair is to his left.
- After the patient comes to a sitting position at the side of the bed, have him grasp the end of the bed for support and come to a standing position. By balancing himself on his unaffected foot, he can grasp the far arm of the chair, pivot, and sit down.

To return to bed:

- Place the chair facing the bed in such a way that the patient has his unaffected arm near the end of the bed.
- Have him grasp the end of the bed and come to a standing position, balancing on his unaffected foot.
- Have the patient balance against the side of the bed, pivoting on his unaffected foot until he can sit on the side of the bed. Then let him release the grasp on the end of the bed, place his good hand beside him on the mattress for support, and slide back onto the bed in a sitting position.
- Have the patient maintain his balance in a sitting position. Then have him lift his affected leg onto the bed, grasp the mattress,

and lie down, at the same time bringing his unaffected leg onto the bed.

POINTS TO REMEMBER ABOUT HELPING THE PARALYZED PATIENT

- Encourage the patient to do as much for himself as he can.
- Stabilize the bed and the chair for safety.
- Teach the patient to support himself by holding on to an end of the bed.
- Have the patient wear low-heeled shoes that give support to the feet when he is standing or walking.

USING CRUTCHES

The purpose of using crutches is to enable a person who has lost all or partial use of one or both legs to move about in an upright position. Walking with crutches is a skill that a patient must learn. First of all, he must want to walk and must have the patience to practice. The physical demands of using crutches are such that the user must have sufficient strength in his arms to be able to move the crutches forward, sufficient strength in his fingers to grasp the hand bar, the ability to straighten his elbow, enough strength to support his body weight on his hands, and enough joint flexibility to extend his hand at the wrist.

The doctor will prepare the patient for crutch walking by prescribing exercises that will strengthen the muscles, assure body balance, and foster self-confidence. The exercises prescribed will depend on the degree of the patient's disability and the muscular strength he must achieve in order to be able to stand and begin to walk. In general, these exercises are those that contribute to the strengthening of the patient's hand, arm, and shoulder muscles and may be started under the guidance of a physical therapist while the patient is hospitalized. In some communities a physical therapist is available for home visits to teach the patient and a member of the family what they are to do. In other communities a public health nurse may perform this service.

Before the patient attempts to use crutches, the doctor usually wishes him to stand first in order to practice or to reestablish his balance. The doctor will assess the patient's body posture. The patient should practice balancing by standing at his bed with one hand on a chair or on the bed, with someone near him for safety.

There are several kinds of crutches and the doctor will prescribe the kind each patient should use. *Crutches must be measured and adjusted for each patient.* If they are too long, the patient's shoulders are pushed up and undue pressue is placed in the axilla; if the crutches are too short, the patient leans forward and his body is in poor alignment. The weight of the body must be supported by the patient's hands rather than by resting the armpits on the shoulder pads of the crutches. The hand grip must be adjusted so that the patient's elbows are slightly flexed.

The way a person walks on crutches is called the "crutch gait." The gait to be taught is determined by the nature and the extent of the patient's disability. The position of the body is called the "crutch stance." To have proper body position the patient should hold his head erect, his back straight, and his pelvis in a straight line with his head and his feet; that is, his body is *not* bent forward. The patient should hold the crutches close against his ribs and flex his elbows slightly, and there should be a space the width of at least two fingers between each crutch top and the axilla.

The normal way for a person to walk is to move his arms and his legs forward alternately, for example, the right arm and the left leg together, and the left arm and the right leg together. On crutches this is called the "two-point gait." The four-point gait is a slow, safe gait for patients who are able to bear at least partial weight on each leg and to advance one leg forward while balancing on the other leg and the two crutches. There are always three points of contact with the floor. The two-point gait is a progression of the four-point gait. It is relatively fast but cannot be used unless the body weight can be borne on either foot. It is faster than the four-point gait but requires greater balance and ability in crutch walking because there are two instead of three points of contact with the floor at any one time. The three-point gait is used by patients with one good leg and one leg that cannot bear full weight. Swinging gaits are used by persons with weakness or paralysis of both lower extremities or by persons with one good leg and one leg that cannot bear any weight.

Equipment

Fitted crutches

Procedures

For the four-point gait:
- Have the patient move the left crutch forward.
- Have the patient move right foot forward.
- Have the patient move right crutch forward.
- Have the patient move the left foot forward.

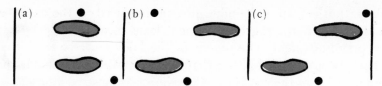

Four-Point Gait: a. Standing position; b. First step; c. Second step.

For the two-point gait:

- Have the patient move the left crutch and the right foot forward simultaneously.
- Have the patient move the right crutch and left foot forward simultaneously.

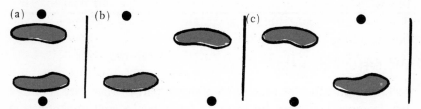

Two-Point Gait: a. Standing position; b. First step; c. Second step.

For the three-point gait:

- Have the patient move both crutches and the affected leg forward together, regulating the amount of weight taken on his leg by the weight taken on the hands.
- Have the patient move the stronger leg forward.

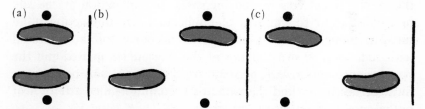

Three-Point Gait: a. Standing position; b. First step; c. Second step

Points To Remember

- Crutches must be individually measured for each person.
- Crutches may need to be adjusted in length with changes in the patient's body posture or as the patient becomes more adept in their use or grows taller.
- For safety the patient should wear low-heeled Oxfords with rubber heels when crutch walking.
- Give the patient necessary support by holding him at the waist from the back. A leather belt around the patient's waist provides a good grasp for the helper.

15

TREATMENTS USING HEAT AND COLD

THE EFFECTS OF HEAT

The application of heat to an affected part of the body is one of man's most common treatments. Heat has a soothing effect, it relaxes muscles, eases tension, frequently relieves pain, promotes healing, and provides warmth. Heat is often used to relieve inflammation caused by a local infection. It increases drainage and softens discharges from an open sore, helping the body to rid itself of the infection and thereby hastening healing.

Heat applied externally raises the temperature of the tissues, dilates the blood vessels, and increases the circulation at the site of and adjacent to the area of application. By this action more blood is brought to the part and this accounts for the increased local redness. The sweat glands of the skin are stimulated and the skin becomes moist with perspiration. For this reason precautions must be taken to avoid the patient's becoming chilled after a heat treatment has been discontinued.

Heat treatments may be either dry or moist. Various forms of dry electric heat, such as electric pads and infrared and sun lamps are frequently used. Chemical pads, which are heated by adding water to the substance in the pad or by being heated to the desired temperature in boiling water, are also used. Hot water bottles or adequate substitutes are devices familiar to everyone. Moist heat treatments that are frequently prescribed are hot tub, foot, and sitz baths; steam inhalations; moist compresses; and irrigations.

Moist heat is more penetrating than dry heat, and a wet substance conducts heat faster than a dry substance. Care must be taken to be sure that hot water bottles do not leak. Pressure should

258

not be exerted on a hot application because the layer of air that acts as an insulator is reduced and the patient's skin may be burned. If the application must be very hot, oil applied to the skin prevents some heat conduction and acts as a deterrent to burning.

Safety precautions must always be taken in the use of heat. Very young, old, and unconscious patients are most likely to be burned because of their lessened sensitivity and their inability to communicate. They must be closely observed and protected against being burned. Confused and very ill patients lack judgment and should also be watched more closely than average patients. In addition, they may be more sensitive to smaller amounts of local heat.

ELECTRIC PADS

An electric pad is convenient and relatively safe when properly used. However, because it can always become a hazard, care must be maintained in its use. An electric pad must never be operated if it is wet or moist or if the cord or the heat regulator shows any evidence of damage or undue wear. The written description attached to the pad should be examined and the underwriter's label, which is the best guarantee of safety, should be present. If possible, a waterproof electric pad should be used, because it lessens the possibility of a short circuit. If the pad has a warning label, "Do not wet," this warning should be precisely observed.

An electric pad usually has a removable washable cotton flannel outer cover to keep the pad itself clean. If the pad is to be used for long periods, extra outer covers should be provided for frequent changes; otherwise, it may become soiled or moist from perspiration and, therefore, potentially dangerous. Before the pad is used, the outer cover should be removed and the pad examined for cracks or other defects. It should never be folded or crushed, because doing so may damage or break the wire heating element. Pins should not be used to fasten the pad in place, because a puncture in the waterproof cover could cause a fire or an electric shock. The appliance should always be disconnected when not in use to prevent its getting overheated. Disconnect by pulling on the plug, not the cord.

ELECTRIC BLANKETS AND SHEETS

The primary purpose of an electric blanket is to provide warmth without weight. The degree of heat can be regulated by setting the heat indicator at the desired temperature. The same general considerations hold for this heating appliance as for the electric pad. Electric blankets usually have an extra length of cloth at one end containing no wiring, which can be tucked under the mattress to hold them in place. Some blankets are made with fitted bottom corners.

HEAT LAMPS

Heat lamps act through radiation of heat generated in a specially manufactured bulb that gives off infrared rays. These lamps have the same effect as other sources of heat; that is, they increase the circulation, relax muscles, and relieve pain. They have an advantage in that they present no problem of weight. For this reason they are quite often used for the treatment of swollen, inflamed joints. The rays can be focused on a small area or a single part of the body, the distance from the bulb to the body being determined by what is comfortable for the patient. There should be a feeling of slight warmth. As with any treatment, the length of time a heat lamp is used should be prescribed by the doctor; usually it is no longer than 20 minutes at a time. Infrared rays produce a dangerous form of heat and, if misused, cause severe burning.

ULTRAVIOLET RADIATION

Ultraviolet rays, which are produced by electricity in electrode and mercury arc lamps, have the same effects and hazards as exposure to rays of the sun. The dosage of ultraviolet radiation, therefore, must be carefully regulated and should not be administered by the inexperienced home nurse unless the doctor prescribes it and gives specific instructions for carrying out the treatment. To prevent damage to the eyes, both the patient and the person giving the treatment must wear dark glasses. The patient should not be left alone because of the danger of his falling asleep and remaining too long under the lamp.

People with fair skin are more apt to receive a burn from ultraviolet rays than are people already tanned by the sun or those who have darker skin. Usually men can tolerate more exposure than women. As with a sunburn, the injurious effects of ultraviolet radiation do not appear for several hours. In the case of a severe reaction, the affected skin area is red, painful, and sometimes blistered, and usually there is local swelling.

CHEMICAL AGENTS

A bag containing a chemical filler that is activated by adding water is the most common device of the several in which dry heat can be chemically produced. Another type, in which a chemical agent is contained in a pliable waterproof plastic bag, is immersed in hot or boiling water until it reaches the temperature desired for application to the body. It can also be chilled or frozen in the refrigerator and used as a cold application or as a substitute for an ice pack. A third type of heating pad has the chemical filler enclosed in a fabric envelope. This type, when immersed in hot water, absorbs some of the liquid and retains the moist heat for a relatively long period of time, about 30 minutes. The fact that this type can be obtained in several sizes adds to its usefulness. Because of its weight, and because it becomes quite hot, this pad must be placed between several layers of heavy cloth before being applied to the skin. Every precaution must be taken to protect the patient against burns.

HOT WATER BAGS

A rubber hot water bag is often used to apply dry heat. The purpose of a dry-heat treatment is to relieve pain, increase the blood supply to an affected part of the body, to give comfort and to promote healing. There are many substitutes for a hot water bag: a cloth bag containing sand, dry oatmeal, or cornmeal that has been heated in the oven; a heated flat stone or brick; a tightly sealed glass jar or bottle containing hot water. Because it is more difficult to regulate the degree of heat of improvised equipment, all such substitutes should be adequately and securely wrapped to protect the patient against burns. The home nurse should test the heat on her own skin, and if it is comfortably warm for her, it will be safe for the patient.

Equipment

Hot water bag with a stopper, washer, and cover
Container, preferably a wide-mouthed pitcher

Supply of hot water
Supply of cold water
Cloth or paper wipes
Waste container

Procedure

- Add hot water to cold water in a container and test the temperature. The water should be momentarily bearable to a clenched fist, or approximately 115° F. to 130° F.
- Fill the bag one-third to one-half full so that it will be light-weight.

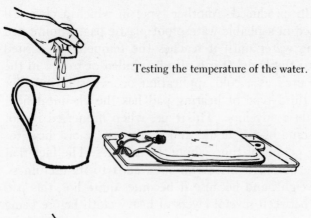

Testing the temperature of the water.

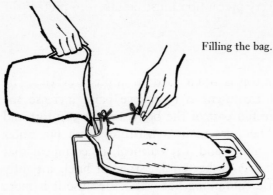

Filling the bag.

Preparing a hot water bag.

- To make the bag pliable, expel the air from the bag by placing the bag on a flat surface and pressing until water appears in the neck. While the water is still in the neck, screw in the stopper.
- Dry the bag and the inside of the neck. Test for leakage by holding the bag upside down.
- Cover it with a bag made of soft material or wrap it in a towel.
- Apply the bag, placing it so that the patient does not lie on the hard neck of the bag.
- Remove the bag when the water has cooled, refill as needed, and continue the applications as ordered by the doctor.
- Note on the daily record where and for how long the bag was applied and what the patient's reaction was.
- Care for the bag after use:
  Allow the bag to drain dry.
  Allow air to enter.
  Screw in the stopper to keep the sides from sticking together.
  Put away in a dry, cool place.

Many gases and drugs are administered by inhalation, for example, oxygen and spirits of ammonia. Some, such as a medicated steam inhalation, have a local effect on the tissues of the respiratory tract, while the effect of others is dependent on their being absorbed from the inspired air into the body tissues. Some medications are volatile; this means that they change readily to a vapor. Others, such as the medications contained in commercial pocket-sized inhalators, which are used to relieve the symptoms of the common cold, are nonvolatile and are added to an agent that will carry them into the lungs. A nonvolatile drug may also be carried in the steam from hot water, and this method of inhalation is often prescribed for hoarseness, a sore throat, or difficulty in breathing. The mist-like spray of an atomizer or a nebulizer is another common method of administering an inhalant. The purpose of giving a steam inhalation is to relieve hoarseness, a sore throat, coughing, or difficulty in breathing. Warm, moist air has a soothing effect on the mucous membranes, tends to soften and make secretions less thick and sticky and easier to cough up, and usually makes the patient more comfortable. Evaporation of water from an open container in the room will add moisture to the air, or hot water taps may be turned on. Modern heating appliances provide for the addition of moisture to room air.

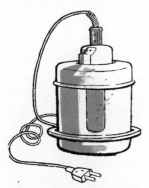

Safety precautions should be observed when an electric inhalator is used.

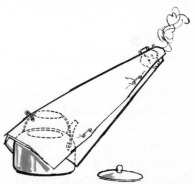

Improvised inhalator made from a newspaper cone placed over the top and spout of a teakettle.

A commercial electric inhalator that produces steam is commonly used to increase humidity at home or in the hospital. These appliances vary in price and in length of time they will operate. Most electric inhalators have a safety device that shuts them off when the water reaches an unsafe level in the container or has evaporated. These appliances are effective because they produce steam over a relatively long period of time and are easy to operate.

Safety precautions should be observed when an electric inhalator is in use, especially if the patient is a child. The apparatus should be inspected before use for evidence of any defect and should be disconnected from the electric outlet when not in use. It should be placed where the steam cannot burn the patient and, if it is used at the bedside, someone should stay with the patient. Usually the inhalator can be placed on the floor, out of the way, so that it will not be overturned and cause harm.

Equipment

Teakettle or other covered container of boiling water or a commercial inhalator, if available
Paper funnel
Medication if ordered, cotton, safety pin
Protected chair, stool, or box

Extra pillow
Umbrella or card table
Blanket to make a tent cover
Towel or blanket for the patient's shoulders
Towel to cover the patient's hair
Paper tissues

Procedures

When using improvised equipment:
- Assemble the equipment.
- Arrange the patient comfortably in bed and protect the working areas.
- If a medication is ordered, saturate an egg-sized ball of cotton with the ordered amount of medication and pin the cotton inside the top of the newspaper funnel. (For instructions on making an improvised funnel, see page 327.) The drug will mix with the steam passing through the funnel and be breathed in by the patient.
- Support the patient's head with the extra pillow, place a towel or a blanket over his shoulders, protect his hair against moisture with a towel, and provide tissues so that he can wipe his face.
- Make a tent by adjusting an opened umbrella or card table over the patient's head and shoulders. Cover it well with the blanket, leaving an open airspace at the near side.
- Bring the kettle to the bedside and place it on a protected surface, with the spout below the level of the mattress for safety. Remove the lid and place the handle, if it is movable, in an upright position.

264

- Hold the funnel over the kettle, secure it firmly to the handle, using a safety pin through the layers of paper, and adjust the wide end of the funnel over the opening.
- Direct the steam toward the top of the tent but not into the patient's face.
- Maintain steam in the kettle by changing the water as necessary. Remain on hand to give assistance as needed.
- Discontinue the inhalation at the time indicated, remove the equipment, and dry the patient's face. To avoid getting chilled, the patient should remain quiet in a warm room for about an hour after the treatment.
- Note on the daily record the time and the length of the treatment, the patient's comments, and any improvements noted, such as easier breathing, less coughing, or less hoarseness.
- Clean and put away the equipment after use.

When using a commercial inhalator:
- Modify the above procedure as follows:
  Have the patient turn on his side with his face near the edge of the bed.
  Protect his head against moisture with a towel.
  Place the inhalator at the side of the bed, with the steam outlet directed so that the vapor rises around the patient's head.

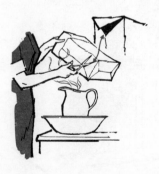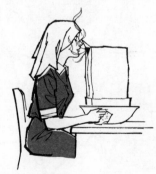

Steam inhalation for the patient able to sit up.

When the patient is sitting up:
- Assemble the following equipment:
  Pitcher or other container of steaming water
  Paper bag in which an opening has been cut on one end
  A basin
  Towels
  Extra blanket, if needed

- Protect the patient's hair and shoulders with towels.
- Make sure that the patient's position during treatment is comfortable. Provide extra warmth if needed to avoid his getting chilled.
- Place the container of steaming water in the basin for safety.
- Invert the paper bag over the container.
- Place the equipment at a comfortable height.
- Have the patient lean forward and breathe in the warm, moist air through the hole in the paper bag.
- Replenish the hot water as needed to provide adequate steam for effective results.

STEAM INHALATIONS FOR CHILDREN

An infant or a child suffering from bronchitis, laryngitis, a cold, or other respiratory ailment often benefits greatly from breathing in warm, moist air. A kettle of simmering water or a commercial inhalator may be placed in the sickroom and operated continuously if necessary. The amount of steam generated is not enough to cause any damage to the furniture or the room decorations.

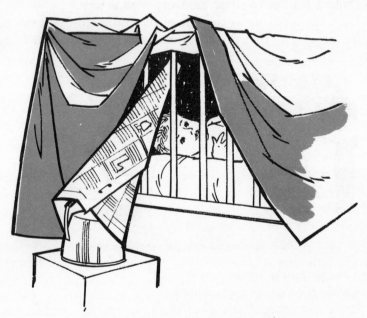

Steam inhalation using improvised equipment.

If the doctor orders steam treatments of greater intensity or of a specific length and frequency, a croup tent can be improvised by draping a cotton blanket over the sides of a crib. Steam, either

266

plain or medicated, can be introduced into the croup tent as described above in the procedure for the patient in bed. An older child can be treated by placing him in the tent made with an umbrella or a card table and a blanket. Safety precautions are the same for all patients and someone must remain in the room while the treatment is being given.

If the child is afraid or restless and has to be held, a satisfactory treatment can be given in the bathroom. The following procedure should be used:

- Turn on the hot water in the tub or the shower, letting it run so that the bathroom fills with warm steam.
- Wrap the baby or the child in a blanket and sit down with him in the bathroom, closing the door.
- Remain in the room for the necessary length of time.
- Protect the child against chilling when he is back in his bed.

POINTS TO REMEMBER ABOUT GIVING STEAM INHALATIONS

- Avoid burning the patient with steam by directing the steam away from his skin.
- Prevent fire when using an electric device at the bedside by keeping the device away from the bedding.
- Stay with the patient.

THROAT IRRIGATIONS

A throat irrigation is a way of applying moist heat directly to the mucous membranes that line the throat. Its purpose is to relieve pain, redness, swelling, and tightness in the throat and to soften and remove throat secretions by applying moist heat directly to the membrane lining the throat. A medicated gargle has essentially the same purpose as a throat irrigation, but the patient may find it difficult to gargle. Irrigation has the advantage of being continuous and it can be prolonged.

A throat irrigation should be given only when ordered by the doctor. A number of solutions may be used, such as plain hot water, salt or soda and water (1 level tablespoonful of either to 1 quart of water), or an antiseptic of the type used for a gargle. The solution should be as hot as the patient can tolerate. The beneficial effects result from the heat of the solution and its cleansing action. If a medicated solution is ordered, the doctor will specify the kind to be used. The solution need not be sterile, but it and all the equipment must be clean.

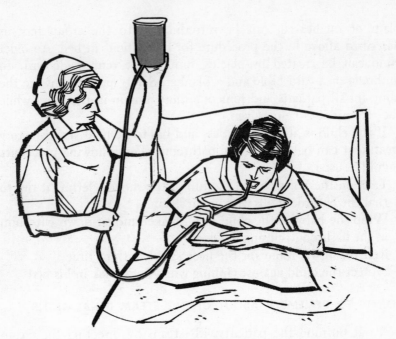

Giving a throat irrigation.

For best results the flow of the solution should be gentle and continuous, with the patient's head tilted forward if he is sitting up, or to the side if he is lying down, so that the solution can flow freely into and out of the mouth. The patient should be instructed not to breathe while the solution is flowing, to avoid his choking or his aspirating some of the fluid into the lungs. If the nozzle touches the back of the patient's tongue or throat, it may cause him to gag. If he can hold the nozzle and direct the flow of the solution himself, he can avoid gagging. He can also stop the flow of the solution at will so that he can breathe.

If the patient cannot sit up while the irrigation is being done, he should be helped to turn to his other side when about half of the solution has been used so that both sides of the throat may be treated.

Equipment

Irrigating can or fountain syringe

Tubing and stopcock

Plastic or glass drinking tube

Rubber or plastic protector for the bed

Waste container

Solution ordered by the doctor, 3 or 4 pints

Paper tissues

268

Procedure

- Explain to the patient what is going to be done and how he can assist.

- Make the patient comfortable, preferably sitting up, or let him lie on his side. Place a container of paper tissues where he can easily reach them.

- Protect the bedding with a waterproof cover.

- Hang or hold the irrigating can so that the top of the solution is approximately 12 inches above the level of the patient's mouth. The flow can be regulated by lowering or raising the can or by closing the stopcock on the tubing.

- Check the temperature of the solution with a candy or bath thermometer if one is available. It should be from 110° F. to 120° F. (43.4° C. to 48.8° C.). The temperature can be tested by putting a small amount of the solution on the inner surface of the wrist. It should be hot enough to sting.

- Allow the patient to operate the flow of the solution with the stopcock, or arrange a signal with him so that you can stop the flow and let him breathe.

- Place a basin so that it will catch the return flow of the solution.

- Permit the patient to hold the irrigating nozzle or the drinking tube and insert it in his mouth, being careful to put it only about two-thirds of the way back so that he will not gag.

- When the treatment is completed, wash and dry the patient's hands and face. Remove the equipment and see that the patient is warm and comfortable.

- Note on the daily record the time the treatment was given, the amount and the kind of solution used, the appearance of the return flow, and observations about the patient's reaction and condition.

- Care for the equipment:
    Wash the irrigating nozzle with hot, soapy water, using friction. Rinse and boil it for 3 minutes, allow it to dry, and store it with the rest of the equipment.
    Wash the irrigating can and the tubing in hot, soapy water. Rinse and dry them before putting away.
    Store any rubber equipment in a cool, dry place because heat and moisture cause rubber to deteriorate. Coil the tubing. Store the fountain syringe flat, stuffing it with dry, crumpled paper to keep the sides from sticking together.

- Have the solution the correct temperature. If it is too hot, it will burn the patient's throat and mouth and injure the tissues. A cool solution is not effective.
- Give this treatment only when ordered by the doctor.
- Clean and put away the equipment as directed after use.

ENEMAS

The cleansing enema is the one most commonly ordered by the doctor, but there are other kinds of enemas given for specific purposes. Food and drugs are sometimes administered to the patient by this method, and certain kinds of enema solutions may be ordered to protect, to soothe, or to irrigate the mucous membrane of the lower bowel.

The purpose of giving a cleansing enema is to stimulate peristalsis as an aid to elimination and to remove feces from the lower bowel. Most people understand the use of the enema and how it is administered. If the patient has never had an enema, explain the procedure to him so that he can cooperate. If he is relaxed, the enema is more likely to be successful. The patient should be in a comfortable position, lying either on his left side or on his back. The sitting position is not satisfactory, because the solution must then flow against the force of gravity, and greater pressure is needed than when the patient is lying down. The home nurse should provide as much privacy as possible and should avoid exposing the patient at all times. He should help with the treatment as much as he can.

If the home nurse prefers to use disposable enema units, they can be obtained at a drugstore. They are easy to use, save time, and have no irritating effect on the lining of the bowel. The unit is complete, even to the lubricant for the nozzle, making all other equipment unnecessary. The plastic tube or sack containing the enema solution can be completely immersed in a basin of warm water until the solution is warm enough to be comfortable to the patient. After the nozzle has been inserted in the patient's rectum, the solution is squeezed out of the plastic container. After use the unit is discarded, and there is no cleaning and storing of equipment. Because this type of enema contains only 4 or 5 ounces of solution, it can be used successfully with infants and children and with adults who find it difficult to retain the quantity of fluid used in giving a plain water enema.

Tray for the equipment
Enema bag, can, or funnel
Connecting tubing, stopcock, and enema nozzle or rectal tube
Enema solution, as ordered by the doctor (if none has been specified, give 1 to 2 pints of plain warm water)
Standard on which to hang the enema bag
Lubricant for the nozzle
or
Disposable enema unit

Extra towel (for a child)
Extra blanket
Warmed bedpan and cover, unless the patient can use a commode or go to the bathroom
Toilet paper
Basin of warm water, washcloth, and towel
Rubber or plastic sheet or bed pad
Newspapers for protection of the furniture
Call bell

Procedures

For an adult:

- Protect the table and the chair. Have the bedpan or the commode at the bedside.
- Cover the patient with the extra blanket and, reaching under it, fold back the upper bedclothes to the foot of the bed.
- Place the bedpad or the rubber sheet under the patient's hips to protect the bed.
- Roll up the gown or remove the pajama trousers.
- Have the patient lie on his side or his back at the near side of the bed with a pillow under his head if desired.
- To permit proper flow of the solution, place the bag so that the top level of the solution will be approximately 18 inches above the upper surface of the mattress.
- Close the stopcock and pour the solution into the bag.
- Open the stopcock and let a small amount of the solution flow into the bedpan to remove air from and to warm the tubing.
- Test the temperature of the solution on the wrist. It should be comfortably warm. Close the stopcock.
- Lubricate the nozzle.
- Insert the tip of the rectal tube 2 to 3 inches into the rectum and hold in place. If a hard rubber nozzle is used, it is inserted to the bulge at its base, usually about 2 inches.
- Rotate the tip slightly but gently. If there is blockage, withdraw the tip a little and try again. If the tube has become clogged,

withdraw the nozzle, allow the solution to run through it, and then reinsert.

- Open the stopcock when the nozzle tip is in place. Allow the solution to flow into the rectum slowly. If the patient complains of pressure or pain, close the stopcock, wait a minute or two, and then start the flow gradually. Gentle pressure against the rectum may help the patient to retain the solution. Instruct him to open his mouth and take long, deep breaths if he feels discomfort or pressure.

- Withdraw the tip gently when there is still a small amount of solution in the container. Allow the remaining solution to flow into the bedpan. Remove the tip from the tubing, wrap it in toilet paper, and place on the tray until it can be cleaned.

- Encourage the patient to retain the solution for a few minutes.

- Place the patient on the bedpan and stay with him or within call while the enema is expelled, or help him to get out of bed to use the commode or go to the bathroom.

- Cleanse the patient after the enema is expelled or let him cleanse himself if he is able. Dry the patient thoroughly to keep his skin in good condition.

- Remove the bedpan and cover it immediately.

- Remove the bed protection, replace the upper bedclothes, and make the patient comfortable. Air the room but do not chill the patient.

- Make sure that the patient's hands are washed.

- Note the contents of the bedpan, and if unusual, save for the doctor to see. Note also the patient's reaction.

- Care for the equipment:
    Empty the bedpan, cleanse it, and put it away.
    Open the stopcock, rinse the enema can or bag and the tubing with clear water, and hang the equipment up to drain and dry. Replace the dry tubing in its box or wrap it in a clean cloth, leaving the stopcock open. If an enema bag was used, stuff it with tissue paper to keep the sides from sticking together. Keep it dry.
    Wash the enema nozzle with hot, soapy water, using friction. Rinse, boil for 3 minutes, dry, and place it with the bag.
    Store any rubber equipment in a cool, dry place to prevent deterioration.

For a child:

- Explain what is going to be done if the child is old enough to understand.
- Have the room warm and free from drafts.
- Have the child lie on his back or his left side on a well-protected bed or table. If the child is very small and the enema is to be given on the lap, use waterproof material and a diaper to protect clothing.
- Place a folded towel under the child's buttocks to raise them slightly to the right level for receiving the enema.
- Give the enema as described above. Use the amount of solution ordered by the doctor, usually about one-half pint. Allow the solution to flow into the rectum gently and very slowly.
- Allow the child to sit on a potty or else he may expel the enema into the diaper.
- Care for the equipment as described above.

For an infant:

- Assemble the following equipment:

Small rubber bulb syringe with a nozzle	Small blanket for warmth
Enema solution ordered by the doctor	Lap or bed protector of waterproof material
Toilet paper	Basin of warm water
Small basin or potty	Soft washcloth
Clean diaper	Skin lotion
	Lubricant

- Have the room warm and free from drafts.
- Place the baby on his back on the lap, a bathinette, or a well protected table. Remove his diaper and fold back his clothes.
- Draw the enema solution into the bulb, hold the nozzle up, and squeeze the bulb gently to expel air. Test the temperature of the liquid on the inner surface of the wrist. It should be comfortably warm. Lubricate the nozzle.
- Lift the baby's legs with one hand, holding them at the ankles with a finger between them to prevent rubbing.
- Gently insert the nozzle of the syringe about 1 inch into the rectum.
- Introduce the solution very gently by slowly squeezing the bulb of the syringe. A small baby can usually be given about 2 or 3 ounces, and a larger baby can be given more.

- Withdraw the nozzle carefully when the bulb is empty and put the syringe aside. Apply gentle pressure to the baby's buttocks and anus with a folded diaper to help him retain the solution for a few minutes.
- Hold the basin, potty, or diaper under the baby's hips to receive the bowel movement. If the enema is expelled without a bowel movement, a second enema may be given.
- After the enema is expelled, wash, dry, and care for the buttocks as after any bowel movement. Put a fresh diaper on the baby and put him to bed.
- Note on the daily record the time the enema was given, the amount of solution given, and the amount and the character of the stool, such as undigested food, blood, or mucus. Indicate whether or not gas was expelled with the enema.
- Note the baby's condition after the treatment.
- Inform the doctor of any unusual condition.
- Care for the equipment:
  Cleanse the potty or the basin.
  Wash the syringe with hot, soapy water. Rinse it with clear water and boil it for 3 minutes. Rinse, drain, and dry it.
  Wrap the syringe in a clean cloth or paper and put it in a cool place.

Points To Remember

- Assure a gentle flow of solution without pressure.
- Lubricate the nozzle well to avoid injury to the rectum.
- Give only the amount of solution ordered by the doctor.
- Have the patient lying down and in a comfortable position.
- Avoid chilling the patient.

HOT MOIST COMPRESSES

The purpose of a hot compress is to relieve pain, to increase the blood supply to the affected part of the body, and to promote healing. The length of time that hot compresses are to be used and the extent of the body surface to be treated will determine to a considerable extent the choice of equipment. Soft woolen fabrics, such as pieces of blanket or heavy flannel, should be used for the compresses. The natural lanolin in wool makes the fabric somewhat water-repellent and also helps it to retain its texture and to trap heat between the woven threads. A cotton fabric, which absorbs and holds more water, is less desirable than wool because it is heavier and less comfortable and the patient is in greater danger of getting burned. Also, cotton does not retain heat for as long a time as wool. Because steam or hot water can burn the patient, compresses must be wrung out as dry as possible and the steam must be shaken out. A thin layer of oil or petrolatum applied to the patient's skin helps to prevent the compress from burning him and is useful if his skin is thin or tender. The cloth for the compress, depending on its thickness, should be cut two or four times larger than the area to be treated and should be folded into either two or four layers before it is heated.

If a drug is to be used in this type of treatment, the doctor will give directions for its use. Ointments are sometimes rubbed gently on the skin. If a liquid drug is prescribed, it can be painted on the skin with a cotton applicator or it can be mixed in the water in which the compress is moistened.

Equipment

Double boiler

2 folded woolen compresses large enough to cover the area to be treated

Binder: a towel or a strip of cloth to hold the compress in place

Safety pins to fasten the binder

Protectors for furniture

To fit inside binder, a piece of dry woolen cloth and a piece of wax paper, plastic, or aluminum foil

Medication, if ordered

Bed cradle, if the bedclothes must be held away from the part being treated

Procedure

- Moisten the folded woolen compresses in water that is comfortably warm to the hands and *wring them out as dry as possible.*
- Place the folded compresses in the empty top of a double boiler, put the lid on, and heat the compresses over boiling water until they are steaming hot. This will take from 5 to 10 minutes.
- Adjust the patient's position so that he is comfortable and in good body alignment.
- Have the binder, which includes the woolen cloth and the wax paper or other protection, ready, with the safety pins in position so that the binder can be fastened as soon as the compress is applied.
- Protect the bedside table against heat and moisture.
- Carry the hot compresses to the bedside table in the top of the double boiler.

- Expose the body area where the compress is to be applied.
- Remove one of the compresses from the top of the boiler and, without unfolding, give it two quick, vigorous shakes to remove steam. Apply it to the area to be treated.
- Quickly place the binder over the compress to hold in the heat and to protect the bedding from moisture.
- Pin the binder securely in place at both ends to keep out cool air and to hold in the heat. Pin it loosely at the center, to allow an airspace and to avoid pressure.
- Place a cradle if needed over the part of the body being treated. Replace the covers.
- Leave the second compress in the top of the boiler and keep it hot until needed.
- Change the hot compress as needed, the first time in about 5 minutes, then every 10 or 15 minutes after that. Continue the treatment for the length of time ordered.

When changing the compress:
- Remove the pins from the binder but leave it in place.
- Bring the heated compress to the bedside as before and remove the steam with two quick, vigorous shakes.
- Open the binder quickly. Lift up the compress and the protective coverings and place the fresh compress on the skin. Pull out the cooled compress, placing it in top of double boiler if it is to be used again.
- Fasten the binder as before.

When discontinuing the treatment:
- Remove the moist compress and the wax paper or other protection.
- Pat the skin dry, cover with the dry wool and leave the binder loosely in place for 10 or 15 minutes to protect the patient against chills.
- Clear away the equipment.
- Note on the daily record the time the treatment was started, the time it was discontinued, any unusual appearance of the skin, the results of the treatment, and any comments made by the patient about the effect of the treatment.
- Wash and rinse the compress cloths and hang them up to dry.

PARAFFIN PACKS

The paraffin pack, another method of applying local heat, is sometimes ordered by the doctor for the treatment of arthritis and other conditions that cause inflammation and pain in the joints.

This treatment often gives comfort and relieves pain. The patient's extremities, especially the hands and the feet, are dipped in a mixture of paraffin and oil until a thick coating is formed. The same result can be obtained by using a clean paintbrush to paint layers of the mixture over and around the affected joint, such as a knee, elbow, or shoulder. Because the paraffin and the oil may be used over and over, the treatment is inexpensive.

Equipment

Paraffin	Aluminum foil or heavy wax paper
Mineral oil	
Large double boiler or a safe substitute	3-inch paintbrush
	Heavy bath towel
Candy or bath thermometer	Safety or electric razor

Procedure

- Remove the hair from the part of the body that is to be treated. Otherwise, removal of the paraffin pack will be painful.
- Put 3 pounds of paraffin and ¾ cup of mineral oil, or 4 pounds of paraffin and 1 cup of oil, into the top of the double boiler and heat until the paraffin melts and mixes with the oil. Check the temperature of the mixture carefully with a candy or a bath thermometer. The mixture should not be hotter than 125° F. to protect the patient against burns.
- See that the patient is in a comfortable position and that the hand or the foot to be treated is properly supported.
- Have the patient dip his hand or his foot in and out of the hot paraffin and oil so that the mixture comes above the wrist or the ankle, forming a thin layer. If the hand is being treated, have the patient bend his fingers and keep them separated. Use the paintbrush to apply the mixture to other joints.
- Wait a few seconds while the paraffin hardens.
- Repeat the dipping or the brushing 8 or 10 times or until about a ¼-inch coat of paraffin is formed over the entire area being treated. Caution the patient not to move the coated area, for movement will cause the paraffin to break and fall off.
- Wrap the treated area first in aluminum foil or heavy wax paper and then in a dry, heavy towel to hold in the heat. A piece of wool wrapped around or over the treated part before the towel is put on will help to keep the pack warm for a long time.
- Leave the paraffin on for 20 or 30 minutes or for as long as the doctor has ordered.

When discontinuing the treatment:

- Remove the towel but leave the foil or the wax paper in place.
- Have the patient move or bend the treated joint to crack the paraffin. The pack will come off in large pieces.
- Wrap the treated area in the towel for 5 or 10 minutes to protect the patient against chills.
- Rinse off the paraffin to remove perspiration and return it to the top of the double boiler for reuse.
- Dry the patient's skin gently because it will be moist from perspiration.
- Apply hand lotion or cream as desired to keep the patient's skin in good condition.
- Record the treatment on the daily record.

POINTS TO REMEMBER ABOUT TREATMENTS USING HEAT

- Use heat treatments only when the doctor prescribes them for the patient.
- Take every precaution to avoid burning the patient when applying heat to the skin, especially if the person is unconscious, paralyzed, very young or very old or has diabetes or edema (excess fluid in the tissues).
- Exercise caution against burning oneself when giving the patient any kind of heat treatment. Wear rubber gloves to protect the hands against moist heat. Use padded mitts or holders when handling hot objects.
- Take good care of electrical appliances. Clean and store them according to the manufacturer's directions. Repair or replace worn parts.
- Dry the hands before grasping and pulling the plug to connect or disconnect electrical equipment.
- Keep electric pads and electric blankets in good condition. Use care in folding them and avoid crushing them so that the heating elements and the thermostats are not damaged.
- Use care in sunbathing until the patient's skin has developed some tolerance to the sun's rays by becoming tanned.
- Use caution when heating paraffin, which is flammable. Do not let it come into contact with an open flame.
- If the patient has open cuts or lesions on the skin where the paraffin is to be applied, consult the doctor before carrying out the treatment.

THE EFFECTS OF COLD

Cold is used to lower the body temperature, to reduce inflammation, to control hemorrhage, and to relieve pain. Its effect is to contract the blood vessels and to reduce the flow of blood in the skin and the adjacent layers of tissues.

ICE BAGS

The device most commonly used to apply cold to a part of the body is an ice bag or an ice collar. Chemical bags are available that can be chilled in the freezing compartment of the refrigerator and used in the same way as an ice bag.

Equipment

Ice bag, complete with cap and washer

Container of finely cracked ice

Cloth ice bag covers

Procedure

- Inspect the ice bag or the ice collar and its cap and washer carefully to see that all the parts are in good condition.
- Fill the bag about half full with ice.
- Squeeze the bag in the hands to expel as much air as possible. Make sure that the washer is in place and screw on the cap securely.
- Dry the outside of the ice bag and place it in the cloth cover.
- Apply to the patient's body as ordered by the doctor.
- Empty the water from the bag and replace the ice as necessary. For the comfort of the patient and the protection of the bedding or the pillow, change the cover as it becomes moist.
- Discontinue the treatment when it has been applied for the prescribed length of time.
- Note the patient's reaction on the daily record.
- Care for the equipment:
  Empty and dry the bag.
  Inflate it with air and screw on the cap to keep the sides from sticking together. Store the bag in a cool, dry place to prevent deterioration of the rubber.
  Dry the covers and put them with the soiled laundry.

COLD MOIST COMPRESSES

Cold moist applications are sometimes ordered as treatment for an eye injury, following the extraction of a tooth, in some unusual skin conditions, and for relief of a headache. The size and the weight of the compress used will depend on where it is to be applied.

Equipment

Two or more compresses of the size and weight needed

Basin of ice with a small amount of water

Waterproof protector for the bed or the pillow

Procedure

- Place the patient in a comfortable position and protect the pillows or the bedding against moisture.
- Moisten a compress in the ice water, wring it out thoroughly to prevent dripping, and apply as ordered.
- Place another compress in the basin of ice and water to cool. If the patient is able to help, place the equipment conveniently near him so that he can change the compresses himself.
- Change the compress as soon as it begins to feel warm to the patient.
- Discontinue the treatment as ordered by the doctor, usually in about 15 or 20 minutes.
- Note on the daily record any reaction of the patient.
- Discard the soiled compresses.
- Empty, clean, and put the basin away.

SPONGE BATHS

The doctor may order a cold water or an alcohol sponge bath to reduce the patient's temperature. If cold water is used, it will probably cause the patient to shiver. If alcohol is used, its rapid rate of evaporation will remove heat very quickly from the body surface, also causing the patient to feel chilly. However, when a solution of equal parts of alcohol and tepid water is used, the sponge bath will be more comfortable for the patient.

Equipment

Waterproof protector for bed
Bath blanket or bath towels
Basin
Washcloths, towels
Hot water bottle (filled)

Ice bag (filled)
Extra blanket
Alcohol
Tepid water

- Prepare a solution of equal parts of alcohol and tepid water.
- Protect the bed with the waterproof sheet covered with a bath blanket or bath towels.
- Place an ice bag at the patient's head and a hot water bottle at his feet to make him comfortable.
- Place moist, cool cloths in the axilla and at the groin over the large superficial blood vessels.
- Bathe the patient's entire body surface, including his back, with the alcohol-water solution.
- Observe the patient closely for any change in color or for an increase in the rate of his pulse and respiration. Stop immediately if he is shivering or appears to be having a chill.
- Stop the bathing after 20 or 30 minutes and remove the wet linens, the ice bag, and the hot water bottle.
- Dry the patient and replace his gown or his pajamas.
- Cover the patient with a light blanket or a sheet and make him as comfortable as possible.

POINTS TO REMEMBER ABOUT TREATMENTS USING COLD

- Cold treatments should be used only when ordered by the doctor.
- The body adjusts to external cold by varying the amount of heat production or heat loss by muscle reaction (shivering) or by constriction of the blood vessels in the skin.
- Body reactions to moderate cold are both immediate and delayed. The immediate reaction causes the skin to become pale and cool, sometimes with the appearance of gooseflesh and shivering. The secondary reaction occurs in about 30 minutes; the skin becomes red and warm and pulse and respiration become slower.
- The effect of the application of cold depends upon the amount of body surface involved. The greater the area treated, the more intense is the reaction.
- Application of cold to the entire body has a sedative effect.
- Lower degrees of temperature can be tolerated if the cold application is dry rather than moist.
- The age of the patient must be considered when cold is being applied because the temperature-regulating mechanism of the body is less stable in the very young and the aged.

16

MEDICATIONS

GENERAL CONSIDERATIONS

When the doctor writes a prescription, it is taken to a pharmacist. The pharmacist fills the prescription and usually includes on the label of the container the following information: name of the patient, name of the doctor, date filled, instructions for taking, and a prescription number. If the prescription contains a narcotic or is one of several medicines that are under regulation by law, the label may indicate that the prescription cannot be refilled.

All medicine should be clearly labeled, and any with no label or an unreadable one should be properly disposed of. Medicine should be kept in a safe place that is known to the responsible adults in the household, away from children, and apart from other bottles and jars. Medicines in dark bottles should be kept in dark places because light causes a chemical change in the contents. Liquid medicines, even those to be kept in the refrigerator, should not be allowed to freeze.

The doctor may order medicine to be taken one time, once a day, several times a day, before or after meals, at bedtime, or at other regular intervals. If the directions for giving a medication are not clearly understood, the home nurse should consult the doctor before giving the medicine to the patient. Any medicine may be unsafe if the wrong dosage is taken. Also, if there is anything unusual about the appearance, smell, or taste of the medicine, if pills are discolored, or if a liquid has crystallized, the medicine should not be taken until its safety has been discussed with the doctor. Medicine taken by mouth may be in the form of a liquid, a powder, pills, tablets, and capsules.

Medicine that has a disagreeable taste may be followed by a cookie, a cracker, fruit, or fruit juice if the doctor permits. However, persons on a restricted or a special diet may not always have such freedom of choice. Also, discretion must be used in this practice, for both adults and children may associate the food with the medicine and acquire a dislike for the food. Medicine that may discolor the teeth or have an adverse effect on the enamel of the teeth is usually taken through a drinking tube or a straw and is swallowed quickly. The patient should then rinse his mouth. Cough syrups should not be diluted if they are to have the desired effect, and therefore they should not be followed by fluids or by food.

The doctor may occasionally order medicine that must be given hypodermically. The doctor, or a public health or other professional nurse can teach someone in the family or the patient himself how to give the medicine in this way. Most patients who need to have medicine regularly by hypodermic injection learn to give their own.

Some other ways of giving medicine are by inhalation, by rectum, and by absorption through the skin.

Unused medicine should be promptly destroyed and the safest way to dispose of it is by burning. Liquid medicine can be poured over crumpled newspapers, which may then be burned. Flushing some medicines down the toilet may discolor the porcelain. Destruction of medicine no longer needed prevents active, dangerous drugs from doing harm to anyone. Also, many medicines deteriorate with age, some becoming weak and therefore ineffective, others becoming stronger and therefore dangerous.

ORAL MEDICATIONS FOR ADULTS

Equipment

Tray of suitable size
Medicine as ordered
Medicine glass or paper cup
Standard-size teaspoon or medicine dropper
Glass of cool, fresh water
Good natural or artificial light for reading directions

Paper wipe or napkin
Something to mask an unpleasant taste, if desired and allowed, such as a piece of fruit, a cracker, or ice
Glass or plastic drinking tube or disposable straw

Procedure

When giving liquid medicine:

- Compare the label on the medicine bottle with the doctor's orders, reading aloud. If the directions so specify, shake the bottle well to distribute the drug equally throughout the solution.
- Remove the cork or the bottle top and place it top side down on the tray for cleanliness.
- Pour the medicine into the spoon or the medicine glass, holding the bottle so that the label is toward the palm of the hand to keep the label clean and readable.
- Measure the amount accurately, holding the medicine glass so that the line measuring the needed amount is at eye level.
- Hold the dropper vertically when measuring drops, to keep the liquid from running into the bulb of the dropper and count aloud. Before giving the medicine to the patient, add a small amount of water if it is allowed.
- Read the label again before giving the medicine to the patient.
- Give him the medicine, making sure that he swallows it. Follow with water or other liquid.

When giving tablets, pills, or capsules:

- Compare the label on the box or the bottle with the doctor's orders.
- Use a spoon to remove the medicine from the container for cleanliness.
- Close the container and read the label again before putting it aside.
- Give the medicine to the patient from the spoon.
- Have the patient place the medicine on the back of his tongue, take a mouthful of water, tilt his head back, and swallow. The medicine should go down easily. The patient should chew a tablet or allow it to dissolve in his mouth, if the doctor so orders.
- Stay with the patient until he has swallowed the medicine. It may be necessary to examine his mouth to be sure that he does not hold the medicine in his mouth and remove it later.
- Note on the daily record the kind and the amount of medicine given, the time it was given, and any effect observed later. If the patient fails to take the medicine as ordered, note also the reason: "Asleep," "Refused," or "Vomited the medicine."
- Care for the equipment:
    Cleanse the glasses and the spoon or the tube.
    Set up the tray for the next use. If medicine is kept on the tray, put the tray in a safe place.

284

Giving medicine to children requires special knowledge and skill. Almost all medicines are ordered in smaller amounts for children than for adults, and the dosages quite often are in proportion to the body weight of the child. Naturally, the home nurse must observe all the safety requirements of giving the right amount in the manner prescribed and at the time ordered.

Most toddlers and some older children will to some extent resist taking any medicine. The principal skill needed by the home nurse is the ability to persuade children to take medication by mouth. Her approach should be positive, calm, and firm but kind. There should be no implication by word, tone of voice, or manner that there is any doubt that the child will take the medicine. He should be helped to understand that the medicine is necessary to help him get well. Such questions as "Does it taste bad?" and "Will this be all?" should be answered truthfully. Some children respond well when they are made to feel that the decision to take medicine rests with them. If the child wishes to take his own oral medicine rather than have it given to him, he should be allowed to do so. Taking the medicine from a special small cup or glass, such as a cup from a set of doll dishes, may appeal to a child. It is common practice to disguise the taste of some medicines in fruit juice or jelly, and every effort should be made to make the taking as pleasant as possible. Even though a child may have shown considerable resistance to taking the medicine, he should be praised for his cooperation.

If the child is not old enough to swallow a pill, tablet, or capsule, the pill or the tablet may be crushed and the capsule emptied into a spoon. Water added will dissolve the powder. A drink of water should follow its administration.

Giving medicine by mouth to babies is comparatively easy, although care must be taken not to choke them, for they may cough out or vomit the medicine. A medicine dropper works well in placing the medicine on the baby's tongue. A small paper cup, such as those used in lining cupcake pans, is also easy to use, because it can be compressed by the fingers and the medicine can be expelled into the baby's mouth as from a funnel. In general, drugs should not be put into the baby's formula. All of the formula may not be taken, and then, too, this practice may cause the baby to refuse the usual formula.

POINTS TO REMEMBER ABOUT GIVING MEDICINES

- Give medicine only to the one for whom it is prescribed.
- Give medicine only when and as directed and in the amounts prescribed by the doctor.
- Have a good light and read the label aloud at least twice, once when taking the bottle from the shelf and once after the medicine is poured or otherwise removed from the container.
- Check with the doctor if anything about the medicine seems unusual.
- Note and record any change in the patient's condition after the medicine has been taken.
- Have a safe place, known to all adults in the family, for keeping the medicines. A first aid book may also be kept with the medicines.
- Keep the doctor's name and telephone number and the telephone number of the nearest hospital in a convenient place near the telephone.
- Dispose of unused medicine promptly.
- Remember the "Five Rights" in giving medicine—
  - The right medicine
  - To the right patient
  - At the right time
  - In the right manner
  - In the right amount

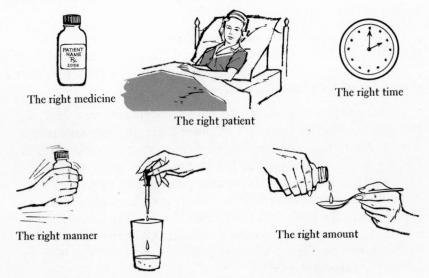

The "Five Rights" in giving medicine.

The right medicine

The right patient

The right time

The right manner

The right amount

EYE DROPS

The purpose of using eye drops is to relieve eye conditions, to dilate the pupils for a doctor's examination, to soothe irritation, or to relieve pain. Putting drops in the patient's eye is a treatment ordered by the doctor that can safely be carried out at home. If the patient has not had this done for him before, his part in the procedure should be explained. He should also be instructed to hold as still as possible while the medicine is being placed in the eye. Some drugs will cause a stinging sensation and blurred vision, but the patient should be cautioned against squeezing his eyes shut tightly, using pressure with the fingers, or rubbing the lids forcefully.

Eye drops are usually dispensed in a small bottle with a dropper attached to the top. The person giving the medicine should make sure that his hands are clean and should take every precaution to keep all equipment clean. If by accident the tip of the dropper touches the eye or anything else, the dropper must be cleaned before it is returned to the bottle. In addition, for cleanliness, any unused medicine in the dropper should be thrown away.

Eye medications usually have an expiration date, after which they should not be used. This date, which appears on the label, should be checked carefully each time the medication is used, and outdated medicine should be destroyed.

Equipment

Drops prescribed by the doctor

Clean medicine dropper

Towel or other shoulder protection

Paper tissues, wipes, or cotton balls

Procedure

- Wash the hands well before starting the treatment.
- Have the patient sit in a comfortable position facing a good light with his head tilted back.
- Loosen the top of the bottle so that the dropper can be removed easily. Have ready a tissue or a cotton ball with which to wipe the patient's cheeks.
- Check the label of the bottle.
- Hold the dropper vertically so that no medicine goes into the bulb.
- Try to draw up only the amount needed. Make sure the dropper contains enough medicine if both eyes are to be treated.

287

- Recheck the label on the bottle.
- Stand in back of the patient or at his side.

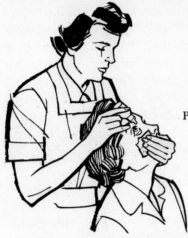

Putting drops in the patient's eyes.

- Hold the dropper in one hand. Draw down the lower lid of the patient's eye gently with the first two fingers of the other hand, using a cotton ball or a tissue. Never press on the eyeball.
- Ask the patient to look up without moving his head.
- Brace the hand holding the dropper by placing the little finger against the patient's cheek. Otherwise, reflex action when the drops are administered may cause the patient to jerk his head and to come in contact with the dropper, with possible injury to his eye.
- Holding the dropper above the lower lid but not touching the eye, the lid, or the lashes with the dropper, gently press out the number of drops ordered by the doctor, letting them fall into the lining of the *lower lid*, never on the eye.
- Tell the patient to close his eye so that the drops are distributed over its surface. Wipe away any medicine or tears from the cheeks.
- Treat the other eye at once if ordered. *Do not allow the dropper to touch anything.*
- Return the dropper to the bottle to keep the tube and the drops absolutely clean if there is a delay before treating the patient's second eye.
- Tell the patient not to rub his eyes after they are treated.
- Dispose of any medicine remaining in the tube. Clean the dropper if the tip of it touched the eye or anything else, and return it to the bottle. If a separate dropper was used, rinse it thoroughly and put it away.

- Note on the daily record the time the drops were administered, the condition of the eyes, and any reaction, immediate or delayed, on the part of the patient.

If it is necessary for the patient to administer the drops himself, he may stand before a mirror so that he can see what he is

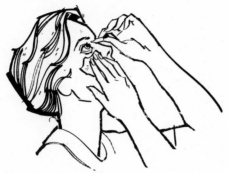

The patient may administer eye drops unassisted.

doing and with one hand draw the lower lid down to form a cup. He then drops the medicine into the cup. Another way to self-administer the drops is for the patient to lie down without a pillow under his head and with one hand pull the lower lid down. He may rest the dropper across the bridge of his nose and use the dropper as a guide to drop the medicine on the lining of the lower eyelid.

Points To Remember

- Keep the hands, the medicine dropper, and all equipment clean. *Never* use the dropper for any other solution until it is properly cleansed and, preferably, boiled for 3 minutes.
- Be very gentle.
- Allow the medicine to drop on the lining of the patient's lower lid.
- Tell the patient to keep his hands away from his eyes.
- Discard any solution left in the dropper. If the dropper has touched anything, clean it before returning it to the bottle.

EYE OINTMENTS

Eye ointments are usually dispensed from a tube. If the ointment is ordered for the inner surface of the eye, a small amount is gently squeezed from the tube into the cupped lower lid in the same manner that drops are administered. Take the same precautions as with the dropper to keep the open end of the tube from becoming soiled and from touching anything.

If the doctor orders an ointment for treatment of the outer surfaces or the edges of the eyelids, they should first be cleansed of any discharge or secretions. He will recommend a cleansing solution and tell the home nurse how it is to be used. The ointment may be applied gently with a cotton applicator at the time and in the amount prescribed.

17

EMERGENCY TREATMENTS

Nearly all emergency treatments in the home relate to injuries caused by accidents, most of which could have been prevented. No age group is immune, but children and old people are particularly prone to accidents for reasons that are self-evident.

Simple objects used every day can become dangerous weapons in the hands of someone in a hurry. It is important to develop the habit of doing household tasks in a safe manner and of being constantly on the alert for dangerous conditions that could cause accident or injury. Cuts and burns are probably the commonest injuries encountered by the home nurse, and they range in importance from a minor wound to one of great severity. Care and attention should be given to all wounds so that healing is promoted and infection prevented. Drugs and household substances that are potential poisons should be safely stored and kept out of the reach of children. Electrical appliances should be kept in working order so that they are not a source of burns or of electrical shock.

The best source of advice on the care of any wound is the family physician. If he is unavailable in an emergency, care must be provided for the protection of the patient. It is usually safe to carry out the procedures described below.

CARE OF MINOR WOUNDS

Equipment

Soap and water
Adhesive tape
Scissors

Sterile dressing
Bandage

291

- Wash the hands thoroughly with clean soap and water.
- Cleanse the injury thoroughly, using a sterile dressing to apply plain soap and cooled boiled water or clean, running tap water. To open the package containing the sterile dressing, tear or cut along one side and handle the dressing by the corner to avoid soiling it.
- Pat the wound dry with a sterile dressing.
- Apply a dry sterile dressing over the wound and bandage or tape it in place.
- See the doctor promptly if there is any evidence of infection.

CARE OF MAJOR WOUNDS

Control of bleeding is of urgent importance, and first aid should be started at once. Most external bleeding can be controlled by a pressure dressing placed directly over the wound. Sterile dressings are preferred, but in an emergency the bare hand may be used. Dressings are applied to prevent infection and the loss of body fluids.

Immediate care should be given to a patient who has suffered extensive thermal burns. Only large, easily separated foreign particles, such as pieces of clothing, should be removed. If the clothing adheres, as much of it as possible should be cut away and fragments of cloth left in place to be removed later by the doctor. Complete removal may cause bleeding, additional injury, or infection.

Equipment

Dressings	Binders or tensile-type bandages
Scissors	Safety pins or adhesive

Procedure

- Apply a dressing large enough to cover the injured area completely.
- Secure the dressing in place with a tensile-type bandage or a binder, using firm, gentle, even pressure to control the loss of body fluid.
- Fasten the bandage or the binder with safety pins, adhesive, or a knot.
- Apply another dressing over the original dressing if blood or drainage soaks through the dressing.

- Apply a label or use lipstick or a crayon to indicate a second dressing, the size of the seepage stain, and the time the dressing was applied.

POINTS TO REMEMBER

- Get medical care for the patient as quickly as possible.
- Stop bleeding promptly.
- Apply pressure directly over the wound and secure the dressing firmly in place.
- Use sterile dressings if possible; otherwise, use cloth as clean as can be obtained.
- Place finely woven cloth or gauze next to the wound.
- Elevate a wounded arm or leg to help control any bleeding.
- Give nothing by mouth if a wound is in the chest or the abdomen.
- Apply no medicine or ointment to a burn *except when ordered by the doctor.*
- Do not break the blisters of a burn.

IMPROVISED DRESSINGS

Heavy bath towels make excellent improvised pressure dressings for large wounds, but there should be a protective layer of finely woven sterile cloth between them and the injured area because the loose threads of the toweling will adhere to the wound. Nor should absorbent cotton be placed next to the injury, because it, too, will adhere to a cut or a burn and its fibers will be difficult to remove. A linen napkin is a good substitute for conventional dressings and can be placed next to the wound before the towel is applied.

Pressure dressings are the recommended treatment in the care of extensive burns to help prevent infection, to relieve pain, to keep the affected area clean, and to prevent the loss of body fluids. Only sterile or clean dressings should be used. If the burn is extensive and sterile dressings are not available, the burned area should be covered with a clean, dry sheet, and a padding of thick, dry bath towels should be applied and held in place with a snug binder.

Sterile dressings may be purchased in sizes suitable for ordinary use. Some are packaged singly; others come in packs of 6 or 12 or more. Sterile dressings are completely free from disease germs and must be carefully handled to avoid their becoming unsterile. Some packages have to be cut open; others are manufactured with a string that, when pulled, slits the package open along one edge. The dressing should be handled by one corner or with sterile forceps or points of scissors so that the surface is kept sterile until placed on the wound.

If sterile dressings are not available, several layers of clean fabric can be placed over the wound. Before the cloth is used, it must be treated to remove some of the germs by being ironed with a very hot iron. A dressing may also be sterilized by being placed, loosely wrapped, in a large covered pan in a 300° F. oven. A large white potato or a large container of water should be put in the oven at the same time. When the potato is done or when the water has boiled for 30 minutes, the dressings may be removed from the oven. Cloth that is to be used as a dressing may also be sterilized by being boiled for 5 minutes in clean water and then dried in the sunlight or with a very hot iron.

ARTIFICIAL RESPIRATION—MOUTH-TO-MOUTH OR MOUTH-TO-NOSE METHOD

Apnea, the stoppage of breathing, may be the result of a disease or an accident. Because the body cannot store oxygen, it must have a continuous fresh supply to carry on life. *Therefore, when breathing has stopped, some form of artificial respiration should be started at once,* and if at all possible someone should send for a doctor.

Any procedure that will create and maintain an open air passageway from his mouth to his lungs *and* provide for an alternate increase and decrease in the size of his chest will move air in and out. When a person is unconscious and not breathing, the base of his tongue tends to press against and block the upper air passageway.

To obtain an open airway:

• Clear the victim's air passageway of any foreign substance.

• Tilt his head back or slightly to the side, with full extension of his neck.

• Hold his lower jaw in a jutting-out position.

The purpose of the oral method of artificial respiration is to cause air to flow into and from the lungs by mechanical means when natural breathing ceases. This method has the advantage of providing immediate inflation of the victim's lungs. The rescuer who does not wish to have direct contact with the victim may hold a thin cloth over the victim's mouth or nose and breathe through it. The cloth does not greatly affect the exchange of air.

294

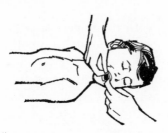

Quickly wipe out the victim's mouth.

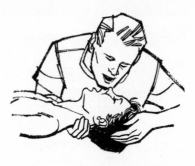

Tilt the head back so that the chin is pointing up.

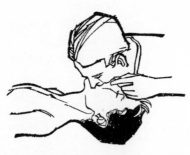

Put open mouth over the victim's mouth. Pinch his nostrils shut and blow into his mouth.

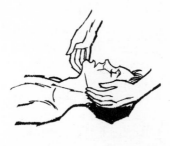

If not getting air exchange, recheck the head and jaw position.

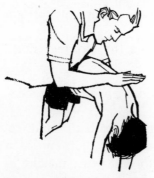

Invert a child over one arm and pat sharply two or three times between the shoulder blades to dislodge obstructing matter.

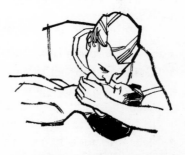

Immediately resume breathing into the victim's mouth.

Mouth-to-mouth resuscitation.

Procedures

For adults and older children:

- Turn the victim's head to the side and, with the fingers or with a cloth wrapped around the fingers, quickly wipe out his mouth to remove any visible foreign matter.
- Tilt the victim's head back so that his chin is pointing upward. Pull or push his jaw into a jutting-out position. These maneuvers should move the base of his tongue away from the back of his throat, thereby relieving obstruction in the airway.
- Open the mouth wide and place it tightly over the victim's mouth. At the same time, pinch his nostrils shut or close them by pressure of the cheek. Blow into the victim's mouth. Air may be blown through his teeth even if they are clenched. Or close the victim's mouth and blow into his nose. The first blowing efforts should determine whether or not obstruction exists.
- Remove the mouth and turn the head to the side to take another breath.
- Repeat the blowing effort. Blow vigorously at the rate of about 12 breaths a minute.
- Recheck the position of the victim's head and jaw if there is no air exchange.
- Try to obtain air exchange by quickly turning the victim on his side and giving him several sharp blows between the shoulder blades as an aid to dislodging any foreign material.
- Again sweep the fingers through his mouth to remove any foreign material.
- Reposition the patient quickly and resume the blowing effort.

For infants and young children:

- Clean out the victim's mouth quickly as described in the procedure above, if foreign matter is visible.
- Place the child on his back, using the fingers of both hands to lift his lower jaw from beneath and behind so that it juts out.
- Place the mouth over the child's *mouth and nose*, making a relatively leakproof seal.
- Breathe into the child, using shallow puffs of air appropriate to the size of the victim. The breathing rate should be about 20 times a minute.
- Recheck the position of the victim's jaw if there is resistance to the blowing efforts.
- Suspend the child momentarily by the ankles if the air passages are still blocked, or invert him over one arm and give him two or

three sharp pats between the shoulder blades in the hope of dislodging the obstructing matter.
- Reposition the child quickly and resume the breathing effort.

Points To Remember

- Begin some form of artificial respiration *at once.*
- Remove any foreign material from the victim's mouth and throat that is obstructing the airway.
- Always be sure that the tongue does not block the air passages.
- Turn the victim on his side without delay if vomiting occurs, and wipe out his mouth. Quickly reposition him and at once resume artificial respiration.
- Continue artificial respiration until the person can breathe for himself or until a physician pronounces him dead or until it is evident beyond any doubt that he cannot be made to breathe.
- Keep a revived victim as quiet as possible until he is breathing regularly. Cover him to conserve body heat, especially if he starts to shiver or if other circumstances indicate the need for additional warmth.
- Make sure that the victim receives medical care during his recovery.

BABY CARE

Nearly everyone has had some experience in handling children and is probably more skilled than he realizes. Many young parents receive so much advice that they begin to believe that caring for a new baby is very complicated. One important ingredient of infant care is common sense. Skill comes with practice, and each time the baby is bathed or clothed, handling him becomes easier. With practice comes confidence, relaxation, and inner security, which are evidenced by the touch of loving hands and one's facial expression. All of this tenderness is reflected in the baby's satisfaction at the attention he receives and in his emotional response to his parents.

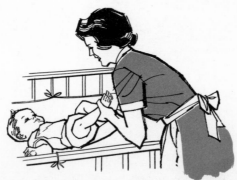

Picking up the baby.

HANDLING THE YOUNG BABY

Because of the great importance of safety in caring for the young baby, the skills necessary in the day-to-day handling of the young baby are illustrated and explained on page 299.

When picking up the baby:

- Grasp the baby's feet at the ankles, placing a finger between his ankles for security and comfort, and lift his buttocks slightly.
- Slip the other hand under his buttocks and up along his back and, with the fingers spread, support his head and his shoulders.
- Shift the hand from his ankles to his buttocks, supporting them in the palm of the hand, and raise the baby gently into the arms. Avoid any sudden motion, which may frighten him. Give support to the heaviest parts of his body: head, back, and buttocks.

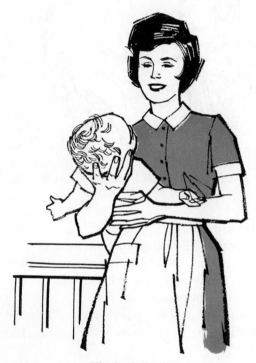

The football hold.

For using the football hold:

- Pick up the baby, supporting his head, back, and buttocks with both hands.
- Holding the baby in the arms, gently move him to one side so that his hip rests on the hip on the same side as the hand that supports his head and his back. Clasp him securely with the elbow. This position will free the other hand and arm.

For using the body-arm hold when bathing the baby:
- Slip one hand under the baby's head and shoulders as the infant lies on his back.

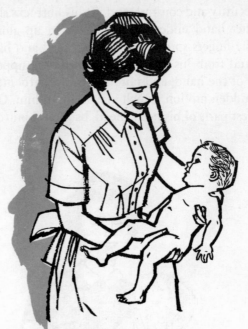

The body-arm hold is used to support the
baby when moving him.

- Grasp his far arm at the shoulder with a firm grip. With the other hand, support his buttocks in the palm of the hand, grasp-in his far leg at the thigh with the fingers and the thumb.
- Lift the baby gently and slowly lower him feet first into the water. Avoid quick motions.
- Maintain a firm grasp of the baby's arm and shoulder, support-ing his head on the wrist, and wash and rinse his chest, abdomen, and legs.
- Shift the grasp on the baby's arm and shoulder to the other hand. Reach across his chest and grasp his far arm at the shoulder. Let his chin rest forward on the wrist and the hand while his back is washed and rinsed.
- Return to the original hold, supporting the baby's head on the wrist, and grasping his arm and his shoulder firmly with the fingers of one hand. Support his buttocks and grasp his far leg at the thigh with the other hand.
- Lift the baby gently and slowly out of the tub.

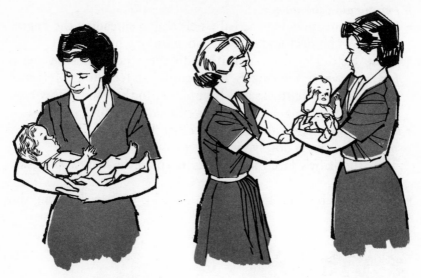

The cradle hold is used to transfer the baby to another person.

For using the cradle hold:

- Cradle the baby in both arms, the bent elbows supporting his head and his feet while he is being transferred to another person.
- Have the other person hold his arms forward, slightly bent, to receive the baby.
- Place the baby in the bend of the receiver's arms.
- So that the baby will feel secure, do not release him until he is safely in the arms of the other person.

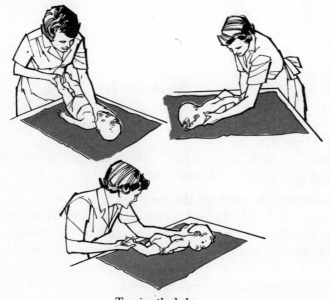

Turning the baby.

When turning the baby:

- Place a forearm along the baby's chest and spreading the fingers to support his neck and his head when turning him.
- Grasp his ankles from beneath with the other hand, placing a finger between the ankles for security and comfort. Lift the baby's legs and buttocks and turn him onto the hand with which his head, neck, and chest are being supported.
- Release his ankles and slip the other hand from beneath his body. The baby is now lying on his abdomen.
- Turn the baby's face to one side and place his hands alongside his head.
- Turn the baby from his abdomen onto his back by reversing the steps above.

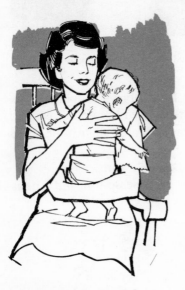

Gently rubbing or patting the baby's back
helps him to release swallowed air.

When burping the baby on the shoulder:

- Place a clean towel over one shoulder. Lift the baby, placing his head on the protected shoulder, with his face to one side so that he can breathe.
- Support his back and his head and gently rub or pat his back to help him to release the swallowed air.

When burping the baby on the lap:

- Use the free hand to reach across the baby's chest and grasp his far arm at the shoulder, supporting his chin on the forearm.
- Bring him to a sitting position, letting him lean forward for support.
- Gently rub his back to help him release the swallowed air.

Points To Remember

- Maintain a secure but gentle grasp when handling the baby.
- Lift the baby gently and slowly to avoid sudden motions, which frighten him.
- Support the baby's back and head at all times.
- Provide an opportunity for the baby to release swallowed air during and after feeding.

BATHING THE BABY

After the cord has dropped off and the umbilicus, or navel, has healed, the baby can be given a tub bath. This will be when he is from 10 days to 2 weeks old. Baths are given to keep the baby clean and his skin in good condition. But bathing is more than that to both the baby and his parents. It is a social experience for the baby and usually one that he enjoys. It has aspects of play as he grows older, and the laughter, talk, and cuddling he receives make it even more pleasant.

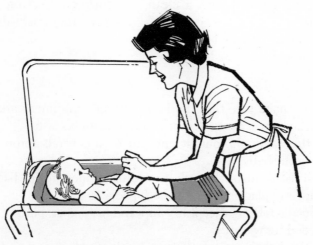

The baby must never be left alone during his bath.

It matters little when the bath is given, except that it should be before a feeding or not sooner than 1 hour afterward because the activity may cause him to spit up his food. The combination of a warm bath followed with a bottle or a meal usually makes the baby sleepy and ready for a nap. Some mothers bathe the baby in the late afternoon so that he is fresh and clean when his father comes home. If the father bathes the baby, he usually does it before the last feeding is given and the baby put to bed for the night.

303

The bath should be given at the same time every day, preferably when it does not conflict with other family activities.

The bath can be given in any room that is warm enough and free from drafts so that the baby does not get chilled. A bathinette is usually kept in the baby's room, for few bathrooms are large enough to accommodate this piece of equipment. The baby may be bathed also in a baby bathtub, in the washbasin in the bathroom, or in the kitchen sink if it is cleaned well both before and after the bath. Even before the baby can sit up, he may be bathed in the family bathtub, which allows him more freedom to kick and splash than does a bathinette or a baby bathtub. During his bath the baby must never be left alone and unprotected in the tub or on a table, from which he might easily fall.

Equipment

Bathinette, tub, basin, or sink	Clean clothing
Bath water of proper temperature, about 100° F.	Bath tray containing: soap, oil or lotion, powder or
Bath pad covered with a clean towel	cornstarch, cotton balls, safety pins, waste disposal bag
Newspaper for soiled clothing	
Bath towel and washcloth	

Procedure

- Check to make sure that the room and all equipment are ready before the baby is undressed or removed from his crib.
- Wash the hands thoroughly and put on a coverall apron before handling the baby.
- Lift the baby out of the crib, providing support to his back and his head, and place him on the bath pad.
- Remove all clothing except his shirt and his diaper, both of which are needed for warmth.
- Clean the baby's nostrils with a small piece of cotton twisted into a wick and moistened with clean water. Use a separate wick for each nostril. If commercial cotton applicators are used to clean his nose, remove the stick to avoid injuring his nose.
- Test the temperature of the water. It should be comfortably warm, about 100° F., when tested on the inside of the wrist.
- Palm the washcloth to prevent dragging and dripping. Wash the baby's eyes from the nose toward the ear. Wash his face without soap. Use a firm, gentle stroke, supporting his head with one hand. Dry his face.

304

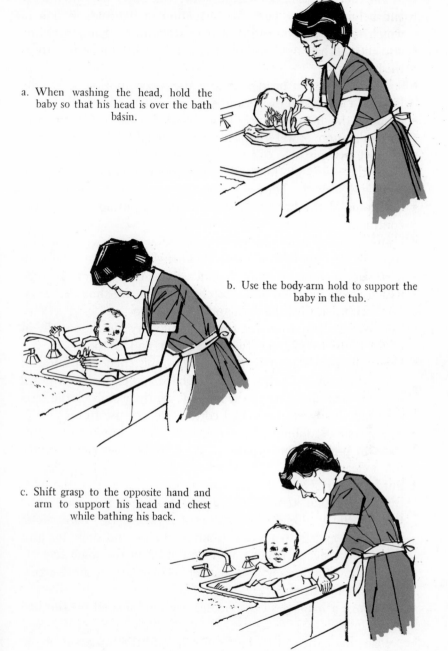

a. When washing the head, hold the baby so that his head is over the bath basin.

b. Use the body-arm hold to support the baby in the tub.

c. Shift grasp to the opposite hand and arm to support his head and chest while bathing his back.

Giving support while bathing the baby.

- Wash the baby's neck, washing only the outer part of his ear and behind it. Give particular attention to the folds of skin in which moisture, lint, and dust may accumulate. Rinse and dry.
- Use the football hold to hold the baby so that his head is over the bath basin.
- Soap and wash his head with a gentle rotary motion, using the hand or a washcloth. Rinse and dry.
- Remove the baby's diaper. If it is soiled, cleanse his buttocks with oil, lotion, or water-moistened cotton balls.
- Remove his shirt.
- Place the soiled clothing on a newspaper or other protection.
- Wet and soap the hands.
- Beginning at the baby's chest and arms and using firm, gentle, continuous strokes, soap his entire body.
- Using the body-arm hold, pick up the baby and slowly slide him feet first into the bath water to avoid frightening him. Maintain a firm grasp on far arm and shoulder. Rinse the front of his body.
- Reach across his chest and grasp his far arm and shoulder. Lean him forward against the wrist and rinse his back.
- Remove the baby from the tub. Carefully dry him, especially in all the folds of skin and between his fingers and his toes.
- Wash the baby's genitals, using cotton moistened with water or oil. If the baby is a girl, separate the labia and cleanse downward once on each side. If the baby is a boy, gently push back the foreskin and wipe with moistened cotton. Do not use force.
- Apply a small amount of powder, baby oil, or lotion to his buttocks to prevent skin irritation. Avoid using excessive amounts.
- Put a clean diaper on the baby.
- Put on a shirt. Open the neck of the shirt wide so that the baby can see through as it is placed over his head. Slip the fingers through the wrist end of the sleeve, grasp the baby's hand, holding all his fingers to prevent injury to them, and draw his arm through the sleeve. A gown may be put on in the same way.
- Wrap the baby loosely in a blanket so that he can move freely and without restraint:

  Arrange a blanket so that it lies diamond-shaped on the bed or a table.

  Place the baby so that his head is toward the top point of the blanket.

  Turn one pointed side loosely across the baby. Cover his feet by folding the bottom point upward and then bring the other point across the baby.

- Put the baby in his crib or in a safe place.
- Clean and dry the bath equipment and put it away.

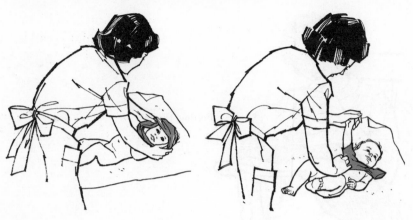

Putting on the baby's shirt.

FEEDING THE BABY

Not only is it simpler, easier, and more economical to breast-feed a baby, but it is a great satisfaction to a mother to feel that she can contribute in this way to her baby's well-being. However, for many good reasons the baby may have to be fed a formula prescribed by the doctor.

Excellent instructions for formula preparation are given in *Infant Care*, a pamphlet published by the Children's Bureau. The method used to prepare a formula will depend somewhat on the ingredients used, but the terminal sterilization method is generally considered to be the easiest and safest way. Its chief disadvantage is that it cannot be used for cultured or "sour milk" mixtures or for formulas to which are added vitamins that are destroyed by or suffer loss from heat. Another way, known as the aseptic method, is to sterilize all the equipment, prepare the feeding mixture, and pour it into the sterilized bottles. Either method is all right. Regardless of how a formula is prepared, scrupulous cleanliness must be observed. All equipment should be assembled for convenience in preparing the formula, washed thoroughly with hot water and soap or detergent, and rinsed thoroughly.

Many hospitals have a nurse demonstrate formula preparation for the mother before she takes the baby home. Upon request, a public health nurse will make home visits to give additional instruction in baby care to those who want this help. Many Red

Cross chapters offer classes for expectant parents where they can observe and practice preparing infant feedings.

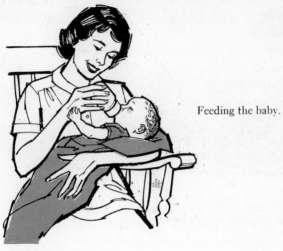

Feeding the baby.

The baby must be held properly during the feeding. The person giving the baby a bottle should sit in a comfortable chair and support the baby's head and back in the bend of the arm, elevating the head so that the baby will have no difficulty swallowing. There should be fluid in the neck of the bottle at all times to prevent the baby from swallowing air, and he should be burped several times during a feeding to release any air he may have swallowed.

TERMINAL STERILIZATION METHOD OF FORMULA PREPARATION

The purpose of sterilization is to cleanse and sterilize bottles, equipment, and formula for infant feeding.

Equipment

Ingredients for formula
Nursing bottles, complete with nipples, caps, and discs
1-quart formula pitcher
Measuring spoon
Can opener

Table knife for leveling powdered milk
Long-handled stirring spoon
Bottle brush
Pencil or similar blunt object to turn nipples inside out
Bottle sterilizer or substitute

Procedure

• Wash the bottles and all other equipment thoroughly in hot water and soap or detergent. Scrub the inside of the bottles with a bottle brush. Rinse everything thoroughly with hot water.

- Turn the nipples inside out with the eraser end of a pencil or other blunt instrument, wash them with hot, soapy water, and rinse them well.
- Squeeze clean water through the holes in the nipples.
- If the nipples contain a metal valve, remove, wash, rinse, and replace each one after the nipples are washed and rinsed. To assure good nursing action, clean the pinhole valves in the base of the nipples.
- Wash the outside of the can and rinse it with boiling water before opening it if canned milk is used.
- Use level measurements for powdered milk and for other dry ingredients.
- Mix the formula in the pitcher according to directions, stirring only long enough to dissolve and mix the ingredients.
- Pour the prescribed amount of the formula into the bottles, filling the number needed for the feedings, usually one day's supply.
- Place the clean nipples on the bottles. If a sealing disc and a cap are used, the tip of the nipple goes into the bottles. If a nipple cover or guard is used, the nipple tip is placed upright and held in place with the screw-on cap. Either method is acceptable.
- Screw the caps on only partway to allow the steam to escape from the bottles.
- Prepare 2 or 3 bottles with water for drinking.
- Put the bottles of formula and of drinking water on the rack in the sterilizer. Pour 2 or 3 inches of water into the sterilizer and cover with the lid.
- Bring the water in the sterilizer to a boil and *boil actively for 25 minutes.* Time the sterilizing period with a clock.
- Remove the sterilizer from the heat after the water has boiled for 25 minutes.
- Let the sterilizer cool without removing the lid until the hands can be placed on its sides without burning.
- Remove the bottles from the sterilizer as soon as they are cool enough to handle, and tighten the nipple caps or the sealing disc.
- Put the bottles in the refrigerator when they have cooled. If for any reason the bottles cannot be refrigerated, leave them in the tightly covered sterilizer. Remove one bottle at a time as needed, making sure to replace the cover.
- Rinse the soiled bottle and nipples with cold water after each use for easier washing later.

WAYS TO FOLD DIAPERS

A diaper is the most ordinary item in a baby's wardrobe, yet it may be selected in a variety of fabrics and may be folded, according to choice, in several ways, depending on the baby's size, body build, and sex. For boys extra thickness is placed in the front, and for girls extra thickness is placed in the back.

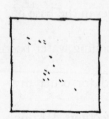 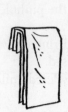 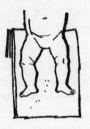 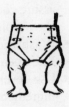

Square fold diaper. Fold first to make three thicknesses. Then fold over about one-third of the end. The extra thickness goes in the back for girls and in the front for boys. (This method of folding is good for new babies.)

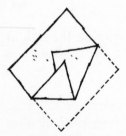 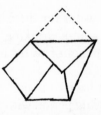 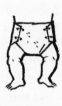

Kite fold with square. Keeping the thumb on one corner, fold over one side diagonally. Fold from bottom toward the top. Turn down top flap. Fold in the other side to cover the points. (This makes a comfortable thick center panel.)

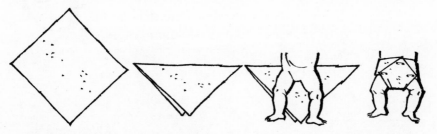

Triangle fold. Fold a square diaper diagonally twice. Best for a boy because the extra thickness comes in front. (This simple method was a favorite in grandmother's day.)

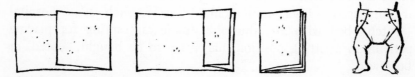

Panel fold. Fold an oblong diaper crosswise, bringing up one end to about 8 inches from the other. Turn back short end to within 2 or 3 inches of folded edge. Turn the other end to the edge of the first fold. (This makes a neat, easily adjusted diaper.)

19

IMPROVISED EQUIPMENT

Sometimes during a short illness or in an emergency, nursing care equipment must be improvised. Some of it can be adapted or made from materials available in the home at much less cost than if purchased. Other equipment, however, such as a hospital (Gatch) bed with an adjustable frame and spring for placing patients in a sitting position, may have to be bought, rented, or borrowed.

Before making, buying, or putting any piece of equipment into use, the following points should be considered: How long will it be needed? Could it be borrowed? Could it be made at home? Would it cost less to make rather than to rent or purchase it? Is someone with the necessary skill and time available to make the article so that it is safe, attractive, and durable for as long as the patient needs it? Does the improvised equipment satisfactorily serve the purpose for which it is needed? Will it bring comfort to the patient? Can it be easily handled? Is it safe for the patient and the home nurse to use? Will there be any danger in its use to children or anyone else in the home? Will it damage furniture or utensils in any way? Is it easy to keep clean?

Ingenuity is a desirable talent for the home nurse to possess. The ideas presented here should suggest other improvisations that will be useful in saving time and energy for the home nurse and that will make the patient more comfortable and hasten his recovery.

BACK RESTS

The purpose of a back rest is to provide support when a patient sits up in bed.

312

Several varieties of back rests, such as a rattan car seat, a triangular lounge pillow, or a bed pillow with arm rests can be purchased. An improvised back rest is often just as effective and can

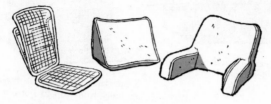

Suggested back rests.

be made easily. Some suggestions are a covered card table, with its legs folded, slanted against the head of the bed and tied securely in place; overstuffed or foam pillows from a chair or a davenport, covered and if necessary tied in place; the seat and the back from a kitchen chair that has had the legs removed; or a cardboard carton back rest.

Equipment

Large cardboard carton approximately 24 by 24 by 18 inches, with cover flaps intact
Sharp knife
Strong cord, several discarded nylon hose, or 2-inch gummed paper tape to fasten back rest
Cloth to cover

Procedure

- Use the broad side of the carton for the front of the back rest. To provide safe support for the patient's shoulders, it should be at least 24 inches in breadth.
- Slit the corners of the front side from top to bottom and let the front side fall forward and lie flat temporarily.
- Score the two sides of the carton diagonally with a knife *on the inner surface* from the back at the top to the lower front corner. Bend the sides inward along the line of scoring.
- Score and bend inward any excess of cardboard at the top of the side cover flaps.
- Bring the cover flap on the back of the carton forward and place it over the folded side flaps. Bring the front side of the carton up over the folded-down back cover flap. To give added strength, crease and bend any excess cardboard from the front side over the back at the top. The resulting form is a triangular back rest.

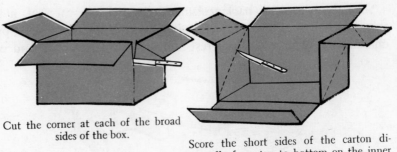

Cut the corner at each of the broad
sides of the box.

Score the short sides of the carton diagonally from top to bottom on the inner
surface.

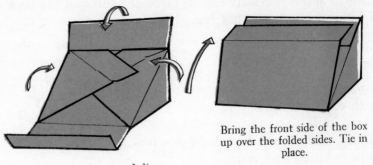

Bend inward on the scored lines.

Bring the front side of the box
up over the folded sides. Tie in
place.

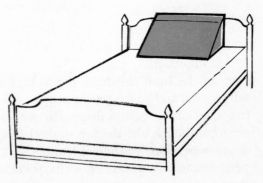

Place on the bed with the slanting side toward
the patient.

Making a back rest from a cardboard box.

- Tie a strong cord or old nylon hose around the back rest, placing the knots so that they will not be under the patient's back. For a smoother finish, the back rest can be fastened with broad gummed paper tape.
- Cover the back rest with a piece of cloth to give it a neat appearance and to keep the bedding clean. Also, the back rest may be covered with plastic or wallpaper or be painted, to improve its appearance.
- Place the back rest on the bed with the slanting side toward the patient and the right-angled corners toward the head of the bed. If the narrow base is against the mattress, the patient will be sitting almost upright. If the broader base is down, the patient's head and shoulders will be lower.

FOOT SUPPORTS

A support that is approximately 2 inches higher than the patient's feet are long should be provided to prevent weight or pressure on his toes and to maintain proper position of the feet. The type of support is determined by the position of the patient, that is, whether he is lying flat or is elevated in bed, and by the nature and the length of his illness. The paralyzed patient or the patient with a long-term illness has special needs that may require a firmer support or one specially adapted to his disability.

Equipment

Strong cardboard carton approximately 9 by 12 by 14 inches, with cover flaps intact
Washable cover made of toweling or other heavy fabric
(for the patient lying flat or sitting up)
Firm support constructed for long-term use (for the patient with special needs)

Procedures

When the patient is lying flat:

- Lock, tape, or tie the cover flaps of the carton in place.
- Cover the carton with a towel or other heavy cloth.
- Adjust the support at the patient's feet, bracing it securely against the foot of the bed. The feet should be in normal walking position, with the heels and the soles of the feet flat against the support and the toes pointing upward.
- Place the top bed clothing over the foot support so that there is no weight on the patient's feet.

When the patient is sitting up:

- Construct a foot support by following directions for making a cardboard back rest.
- Cover the carton.
- Place the slanted side of the support against the patient's feet, bracing the straight side firmly against the foot of the bed.
- Place a thin, firm pad such as a folded bath towel under the patient's knees if it is needed for support.
- Place the top bed clothing over the foot support if needed to keep the weight off the patient's toes.

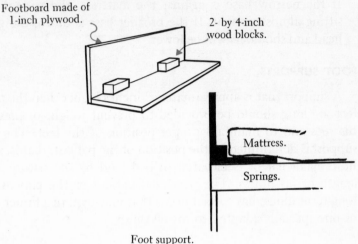

Footboard made of 1-inch plywood.

2- by 4-inch wood blocks.

Mattress.

Springs.

Foot support.

When the patient has special needs:

- Place the foot support against the footboard of the bed as shown in the illustration.
- Anchor the support firmly under the mattress so that the mattress is held away from the end of the bed to provide space at the end of the mattress for the patient's toes or heels.
- Position the patient's feet firmly against the support, maintaining his good body alignment.
- Place the top covers over the footboard to keep their weight off the patient's feet.

BED BLOCKS

Raising the patient's bed to a convenient height lessens the strain on the home nurse's back and shoulder muscles and reduces the fatigue she would otherwise feel. The bed is a suitable working height when the home nurse has to neither drop nor raise her shoulders when she places the palm of her hand flat on the mattress.

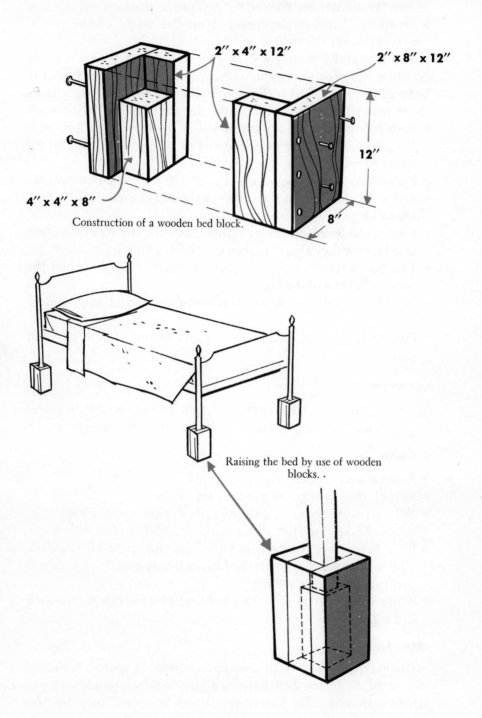

2″ x 4″ x 12″

2″ x 8″ x 12″

12″

8″

4″ x 4″ x 8″

Construction of a wooden bed block.

Raising the bed by use of wooden blocks. .

The distance from the floor to the top of the mattress will average from 30 to 32 inches, depending upon the height of the person who is caring for the patient in bed.

The resourceful person will be able to think of several ways to elevate a bed. For safety the casters should be removed from the bed legs before the bed is elevated. Following are some suggestions about materials for bed blocks and the way they are to be used.

- Four blocks of wood approximately 8 by 8 by 12 inches, with a 3- or 4-inch depression in one end of each to hold the bed leg securely.
- Four stacks of old magazines or folded newspapers, tied securely and with a hole cut in the center of the top of each stack to hold the bed leg.
- Four broad-based cinder or cement blocks (salt blocks are unsafe because they absorb moisture and may crumble).
- Two low sawhorses placed crosswise beneath the bedframe at the top and bottom of the bed.
- Four sturdy kitchen chairs, two under the rail at each end of the bed.
- Four large tin cans, each about two-thirds full of sand or small pebbles

Equipment

4 cans, No. 10 or larger, complete with tops and bottoms

Sand, small pebbles, or gravel to put in the cans

Procedure

- Remove and save the tops of the cans.
- Smooth the cut edges of the cans for safety.
- Fill each can about two-thirds full of sand, small pebbles, or gravel. Make sure that all four cans are filled to the same level.
- Place the tops of the cans on top of the sand, pebbles, or gravel. This arrangement gives the bed legs a steady base to rest on and prevents them from sinking.
- Remove the casters from the bed and place a can under each bed leg.

BED TABLES

Many types of bed tables may be purchased or rented. Some are placed on the bed; others have an adjustable floor stand, with the table on an adjustable arm so that it can be moved into position over the patient's lap. Others, like those used in most hospitals, reach completely across the bed, are on rollers, and can be adjusted in height. Most tables of this type have a concealed compartment for toilet articles and a mirror to aid the patient who is able to take care of his personal grooming. When suitably adjusted, the lid of the compartment converts to a writing surface or a support for reading matter.

A bed table can be improvised by placing the free end of an opened ironing board across the bed. Also, a wooden box or crate, such as an orange box, from which the two wide sides have been removed can be placed across the patient's lap. A satisfactory bed table can also be made from a cardboard carton.

Equipment

Clean, heavy cardboard carton approximately 10 by 12 by 24 inches

Sharp knife
Suitable cover

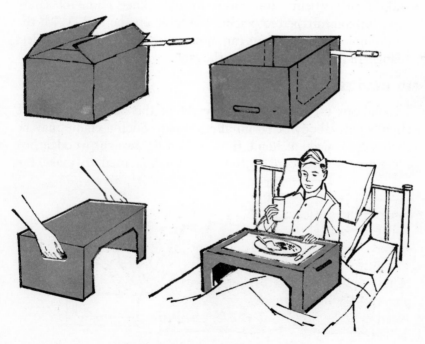

Making a bed table from a cardboard carton.

Procedure

- Cut away the top cover flaps from the carton. For safety, always turn the knife blade away from the body when cutting.
- Cut curved pieces out of the two wide sides of the carton to allow the table to fit comfortably over the patient's thighs. Leave at least 2 inches on each side and the top to support and strengthen the table top.
- Adjust the height of the table according to the size of the patient. With his shoulders level, he should be able to rest his arms comfortably on the table top.
- Cut a narrow opening near the top on each closed side so that the fingers may be inserted to lift and carry the table.
- Cover the cut edges of the carton with adhesive cellophane or gummed paper tape to strengthen the table.
- Cover the table with cloth, paint, wallpaper, or adhesive-backed plastic to improve its appearance.
- Adjust the patient's top covers to allow knee room for safety and for comfort before placing the table on the bed. With the bedding loose, the patient can move more easily and there is less danger of upsetting articles on the table.

BED CRADLES

A cradle is used to keep the weight of the bedclothes off the patient's entire body or off an affected part. Such a cradle may be purchased or made at home from wire, a lightweight wooden box or crate or a cardboard carton. The method used to make the

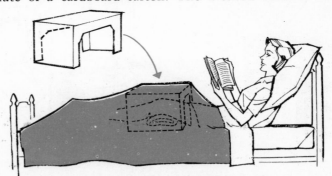

A bed cradle made from a cardboard carton.

cardboard bed table may also be used to make the bed cradle. The part of the body to be protected will determine the size of the cradle needed.

Because there is an airspace beneath the bedcovers when the cradle is in place, the patient may complain of being chilly. If more warmth is needed, it is probably better to warm the room than to put more blankets over the patient, because the additional weight of the covers is uncomfortable to the patient. Usually a well-wrapped hot water bottle placed at the patient's back or abdomen will provide the necessary extra warmth. If the patient's feet are cold, loose woolen socks will provide warmth and comfort.

BLANKET BATHROBES

When a patient has been in bed for some time, getting up becomes quite an occasion. The home nurse will need to see that the patient does not become chilled and that he is comfortably protected. Some type of bathrobe will be necessary and, in an emergency, a blanket may be used to improvise one.

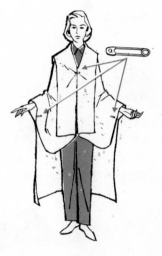

A blanket bathrobe provides warmth and protection.

Equipment

Single blanket of a weight suitable to the room temperature
3 large safety pins

Procedure

- Make a fold along the length of the blanket to form a collar, the width of the fold depending on the size of the blanket and the height of the patient. When finished, the improvised robe should be long enough to cover the patient's legs.
- Adjust the blanket around the patient's shoulders, center it at the back of the neck with the fold on the outside, and pin it together in front.

- Center one width of the blanket on the patient's wrist, turn the overhanging end into a cuff, and pin the material together to form a sleeve. The width of the cuff will depend on the size of the blanket and the length of the patient's arm.
- To make the second sleeve, repeat the preceding step, using the other wide edge of the blanket.
- Adjust the improvised robe for comfort, security, and appearance.
- Bring the collar forward over the patient's head to form a hood for additional warmth and protection.

SHOULDER SHAWLS

A shoulder shawl is used to provide a cover that will protect the patient against chilling. It is a substitute for a bed jacket.

Equipment

Large bath towel   Safety pin

Procedure

- Grasp the diagonally opposite corners of the towel and pull lengthwise so that the towel is folded diagonally.
- Locate the V that is formed by the fold.

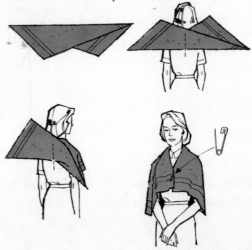

Steps in making a shoulder shawl from a large
bath towel.

- Place the towel on the patient's shoulders and bring the V to the back of his neck.
- Bring the two points over the patient's shoulders and pin them together evenly in front.

322

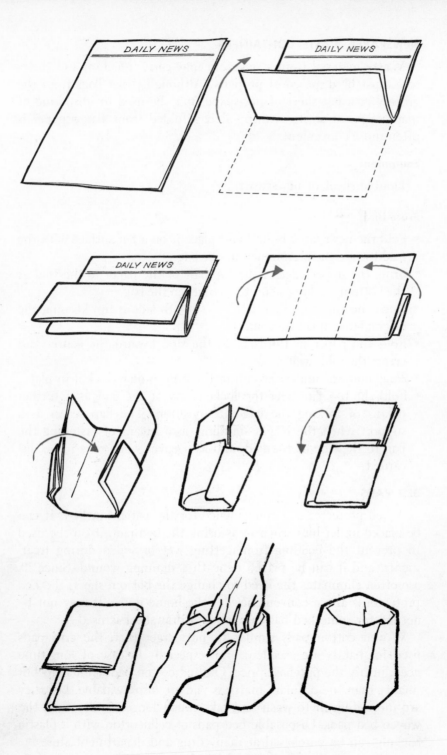

Steps in making a newspaper bag for waste disposal.

NEWSPAPER WASTE CONTAINERS

Waste material from a sickroom may carry infection and therefore must be disposed of properly. Although paper bags from the grocery or a flat sheet of newspaper may be used for disposing of many types of waste, a disposal bag folded from a newspaper is often more convenient.

Equipment

Double sheet of newspaper

Procedure

- Fold the newspaper in half and place it on a flat surface with the fold toward the person making the bag.
- Bring the upper edge of the top half of the paper to the fold at the bottom, making a cuff to strengthen the bag.
- Turn the paper over so that the smooth side is up, keeping the original fold at the bottom.
- Fold the paper in thirds from the side toward the center and crease the folds well.
- Tuck one side under the cuff of the other side to lock it in place.
- Fold the top flap over the locked side of the cuff as a further means of locking the bag into position. The flap serves as a support when the bag is standing, as a means of fastening the bag to the side of the bed, and as a cover when it is to be discarded.

BED PADS

A bed protector is a convenience for the patient in bed. It can be placed under him when he is using the bed pan; it can be used to prevent the bedding from getting wet or soiled during treatments; and it can be placed beneath a draining wound. Since its use often eliminates the need to change the bottom sheet, the bed protector is also a convenience for the home nurse. It may not be needed for some bed patients when a drawsheet is used.

Woven cotton pads similar to but larger than the crib pads used for babies are excellent and, especially in case of long-time need, justify the purchase price. Quilted cotton pads similar to but smaller than the ordinary mattress pad are also available, but they are more difficult to wash and take much longer to dry than the woven bed pads. Disposable bed pads of cellucotton with a plastic backing can be purchased at many drug and department stores.

An improvised protector made of cloth and newspapers protects the bed as effectively as a commercial pad. Because this kind of pad can become wet all the way through, the lower bedding should be further protected with a waterproof drawsheet if the patient is incontinent. Several of these pads are required so that there will be a supply on hand while the soiled cloth covers are being laundered.

Equipment

Cloth, approximately 25 by 36 inches

Newspapers, approximately 15 by 23 inches

Needle and thread or safety pins

Procedure

- Lay the cloth on a table with the long side parallel to the near table edge.
- Place several thicknesses of newspaper in the center of the cloth so that approximately 11 inches of cloth are left exposed on either side of the paper.
- Fold the two 11-inch sides of cloth over the newspaper, forming a 6-inch overlap of material.
- Pin or baste a seam along the short sides of the cloth. Remove the newspaper through the center opening in the cloth.
- Stitch the seams and turn the cover inside out for a smooth, flat finish.
- Prepare the pad for use by placing approximately six double sheets of newspaper inside the cloth cover.
- Place the smooth side of the pad next to the patient. When removing the pad, fold the smooth side in for cleanliness.
- Discard the newspapers and launder the cloth cover when they become wet or soiled.

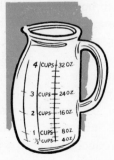 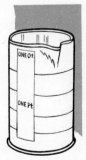

A commercial type (left) and an improvised (right) urinal.

325

BEDPANS AND URINALS

A urinal is usually a bottle-shaped receptacle that male patients use when urinating. A substitute for it during a short illness or in an emergency may be an empty tall fruit juice can, 42-ounce size, from which one end has been removed. There should be no sharp or rough edges on the can. An empty clean paper milk carton with the top cut off or a quart glass jar or pitcher may also be used. All of these items should be discarded when no longer needed.

If the illness is prolonged, it is more satisfactory to use a commercially manufactured urinal made of glass or metal. This piece of equipment can be purchased and sometimes borrowed or rented.

Because it is more difficult and less satisfactory to improvise a bedpan, it is better to borrow, rent, or buy one. However, in an emergency, a bedpan can be improvised. A flat pan approximately 2 by 8 by 12 inches can be placed in a flat cardboard box, and an oval opening can be cut in the top surface of the box to form a seat.

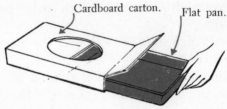

Cardboard carton.   Flat pan.

Improvised bedpan.

COTTON APPLICATORS

A cotton applicator is used to apply an antiseptic to simple wounds or to use for other purposes, such as cleansing the mouth. Cotton-tipped applicators can be purchased in drugstores and in most food markets and are relatively inexpensive. Some applicators have as a safety device cotton tips attached to flexible paper or plastic sticks. Satisfactory applicators can be made quickly for immediate use or prepared in quantity when a need is anticipated.

Equipment

Absorbent cotton
Round toothpicks or wooden
applicator sticks

Clean water
Clean towel
Clean, covered glass jar

Procedure

- Wash the hands well before starting.
- Place the equipment on a clean towel.

326

- Select a piece of cotton, the amount depending upon the size of the applicator desired.
- Wet the end of the toothpick or the applicator stick to make the cotton adhere.
- Place the moist end of the stick at the center of the piece of cotton so that it will be well covered for the protection and the comfort of the patient.
- Roll the stick between the fingers of one hand, holding and shaping the cotton with the fingers of the other hand to bind it securely to the tip.
- Store in a clean, covered container, placing the cotton end down for cleanliness when handling.

FUNNELS FOR STEAM INHALATIONS

A funnel is used to direct live steam to the inside of a croup tent. When a commercially manufactured inhalator is not available or when a concentrated flow of steam within the croup tent is desired, a funnel or a tube of paper may be used to direct the steam from the hot water to the inside of the tent over the patient. Any type of tent may be used: an umbrella or a card table covered with a bath blanket or a blanket placed over a baby's crib.

Equipment

Clean newspapers   Several large safety pins
Teakettle or other container

Procedure

- Open six double sheets of newspaper, placing one on top of another.
- Bring one corner of the newspaper to the center fold and crease the diagonal corner fold.
- Place the teakettle or other container on a table or other work surface. Fit the corner fold of the newspaper around the bottom of the kettle under the spout and adjust the paper to form a cone or a funnel.
- Remove the paper funnel from around the kettle. Pin the paper in several places along the length of the cone to hold it in shape. Leave an opening at the top of the funnel to allow steam to escape. (See illustration on page 263.)

BABY CRIBS

A place must be provided for a baby to sleep and it can be quite elaborate or very simple. In either case the requirements are the same: The sides must be high enough to keep the baby from rolling out, the mattress should be firm and be covered with waterproof material, and adequate length and width should be provided to allow for change of position. A crib made so that both the sides and the springs can be raised and lowered, and large enough to be used until the child can safely sleep in a youth bed, is convenient and economical in the long run. Foam rubber is probably better than any other kind of mattress, although somewhat more expensive than cotton or synthetic foam.

A bassinet may be used, and it can be purchased, borrowed, or improvised. In an emergency a large cardboard carton, an oval clothes basket, or a deep dresser drawer can be used. A crib may be improvised by using chairs.

Equipment

2 straight chairs	1 large sheet or cotton blanket
Strong cord or old nylon stockings	10 large safety pins

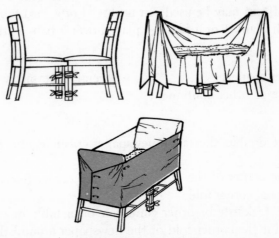

Making an improvised crib.

Procedure

- Place two straight chairs so that the seats face each other and tie the chairs together, using strong cord or discarded nylon stockings.
- Place a large bedsheet or blanket over the chairs lengthwise so that the center of the sheet comes down the center of the backs of the chairs and across the chair seats. Place in a pillowcase a

bassinet mattress, a folded blanket, or other firm pad protected with waterproof material. Put the pad on the sheet over the seats of the chairs. The weight of the mattress or the pad will hold the sheet in place. Pick up the sides of the sheet and bring them up and behind the chair backs, making sides for the bed approximately 15 inches high.

- Pin through the sides of the sheet that form the sides of the bed and also through both layers of the sheet that fall over the center of the chair backs. This will make the bed more secure. Pin the lower parts of the sheet at the back of the chair and tuck the hanging ends up under the sheet to give the crib a neat appearance. Pin the sheet securely at each of the four upper corners for safety.

DOOR SILENCERS

Noise, and especially a recurring, not very loud noise, can be very annoying to a sick person. Also, the home nurse must be able to open and close the sickroom door quietly without disturbing the patient's rest and sleep. The hinges of the door should be lubricated and there should be a silencer on the door latch.

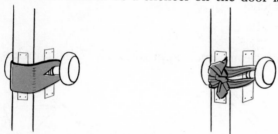

The sickroom door can be closed quietly when a silencer
is placed over the latch.

Equipment

Piece of denim or other strong, fairly heavy fabric, 3 by 24 inches (Method No. 1)
2 discarded nylon stockings (Method No. 2)

Piece of flat rubber from a discarded inner tube, 3 by 10 inches (Method No. 3)

Procedures

Method No. 1:

- Tear a 3-by-24-inch piece of fabric lengthwise from each end toward the center to form 1½-by-10-inch ties and a 2-inch center section.

329

- Place the center section of the strip across the door latch.
- Tie the two ends securely around both doorknobs.

Method No. 2:

- Place 2 stockings together lengthwise.
- Hold the stockings at each end and center them across the door latch. Loop the ends of the stockings around the knob on each side of the door.
- Bring the two ends of the hose together and tie them securely over the latch.

Method No. 3:

- Cut a lengthwise slit near one end of a 3-by-10-inch piece of rubber and slip the doorknob through the opening.
- Stretch the rubber tightly across the latch to the other knob.
- Determine the proper position for a corresponding slit in the rubber for the doorknob and cut an opening.
- Put the rubber strip in place over each doorknob.

PAPER DRINKING CUPS

Knowing how to improvise a paper drinking cup may be valuable in an emergency.

Equipment

Square of clean paper, approximately 7 by 7 inches.

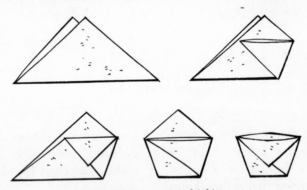

Steps in folding a paper drinking cup.

Procedure

- Fold the square of paper in half diagonally.
- Place the paper with the folded edge parallel to the edge of the table.
- Fold the lower right-hand corner up toward the left until the point touches the left-hand edge of the paper, and make a crease.

- Fold back the top half of the upper corner to lock the side and crease the edge to hold in shape.
- Turn the paper over. Fold the lower right-hand corner up to the left until the point touches the left-hand edge of the paper, and make a crease.
- Fold the flaps on each side toward the bottom to lock the side and crease the edge to hold in place.
- Pick up and press the sides to open the cup.

ACCESSORY BAGS

A convenient item for the patient in bed is a cloth bag attached to the side of the bed in which he can keep small articles, such as a comb and a brush, a mirror, an eyeglass case, a nail file, or paper and pencil.

Although the bag may be made from any kind of material, durability and washability should be considered. The over-all completed dimensions are approximately 12 by 20 inches. On the outer side of one end there should be a pocket about 6 inches. deep which may be divided in vertical sections. At the other end of the bag there should be a double fold of material into which a piece of cardboard is inserted (about 10 by 12 inches) before the material is placed between the mattress and springs. The cardboard helps to keep the bag extended to its full width.

The illustration below shows how to design and complete this piece of equipment.

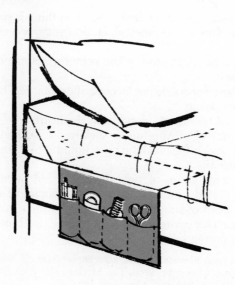

ABRASION. A spot stripped of skin by rubbing or scraping.

ABSCESS. A localized collection of pus in any part of the body.

ADOLESCENCE. The youth period, extending from puberty to maturity.

AIR HUNGER. Shortness of breath caused by insufficient oxygen, usually evidenced by rapid, labored breathing.

AIRWAY. A respiratory passage.

ALLERGIC REACTION. The abnormal reaction to substances such as pollens and certain foods, which ordinarily have no adverse effects on other people.

ANEMIA. A condition of the blood characterized by a reduction in the number of red cells or by a deficiency in the hemoglobin content of the cells or by both.

ANEMIA, NUTRITIONAL. That anemia caused by faulty or inadequate diet or nutrition. Also called *deficiency anemia*.

ANTIBODY. A substance in the blood plasma that reacts in a highly specific way with a foreign substance (called an antigen) introduced into the body.

ANTIDOTE. Any agent administered to prevent or counteract the action of a poison.

ANTITOXIN. A substance found in small amounts in the blood and body fluids and formed to act against a specific toxin; a serum injected into a person to prevent a specific disease, such as diphtheria or tetanus; an antibody that neutralizes a toxin or is antagonistic to a toxin.

ANUS. The termination of the rectum; the outlet of the alimentary canal.

ANXIETY. A state of apprehension and fear, accompanied by restlessness and uncertainty.

APNEA. A temporary period of time when breathing is suspended, such as may occur in asphyxia, deep anesthesia, drowning, or a newborn infant at birth.

APPENDICITIS. Inflammation of the vermiform appendix which may be acute or chronic.

APPETITE. Desire for food, not necessarily prompted by hunger; any natural desire or craving.

ARTERY. A vessel conveying blood from the heart.

ASPIRATION. Act of sucking up or sucking in; inspiration.

ATOMIZER. A device for breaking up a liquid into a fine spray.

AXILLA. The armpit.

BACTERIA. A large group of typically one-celled microscopic organisms widely distributed in air, water, soil, the bodies of living animals and plants, and dead organic matter, some of which cause disease.

BIRTH CANAL. The cavity or canal of the pelvis through which the infant must pass during labor.

---

* Based on material from *Blakiston's Illustrated Pocket Medical Dictionary*, 2nd ed., edited by Hoerr & Osol. Copyright, 1960. The McGraw-Hill Book Company, Inc., by permission of the McGraw-Hill Book Company, Inc.

BLADDER. The hollow organ that serves as a reservoir for the urine.

BLAND DIET. Foods modified in consistency, flavor, and method of preparation to eliminate irritation to the digestive tract.

BLISTER. An elevation of the top layer of the skin, usually circular in shape, containing a clear watery fluid.

BLOOD PRESSURE. The pressure exerted by the blood within the arteries, depending upon the force of the heartbeat, elasticity of the vessel walls, resistance of the capillary bed, and volume and viscosity of the blood.

BLOOD GROUP (TYPE). Inherited patterns into which human blood may be divided for scientific purposes. There are four major blood groups: A, B, AB, and O.

BODY MECHANICS. The coordinated use of the muscles, joints, ligaments, and related structures to produce motion and maintain equilibrium.

BOOSTER DOSE. The injection of a vaccine given at a suitable interval following initial immunization for the purpose of supporting and maintaining immunity.

BRONCHITIS. Inflammation occurring in the mucous membrane of the bronchi.

BRUISE. An injury in which the skin is not broken, but causing discoloration.

BUTTOCKS. One of the two fleshy parts of the body posterior to the hip joints, formed by the masses of the gluteal muscles.

CALORIE. A heat unit; the unit used to measure the amount of energy (heat) produced by food in the body.

CARRIER. A normal person or one convalescing from an infectious disease who shows no signs or symptoms of the disease but who harbors and eliminates the microorganism, and so spreads the disease.

CATHARTIC. A medicine used to produce evacuations of the bowels; a purgative.

CHILL. A sensation of cold accompanied by shivering; frequently the initial symptom of acute infections, as pneumonia; a prominent symptom of various forms of malarial fever. The subjective sensation of chilliness results from constriction of the blood vessels of the skin and is accompanied by a rise of body temperature.

CHRONIC ILLNESS. See Long-term Illness.

CIRCULATORY SYSTEM. The complex of the heart, arteries, veins, and capillaries through which the blood circulates throughout the body.

CLAVICLE. The collarbone.

CLINICAL THERMOMETER. A thermometer used to measure the body temperature.

COLOSTRUM. The first milk from the mother's breasts after the birth of the child. It is laxative, and assists in the expulsion of the meconium (the first fecal discharge of the newborn).

COMMODE. A toilet chair with a removable waste basin for use by the bedside.

COMMUNICABLE DISEASE. Transmissible from one person to another.

333

CONCEPTION. The fertilization of the ovum by the sperm, occurring in humans usually about the twelfth to fifteenth day after the first day of menstrual flow.

CONCUSSION. A condition produced by a fall or blow on the head, and marked by unconsciousness, feeble pulse, cold skin, pallor, at times the involuntary discharge of feces and urine; this condition is followed by partial stupor, vomiting, headache, and eventual recovery.

CONSTIPATION. A condition in which the bowels are evacuated at long intervals or with difficulty.

CONTAMINATION. The presence of an infectious agent on a body surface or on or in an inanimate article or substance.

CONTRACTION (in labor). The shortening and thickening of the muscle fibers of the uterus during labor. Commonly known as labor pains.

CONTRACTURE DEFORMITY. Shortening, as of muscle or scar tissue, producing distortion or deformity.

CONVALESCENCE. The restoration of health after disease. The time spent in recovery.

CONVULSION. An involuntary, usually violent, general contraction or spasm of the muscles.

CRADLE, BED. A support of wood, metal or other material placed over some body part for protection and to relieve the weight of the bedclothes.

CROUP. An inflammation of the respiratory passages seen in children, characterized by a harsh, brassy cough and crowing, difficult breathing.

CYANOSIS. A bluish tinge in the color of mucous membranes and skin, caused by lack of oxygen in the blood.

CYSTITIS. Inflammation of the urinary bladder.

DECUBITUS ULCER. A bedsore; an ulceration caused by pressure against the bed, generally occurring in those confined to bed for long periods.

DEHYDRATE. Remove water as from the body or a tissue.

DELIVERY. The act of giving birth; childbirth.

DENTURE, ARTIFICIAL. Artificial teeth of an individual considered as a unit—complete artificial replacement of either the upper or the lower teeth.

DEPRESSION. An emotional state of dejection, characterized by anxiety, discouragement, and a feeling of inadequacy.

DIAGNOSIS. The art or the act of determining the nature of a disease. The decision reached.

DIARRHEA. A common symptom of gastrointestinal disease; characterized by increased frequency and more or less fluid consistency of the stools.

DIET, LIGHT. Plainly cooked foods that are easy to digest. Fat rich foods, raw and coarse vegetables and fruits, spices, and concentrated sweets are restricted.

DIET, LIQUID. Foods in liquid form, or which have been liquefied to make them smooth in texture and easy to digest.

DIET, REGULAR. The full, well-balanced diet.

DIET, SOFT. Consisting of easily consumed, easily digested foods, modified to leave little residue in the digestive tract.

DISASTER. A situation, usually catastrophic in nature, in which numbers of persons are plunged into helplessness and suffering, and, as a result may be in need of food, clothing, shelter, medical and nursing care, and other basic necessities.

DISORIENTED. Mentally confused. The loss of the ability to locate one's position in the environment.

DROPLET. A minute particle of moisture expelled by talking, sneezing, or coughing, which may carry infectious microorganisms from one individual to another.

DYSPNEA. Difficult or labored breathing.

DYSURIA. Difficult or painful urination.

ECLAMPSIA. A convulsive seizure; a convulsion occurring toward the end of pregnancy, or during or after labor, associated with uremia or other toxic states.

EDEMA. Dropsy; excessive accumulation of fluid in the tissue spaces.

ENEMA. A rectal injection for therapeutic, diagnostic, or nutritive purposes.

EPIDEMIC. Unusual prevalence of a disease, ordinarily affecting large numbers or spreading over a wide area.

EPIDEMIOLOGY. The study of occurrence and distribution of disease.

ERUPTION. Lesions on the skin, especially applied to those of such diseases as measles or scarlet fever; a rash.

EUSTACHIAN TUBE. The auditory tube that leads from each middle ear to the throat.

EXCRETORY SYSTEM. The parts of the body that discharge its waste products; the lungs, the bowels, and the kidneys.

EXPIRATION. Act of breathing forth or expelling air from the lungs.

EXUDATE. The material that has passed through the walls of vessels into adjacent tissues or spaces in inflammation; the purulent or serous fluid that collects in the tissues when inflammation is present.

FALLOUT. The descent to earth of radioactive particles following a nuclear explosion.

FECES. The excretions of the bowels; the excretions from the intestine of unabsorbed food, indigestible matter, and intestinal secretions.

FEVER. Elevation of the body temperature above the normal.

FIRST AID. Emergency treatment given before regular medical care can be obtained in cases of accident, injury, or illness.

FORCEPS. A surgical instrument with two opposing blades, controlled by handles or by direct pressure on the blades. Used to grasp, compress, and hold tissue, a part of the body, needles, or other surgical material.

FOREIGN BODY. A substance occurring in any part of the body where it is not normally found and usually introduced from without; for example, a cinder in the eye.

FORESKIN. A fold of skin that covers the end of the penis; the prepuce.

FRACTURE. The breaking of a bone or of cartilage.

FULL-TERM INFANT. An infant born at the end of the tenth lunar month of pregnancy. Not born prematurely.

GAMMA GLOBULIN. The part (fraction) of human blood plasma that contains disease-fighting antibodies.

GANGRENE. Mortification or death of a part; due to failure of the blood supply, to disease, or to injury. The putrefactive changes in dead tissue. Decay of tissue in a part of the body; caused by failure of the blood supply, to disease or to injury.

GENE. Any hereditary factor; the ultimate unit in the transmission of hereditary characteristics, regarded as an ultramicroscopic particle, capable of self-reproduction and imitation, which occupies a definite place on a chromosome.

GENITALIA, INTERNAL, EXTERNAL. The organs of generation. The male has two testes or seminal glands, with their excretory ducts, the prostate, the penis, and the urethra. The female genitalia include the vulva, the vagina, the ovaries, the uterine tubes, and the uterus.

GROIN. The depression between the abdomen and the thigh; also called inguinal region.

HALLUCINATION. A false sense perception; perception of objects that have no reality and of sensations that have no external cause.

HEMIPLEGIA. Paralysis of one side of the body.

HEMOGLOBIN. The red coloring matter of the red blood corpuscles which carries oxygen from the lungs to the tissues and carbon dioxide from the tissues to the lungs.

HEMORRHAGE. An escape of blood from the vessels; bleeding.

HEREDITY. The inborn capacity of the organism to develop ancestral characteristics; the transmission from parent to child of certain characteristics, such as color of eyes, hair, bony structure, or facial resemblance.

HISTAMINE. A substance released by the tissues in allergic reactions that lowers blood pressure by dilating the blood vessels.

HORMONE. A specific chemical product of an organ, or of certain cells of an organ, transported by the blood or other body fluids and having a specific regulatory effect upon cells remote from its origin.

HOST. The organic body upon or in which parasites live.

HUNGER. A sensation of emptiness of the stomach, with a longing for food.

HYPODERMIC. Placed or introduced beneath the skin. Injection under the skin.

IMMUNITY, ACTIVE. That immunity possessed by an organism as the result of disease or of unrecognized infection or that is induced by immunization with bacteria or products of bacterial growth.

IMMUNITY, ARTIFICIAL. Immunity obtained by vaccination or inoculation with the killed or modified form of the disease-causing agent. *See* Immunity, Active.

IMMUNIZATION. The act or process of rendering immune.

IMPACTION, FECAL. A hard, firm mass of stool lodged in the intestine, usually in or near the rectum; occurs in constipation and bowel obstruction when the feces are not eliminated by normal bowel movement.

INCONTINENCE. Inability to control the excretion of feces or urine; involuntary evacuation.

INFECTION. The communication of disease from one subject to another.

INFLAMMATION. The reaction of the tissues to injury. The essential process, regardless of the causative agent, is characterized clinically by local heat, swelling, redness, and pain.

INGESTION. The act of taking substances, especially food, into the body.

INHALATION. The breathing in of air or other vapor.

INSPIRATION. The drawing in of the breath; inhalation.

INTESTINAL TRACT. The intestinal canal, including the digestive and the excretory passages.

LABIA. The female external genital organs surrounding the vulval entrance.

LABOR. Childbirth.

LACERATION. A tear; a wound.

LARYNGITIS. Inflammation of the larynx.

LARYNX. The organ of the voice, situated between the trachea and the base of the tongue.

LAXATIVE. Mildy cathartic. An agent that loosens the bowels; a mild purgative.

LAYETTE. A full outfit of garments, bedding, etc., for a newborn child.

LONG-TERM ILLNESS. Illness that is long continued or of long duration; opposed to *acute illness.*

LYMPH NODES (GLANDS). A usually small, bean-shaped aggregation of lymph nodules and cords lying in groups along the course of the lymphatic vessels.

MALAISE. A general feeling of illness, sometimes accompanied by restlessness and discomfort.

MENINGITIS. Inflammation of the membranes of the brain or the spinal cord.

MENSTRUATION. A periodic discharge of a sanguineous fluid from the uterus, occurring during the period of a woman's life from puberty to the menopause.

METABOLISM. The sum of the chemical changes that go on in the body as food is made into body tissues, energy is produced, and bony tissue is broken down.

MICROORGANISM. A microscopic organism, either animal or plant, especially bacteria and protozoa.

MICROSCOPE. An apparatus through which minute objects are rendered visible. It consists of a lens, or group of lenses, by which a magnified image of the object is produced.

MORNING SICKNESS. Nausea and vomiting occurring during the early months of pregnancy.

MUCOUS MEMBRANE. A mucus-secreting membrane lining body cavities (such as the mouth and throat) that connect with the external air.

MUCUS. The viscid liquid secreted by mucous glands. It consists of water, mucin, inorganic salts, with epithelial cells, leukocytes, etc., held in suspension.

NARCOTIC. A drug that produces stupor, complete insensibility, or sleep. There are three main groups: the opium group, which produces sleep; the belladonna group, which produces illusions and delirium; and the alcohol group, which produces exhilaration and sleep.

NAUSEA. A feeling of discomfort in the region of the stomach, with aversion to food and tendency to vomit.

NEBULIZER. *See* Atomizer.

NOSTRIL. One of the external orifices of the nose.

NUTRIENT. A nourishing food. Generally classified as proteins, carbohydrates, fats, minerals, and vitamins; nutrients build and repair body tissue, provide heat and energy, and regulate the body processes.

NUTRITION. The sum of the processes concerned in the growth, maintenance, and repair of the living body as a whole, or of its constituent parts as related to the consumption and utilization of food.

NUTRITIONAL GOITER. That occurring commonly in iodine-poor geographic areas from failure to get adequate amounts of iodine from foods; endemic goiter.

NUTRITIONIST. A professionally trained person who applies the science of nutrition and related subjects in research, teaching, or advisory services.

OBSESSION. An idea or an emotion that persists in an individual's mind in spite of any conscious attempts to remove it; an imperative idea, as in psychoneurosis.

OBSTETRICIAN. One who practices obstetrics.

OBSTETRICS. The branch of medicine that cares for women during pregnancy, labor, and the puerperium (following childbirth).

PAIN THRESHOLD. The lower limit of pain capable of producing an impression upon consciousness or of arousing a response.

PALLOR. Paleness, especially of the skin and mucous membranes.

PATENT MEDICINE. A trade-marked medical preparation, packaged for sale to the public and carrying directions for its use. As opposed to prescription drugs.

PEDIATRICIAN. A specialist in children's diseases.

PEDIATRICS. The branch of medicine dealing with children's diseases.

PELVIS. The bony ring formed by the two innominate bones and the sacrum and the coccyx; the cavity bounded by the bony pelvis.

PERISTALSIS. A progressive, wavelike motion of the walls of the alimentary canal consisting of alternate muscular contractions and dilations. By means of this movement the contents are forced toward the opening.

PHARMACOPEIA. A collection of formulas and methods for the preparation of drugs, especially a book of such formulas recognized as a standard, as the United States Pharmacopeia.

PHYSICAL THERAPIST. One trained to administer treatment of disease by physical means, such as light, heat, cold, electricity, regulated exercise, and massage. Such treatment is usually prescribed and supervised by a physician.

PICA. A desire for strange foods; a craving to eat strange articles, as hair, dirt, or sand.

PLACENTA. The organ on the wall of the uterus to which the embryo is attached by means of the umbilical cord and through which it receives its nourishment.

PLASMA. The fluid portion of the blood in which the red cells, the white cells, and the platelets are suspended.

POSTURE. Position or bearing of the body when the individual is standing, at rest, or in movement.

PREGNANCY. Being with child; the state of the woman from conception to childbirth.

PREMATURE INFANT. An infant capable of living delivered before term.

PRENATAL. Existing or occurring before birth; preceding birth.

PRESCRIBED MEDICINE. One ordered by a physician.

PRESSURE SORES. *See* Decubitus Ulcer.

PSYCHIATRIST. A specialist in the treatment of diseases of the mind.

PUBERTY. The period at which the generative organs become capable of exercising the function of reproduction.

PUBES. The hairy region at the lower part of the abdomen.

PUBLIC HEALTH. The state of well being of the community; public health is the science and art of preventing disease, prolonging life, and promoting mental and physical health.

PULSE. The throbbing of blood vessels caused by contractions of the heart muscle as they force blood through the arteries.

PUNCTURE WOUND. Produced by a prick, or a piercing instrument, weapon, or missile.

RABIES. An acute infectious disease of animals caused by a filtrable virus transmitted to other animals and man by the bite of an infected animal.

RADIATION, NUCLEAR. Radiant energy in the form of alpha and beta particles, gamma rays, and neutrons released by nuclear fission and atomic weapons detonations.

RANGE OF MOTION. The physical limits of the movement of the joints.

RASH. A lay term used for nearly any skin eruption but more commonly for acute inflammatory diseases of the skin. *See* Eruption.

RECTUM. *See* Anus.

REHABILITATION. The rendering of a physically or mentally handicapped person fit to engage in a remunerative occupation; restoring to optimum health.

RESISTANCE, ACQUIRED. The resistance to disease developed by frequent exposure to disease germs, or by exposure to small numbers of germs over a long period of time.

RESPIRATION. The act of breathing with the lungs; the taking of air into, and its expulsion from, the lungs.

RIB CAGE. The 12 pairs of long, flat, curved bones forming the semirigid wall of the chest.

ROUGHAGE. Foods rich in cellulose which contain relatively large amounts of residue, such as cereals, unpared fruits, and most vegetables.

SALIVA. The mixed secretions of the parotid, submaxillary, sublingual, and other glands of the mouth whose functions are to moisten and lubricate the food, to dissolve certain substances, to facilitate tasting, to aid in swallowing and to digest starches.

SALMONELLA. A large and complex genus of bacteria capable of causing acute intestinal inflammations.

SCLERA. The firm, fibrous, white outer layer of the eyeball.

SEBACEOUS GLANDS. Glands in the skin that secrete oil (sebum).

SENSORY PERCEPTION. Recognition in response to stimuli from the senses (sight, touch, smell, hearing, and taste).

SHOCK. A general term used to describe disturbed body functions resulting from circulatory failure and most commonly associated with injury.

SORDES. Filth, dirt, especially the crusts that accumulate on the teeth and lips in continued fevers.

SPASM. A sudden muscular contraction.

SPUTUM. Material discharged from the surface of the air passages, throat, or mouth, and removed chiefly by spitting.

STERILE. Aseptic; free from living microorganisms.

STERNUM. The flat, narrow bone in the median line in the front of the chest.

STOOL. *See* Feces.

STRESS. The forces that tend to upset the physiologic or psychologic equilibrium of an individual, thus making it difficult for him to fit his environment.

STRIDOR. A peculiar, harsh, vibrating sound produced during respiration.

STUPOR. The condition of being but partly conscious; lethargy; insensibility.

SUPINE. Lying on the back, face upward.

SUPPURATE. To form pus.

SUSCEPTIBLE. Denoting a person who has neither natural nor acquired immunity to a disease and for that reason is liable to contract it if exposed.

SYMPTOM. One of the evidences of disease that serves as an aid in diagnosis. It may be evident to others (objective) or only to the patient (subjective).

TENSION. *See* Anxiety.

TETANUS. An infectious disease, usually fatal, characterized by tonic spasm of the voluntary muscles, an intense exaggeration of reflex activity, and convulsions.

THERMAL BURNS. Burns caused by heat.

TOXEMIA. A condition in which the blood contains poisonous products, either those produced by the body cells or those due to the growth of microorganisms. It is a general involvement in which the blood contains toxins but not bacteria.

TOXIN. A poisonous product of animal or vegetable cells that, on injection into animals or man, causes the formation of antibodies, called antitoxins.

TOXOID. A product formed by the treatment of toxin with physical or chemical agents. A toxoid is nontoxic but maintains the antigenic properties of the toxin. Toxoids are frequently used for immunization, particularly against diphtheria and tetanus.

TRACE MINERALS. Minerals essential to nutrition and biological function found in minute quantity in living tissue.

TRAUMA. A wound or injury. In psychiatry, an emotional shock leaving a deep psychologic impression.

TRIMESTER. A stage or period of 3 months.

UMBILICAL CORD. The cord that connects the baby to the placenta. It contains veins and arteries through which the fetus is nourished and which carry away waste products.

URINAL. A vessel for receiving urine.

URINALYSIS. Analysis or examination of the urine.

URINATE. To discharge urine from the bladder.

URINE. The fluid excreted by the kidneys.

UTERUS. The womb; the organ that receives and holds the fertilized ovum during the development of the fetus and becomes the principal agent in its expulsion during delivery.

VAGINA. The canal leading from the vulva to the uterus.

VOID. To empty the contents of, for example the bladder or bowels; to evacuate.

VOLATILE. Readily vaporizing; quickly evaporating.

VOMITUS. Vomited matter.

WOUND. An injury to the body in which the tissue is damaged.

WOUND, INCISED. Caused by a cutting instrument.

WOUND, PUNCTURE. One made by a pointed instrument.

VOLUNTARY HEALTH AND WELFARE ORGANIZATIONS

AMERICAN ACADEMY OF GENERAL PRACTICE, Volker Boulevard at Brookside, Kansas City 12, Mo.

AMERICAN CANCER SOCIETY, 521 West 57th St., New York 19, N.Y.

AMERICAN DENTAL ASSOCIATION, 222 East Superior St., Chicago 11, Ill.

AMERICAN DIETETIC ASSOCIATION, 620 N. Michigan Avenue, Chicago 11, Ill.

AMERICAN FOUNDATION FOR THE BLIND, 15 West 16th St., New York 11, N.Y.

AMERICAN GERIATRICS SOCIETY, 2907 Post Road, Warwick, R.I.

AMERICAN HEART ASSOCIATION, 44 East 23rd St., New York 10, N.Y.

AMERICAN MEDICAL ASSOCIATION, 355 North Dearborn St., Chicago 10, Ill.

AMERICAN NATIONAL RED CROSS, 17th and D Sts., N.W., Washington 6, D.C.

AMERICAN NURSES ASSOCIATION, 10 Columbus Circle, New York 19, N.Y.

AMERICAN NURSING HOME ASSOCIATION, 1346 Connecticut Ave., N.W., Washington, D.C.

AMERICAN PHYSICAL THERAPY ASSOCIATION, 1790 Broadway, New York 19, N.Y.

AMERICAN PODIATRY ASSOCIATION, 3301 16th St., N.W., Washington 10, D.C.

AMERICAN PUBLIC HEALTH ASSOCIATION, 1790 Broadway, New York 19, N.Y.

AMERICAN SOCIAL HYGIENE ASSOCIATION, 1790 Broadway, New York 19, N.Y.

ARTHRITIS AND RHEUMATISM FOUNDATION, 10 Columbus Circle, New York 19, N.Y.

CHILD STUDY ASSOCIATION OF AMERICA, 9 East 89th St., New York 28, N.Y.

COUNCIL OF JEWISH FEDERATIONS AND WELFARE FUNDS, 729 Seventh Avenue, New York 19, N.Y.

EYE-BANK FOR SIGHT RESTORATION, 210 East 74th St., New York 21, N.Y.

FAMILY SERVICE ASSOCIATION OF AMERICA, 215 Park Avenue, South, New York 3, N.Y.

FLORENCE CRITTENTON HOMES ASSOCIATION, 608 S. Dearborn St., Chicago, Ill.

GENERAL SERVICE BOARD OF ALCOHOLICS ANONYMOUS, P.O. Box 459, Grand Central Annex, New York 17, N.Y.

MATERNITY CENTER ASSOCIATION, 48 East 92nd St., New York 28, N.Y.

NATIONAL ASSOCIATION FOR MENTAL HEALTH, 10 Columbus Circle, New York 19, N.Y.

NATIONAL ASSOCIATION FOR PRACTICAL NURSE EDUCATION, 654 Madison Avenue, New York 21, N.Y.

NATIONAL CONFERENCE OF CATHOLIC CHARITIES, 1346 Connecticut Avenue, N.W., Washington, D.C.

NATIONAL FOUNDATION, 301 East 42nd St., New York 17, N.Y.

NATIONAL HEALTH COUNCIL, 1790 Broadway, New York 19, N.Y.

NATIONAL LEAGUE FOR NURSING, 10 Columbus Circle, New York 19, N.Y.

NATIONAL SAFETY COUNCIL, 425 N. Michigan Ave., Chicago 11, Ill.

NATIONAL SOCIETY FOR CRIPPLED CHILDREN AND ADULTS, 11 S. LaSalle St., Chicago 3, Ill.

NATIONAL SOCIETY FOR PREVENTION OF BLINDNESS, 16 E. 40th Street, New York 16, N.Y.

NATIONAL TUBERCULOSIS ASSOCIATION, 1790 Broadway, New York 19, N.Y.

BIBLIOGRAPHY

Books

AMERICAN NATIONAL RED CROSS. *First Aid.* 4th ed. Washington, D.C.: the Red Cross, 1957. 241 pp. 75 cents.

AMERICAN PUBLIC HEALTH ASSOCIATION. *Control of Communicable Diseases in Man.* 9th ed. New York: the Association, 1960. 235 pp. $1.00.

ARMSTRONG, INEZ L., and BROWDER, JANE J. *Nursing Care of Children.* Philadelphia: F.A. Davis Co., 1958. 616 pp. $5.50.

ARTHUR, JULIETTA K. *You and Yours; How to Help Older People.* Philadelphia: J.B. Lippincott Co., 1960. 315 pp. $1.95.

BIRREN, JAMES E., ed. *Handbook of Aging and the Individual.* Chicago: University of Chicago Press, 1959. 939 pp. $12.50.

BOWER, ALBERT G.; PILANT, EDITH B.; and CRAFT, NINA B. *Communicable Diseases, A Textbook for Nurses.* 8th ed. Philadelphia: W.B. Saunders Co., 1958. 704 pp. $7.50.

BROWN, AMY FRANCES. *Medical Nursing.* 3rd ed. Philadelphia: W.B. Saunders Co., 1957. 947 pp. $7.00.

BROWNELL, KATHRYN OSMOND, and CULVER, VIVIAN M. *The Practical Nurse.* 5th ed. Philadelphia: W.B. Saunders Co., 1959. 899 pp. $6.00.

BUCHWALD, EDITH. *Physical Rehabilitation for Daily Living.* New York: McGraw-Hill Book Co., Inc., 1952. 183 pp. $8.00.

COOPER, LENNA F.; BARBER, EDITH M.; MITCHELL, HELEN S.; and RYNBERGEN, HENDERIKA J. *Nutrition in Health and Disease.* 13th ed. Philadelphia: J.B. Lippincott Co., 1958. 734 pp. $6.00.

COWDRY, E.V., ed. *The Care of the Geriatric Patient.* St. Louis: C.V. Mosby Co., 1958. 438 pp. $8.00.

FISHBEIN, MORRIS, ed. *Modern Family Health Guide.* New York: Doubleday & Co., Inc., 1959. 1001 pp. $7.50.

FITZPATRICK, ELISE and EASTMAN, NICHOLSON J., eds. *Obstetrics for Nurses* by Louise Zabriskie. 10th ed. Philadelphia: J.B. Lippincott Co., 1960. 571 pp. $6.00.

FRAIBERG, SELMA H. *The Magic Years.* New York: Charles Scribner's Sons, 1959. 305 pp. $3.95.

FREEMAN, RUTH B., and HOLMES, EDWARD M. *Administration of Public Health Services.* Philadelphia: W.B. Saunders Co., 1960. 507 pp. $6.75.

FEURST, ELINOR V., and WOLFF, LuVERNE. *Fundamentals of Nursing.* 2nd ed. Philadelphia: J.B. Lippincott Co., 1959. 662 pp. $5.50.

GRAFFAM, SHIRLEY. *Care of the Surgical Patient.* New York: McGraw-Hill Book Co., Inc., 1960. 311 pp. $6.00.

GUTTMACHER, ALAN F. *Pregnancy and Birth.* New York: Viking Press, 1957. 335 pp. $4.50.

HARMER, BERTHA, and HENDERSON, VIRGINIA. *Textbook of the Principles and Practice of Nursing.* 5th ed. New York: Macmillan Co., 1955. 1250 pp. $7.75.

HILLEBOE, HERMAN E., and LARIMORE, GRANVILLE W., eds. *Preventive Medicine, Principles of Prevention in the Occurrence and Progression of Disease.* Philadelphia: W.B. Saunders Co., 1959. 731 pp. $12.00.

JEANS, PHILIP C.; WRIGHT, F. HOWELL; and BLAKE, FLORENCE G. *Essentials of Pediatrics.* 6th ed. Philadelphia: J.B. Lippincott Co., 1958. 714 pp. $6.25.

LEVERTON, RUTH M. *Food Becomes You.* Ames, Iowa: Iowa State University Press, 1960. 198 pp. $3.50.

MONTAG, MILDRED L., and SWENSON, RUTH P. STEWART, *Fundamentals in Nursing Care.* 3rd ed. Philadelphia: W.B. Saunders Co., 1959. 581 pp. $5.00.

MORRISSEY, ALICE B. *Rehabilitation Nursing.* New York: G. P. Putnam's Sons, 1951. 299 pp. $6.00.

MUSTARD, HARRY S., and STEBBINS, ERNEST L. *An Introduction to Public Health.* 4th ed. New York: Macmillan Co., 1959. 358 pp. $5.00.

NEWTON, KATHLEEN. *Geriatric Nursing.* 3rd ed. St. Louis: C.V. Mosby Co., 1960. 483 pp. $6.50.

OTTO, JAMES H.; JULIAN, CLOYD J.; and TETHER, J. EDWARD. *Modern Health.* New York: Henry Holt & Co., 1955. 566 pp. $3.96.

PETRY, LUCILLE, ed. *The Encyclopedia of Nursing.* Philadelphia: W.B. Saunders Co., 1952. 1011 pp. $4.75.

PRICE, ALICE L. *The Art, Science and Spirit of Nursing.* 2nd ed. Philadelphia: W.B. Saunders Co., 1959. 864 pp. $5.50.

ROBERTSON, JAMES. *Young Children in Hospital.* London: Tavistock Publications, Ltd., 1958. 104 pp. 9s/6d.

RUSK, HOWARD A., and TAYLOR, EUGENE J. *Living with a Disability.* Garden City, N.Y.: The Blakiston Co., Inc., 1953. 207 pp. $4.00.

RUSK, HOWARD A., et al. *Rehabilitation Medicine.* St. Louis: The C.V. Mosby Co., 1958. 572 pp. $12.00.

SHAFER, KATHLEEN N.; SAWYER, JANET R.; McCLUSKEY, AUDREY M.; and BECK, EDNA E.L. *Medical-Surgical Nursing.* 2nd ed. St. Louis: The C.V. Mosby Co., 1961. 876 pp. $8.75.

SPOCK, BENJAMIN. *Baby and Child Care.* New York: Pocket Books, Inc., 1957. 627 pp. 50 cents.

STUART, HAROLD COE, and PRUGH, D.G., eds. *The Healthy Child.* Cambridge: Harvard University Press, 1960. 507 pp. $10.00.

U.S. DEPARTMENT OF AGRICULTURE. *Food,* 1959 Yearbook of Agriculture. Washington, D.C.: Government Printing Office (1959). 736 pp. $2.25.

ZIFFREN, SIDNEY EDWARD. *Management of the Aged Surgical Patient.* Chicago: The Year Book Medical Publishers, Inc., 1960. 219 pp. $7.50.

Periodicals

American Journal of Nursing
Official magazine of the American Nurses Association. Published by American Journal of Nursing Co., New York, N.Y.
American Journal of Public Health
Official monthly publication of the American Public Health Association, Albany, N.Y.
Children
Published by Children's Bureau, U.S. Department of Health, Education, and Welfare, Government Printing Office, Washington 25, D.C.

Geriatrics
Lancet Publications, Inc., Minneapolis, Minn.
Journal of the American Medical Association
Published by the American Medical Association, Chicago, Ill.
Paul D. White, M.D. "The Role of Exercise in the Aging," 165, No. 1: 70-71, Sept. 7, 1957.
Nursing Homes
Official journal of the American Nursing Home Association. Published by the American Journal of Nursing Co., New York, N.Y.
Nursing Outlook
Official magazine of the National League for Nursing. Published by the American Journal of Nursing Co., New York, N.Y.
Parents' Magazine
Published by Parents' Institute Inc., 52 Vanderbilt Ave., New York 17, N.Y.
Public Health Reports
Published by Public Health Service, U.S. Department of Health, Education, and Welfare, Washington 25, D.C.
Sight Saving Review
Published quarterly by the National Society for the Prevention of Blindness, 16 E. 40th Street, New York 16, N.Y.
Lois A. Federico, R.N. "Eye Care Procedures in the Home" 30:27, Spring 1960.
Today's Health
Published by American Medical Association, Chicago, Ill.

Pamphlets

Children's Bureau, Social Security Administration, U.S. Department of Health, Education, and Welfare, Washington 25, D.C.
A Healthy Personality For Your Child. Pub. No. 337. 1952. 24 pp. 20 cents.
Infant Care. Pub. No. 8. 1955. 106 pp. 15 cents.
Prenatal Care. Pub. No. 4. 1962. 92 pp. 20 cents.
Your Child From One to Six. Pub. No. 30. Rev. 1961. 148 pp. 20 cents.
Your Child From Six to Twelve. Pub. No. 324. 1949. 141 pp. 20 cents.
Your Children's Bureau; Its Current Program. Pub. No. 357. 1956. 48 pp. 20 cents.
When Your Baby Is On the Way. Pub. No. 391. 1961. 28 unnumbered pp. 15 cents.
U.S. Department of Agriculture, Washington, D.C.
Family Food Stockpile for Survival. Home and Garden Bulletin No. 77. 1961. 16 pp. 10 cents.
Food for Fitness, A Daily Guide. Leaflet No. 424. 1958. unnumbered. 5 cents.
Public Health Service, U.S. Department of Health, Education, and Welfare, Washington 25, D.C.
Health Manpower Source Book. Section 9, Physicians, Dentists, Nurses. Pub. No. 263. 1959. 80 pp. 50 cents.

Public Health Service Action in Poliomyelitis Control, 1961; Based on Recommendations of the Surgeon General's Committee on Poliomyelitis Control. 1961. 14 unnumbered pp.

Report of the Committee on the Control of Infectious Diseases. Evanston, Ill.: American Academy of Pediatrics, 1961. 132 pp.

SUGGESTED READING REFERENCES

Books

American National Red Cross. *First Aid.* 4th ed. Washington, D.C.: the Red Cross, 1957. 241 pp. 75 cents.

Arthur, Julietta K. *You and Yours; How to Help Older People.* Philadelphia: J.B. Lippincott Co., 1960. 315 pp. $1.95.

Fraiberg, Selma H. *The Magic Years.* New York: Charles Scribner's Sons, 1959. 305 pp. $3.95.

Spock, Benjamin. *Baby and Child Care.* New York: Pocket Books, Inc., 1957. 627 pp. 50 cents.

U.S. Department of Agriculture. *Food,* Yearbook of Agriculture. Washington, D.C.: U.S. Government Printing Office, 1959. 736 pp. $2.25.

Pamphlets

Children's Bureau, Social Security Administration, U.S. Department of Health, Education, and Welfare, Washington 25, D.C.

A *Healthy Personality for Your Child.* Pub. No. 337. 1952. 24 pp. 20 cents.

Infant Care. Pub. No. 8. 1955. 106 pp. 15 cents.

Prenatal Care. Pub. No. 4. 1962. 92 pp. 20 cents.

Your Child From One to Six. Pub. No. 30. Rev. 1961. 148 pp. 20 cents.

Your Child From Six to Twelve. Pub. No. 324. 1949. 141 pp. 20 cents.

When Your Baby Is On the Way. Pub. No. 391. 1961. 28 pp. unnumbered. 15 cents.

Public Health Service, U.S. Department of Health, Education, and Welfare. *Strike Back at Stroke.* Pub. No. 596. Washington 25, D.C.: U.S. Government Printing Office, 1958. 37 pp. 40 cents.

U.S. Department of Agriculture, Washington 25, D.C.

Food for Fitness, A Daily Food Guide. Leaflet No. 424. 1958. unnumbered. 5 cents.

Family Food Stockpile for Survival. Home and Garden Bulletin No. 77. 1961. 16 pp. 10 cents.

Periodicals

Parents' Magazine. Published monthly by Parents' Institute, Inc., 52 Vanderbilt Ave., New York 17, N.Y. Subscription price $3.50.

Today's Health. Published monthly by the American Medical Association, 535 Dearborn St., Chicago 10, Ill. Subscription price $3.00.

347

INDEX

Abdominal pain
  as symptom of illness, 50, 157
  precautions to observe, 50, 157
Abrasions (*see* Wounds, types of)
Accessory bag, how to make, 331
Accidents
  emergency treatment of, 291–7
  general procedure in, 147
  prevention of, 103, 145, 170, 246
  stress as a cause of, 124
  what to do in, 147
Aged persons
  change, adjustment to, 2, 116
  chronic illnesses of, 116, 129–43
  disease resistance, lack of, 55
  heat stroke, susceptibility to, 154
  later years, 115–28
  mental health problems of, 116
  pain, sensitivity to, 49
  personality changes of, 116–17
  physical changes to expect, 117–20
  protection of, 223, 259
  sleep requirements of, 46
Aging
  biological, 117
  changes
    personality, 126
    physical, 115, 117, 125
  chronological, 117, 123
  factors, contributing to, 115
  health practices, 121–8
    attitudes mental and emotional,
      influences of, 126–8
    diet, influence of, 121–2
    exercise, influence of, 123–4
    medical supervision, influence
      of, 125–6
    personal safety, influence of,
      124–5
    posture, influence of, 122–3
  illness in, 125–6, 129–32
  long-term illness in, 129–43
  process, 115, 117–20, 211
    chart of, 117–20
  psychological, 117
  social, 117
  stress, relief of, guides for, 128
Aging population, increase in, 1, 16,
  129
Agriculture, U.S. Department of,
  22n, 23, 167n
Aid, mutual (*see* Disaster, preparation for)
Air mattress, 134, 142

Air passage
  breathing, maintenance of, 168,
    171, 294
  foreign body in, 159–60
Alternating pressure mattress (*see*
  Air mattress)
American Academy of Pediatrics, 59
American Cancer Society, 18
American Medical Association, 9
American National Red Cross, 18,
  145, 164–5, 244, 307–8
American Public Health Association,
  18
Anemia, 81
Anesthesia
  care of disaster patients under,
    171–2
  instructions to home nurse, 172
Anger, 128
Animal
  bites, 161–2
  carrier (*see* Communicable
    diseases, carrier, animal)
Antibodies
  body defense against disease, 58
  in gamma globulin, 58
Antitoxin, 58
Anxiety (*see* Stress, emotional)
Appearance
  as a nursing fundamental, 6, 181,
    312
  of food, 27, 37, 45, 122, 233
  of patient's tray, 27
  personal, 6, 216, 222
Appendicitis, 50, 157
Appetite
  abnormal, 45
  definition of, 45
  factors that influence, 27, 40, 122,
    233, 236
  loss of in illness, 37, 45, 47
  recording of for the doctor, 234
  of sick child, 39, 109
  of toddler, variability, 106
Applicators, cotton, how to make,
  326–7
Apprehension, in shock, 148
Arthritis, 129, 138
Artificial respiration, 294–7
  how to give, 294–7
    to adults and older children, 296
    to infants and young children,
      296–7
  point to remember, 297
  purpose of, 294
  when foreign body lodges in air
    passage, 159

349

351

Communicable diseases
(*continued*)
complications, possible, 63, 65, 67, 69, 71, 73, 75
control, 11–12, 15, 18, 54, 60–1, 91
dishes and eating utensils, care of, 235
how long communicable, 63, 65, 67, 69, 71, 73, 75
how spread, 55–6, 62, 64, 66, 68, 70, 72, 74, 168
immunity to (*see* Diseases, immunity to)
incubation period, 62, 64, 66, 68, 70, 72, 74
patients with, care of, 60–1
prevention, 54, 56–7, 60, 62, 64, 66, 68, 70, 72, 74
protection against, 57–60
resistance to (*see* Disease, resistance to)
symptoms of, 57, 63, 65, 67, 69, 71, 73, 75, 144
treatment, advances in, 54
Compresses, 274–6, 279–80
cold, 279–80
equipment, 280
procedure for applying, 280
purposes, 279
snowburn, treatment of, 153
hot, 274–6
croup, treatment for, 158
equipment, 275
precautions in giving, 275
procedure for giving, 275–6
purposes, 274
Concussion, 167, 176–7
Consciousness, loss of (*see* Fainting)
Constipation, 139
corrective foods, 29
Contour sheets (*see* Bedding, sheets)
Contractions of uterus during labor, 86
Contracture deformities, 5, 136–7, 200, 211, 249
Convalescent
adult, 133
child, 112
diet (*see* Diet, convalescent)
homes (*see* Nursing homes)
Convulsions
adults, 154
children, 154
Cookbooks, 26
Cooper, Lenna F., 31*n*
Cord (*see* Umbilical cord)
Coughing and sneezing, transmitting infection by, 54, 56

Coverall apron
how to use, 61, 184–5
worn when handling baby, 304
Crib, baby, how to improvise, 327–9
Crippled children. (*see* Handicapped child)
Critical minerals (*see* Minerals, essential nutrients)
Croup, 157–8
tent for, 264, 266, 325, 327
Crutches
kinds of, 255
measurement of, 255–6
need for, 236
special appliance, 237
Crutch walking, 255–7
gaits, 256–7
points to remember, 257
preparation for, 255
stance, 256
support of the patient, 257
Cuddling (*see* Baby, cuddling of)
Cyanosis, 170–1

Daily record, patient's
sample form, 8
what to record, 6–7
Danger signals
in aging, 125–6
bleeding from body openings, 151
convulsions, 154
during pregnancy, 82, 151, 154
unusual conditions, 216
in urinary disturbance, 51
Decubiti
causes of, 131–2, 141
nursing care of, 141–3
prevention of, 132, 141–3, 201, 216
symptoms of, 141
what to report to the doctor, 142
Deformities, contracture (*see* Contracture deformities)
Delirium of elderly patients, 52
Delivery
care of baby after, 87–9
emergency
of baby, 86–90, 168
essentials to remember, 89–90
length of labor, 86–7
position of baby, 86–7
stages of labor, 86–8
Dental care
during pregnancy, 76, 80
record of, 9
Dentition, poor, 39
Dentures, care of, 221
when the patient can help, 221
when the patient is helpless, 221

357

Improvised equipment (*continued*)
commode chair, 244
door silencers, 329–30
dressings, 293–4
drinking cup, paper, 330–1
foot supports, 315–16
for patient lying flat, 203, 210, 315
for patient sitting up, 205, 316
for patient with special needs, 316
incubator for premature baby, 96
inhaltor, steam, 264–7
funnel for, 327
need for, during disaster, 3, 169
points to consider about, 312
shoulder shawl, 322
urinal, 326
waste container, newspaper, 323–4
wheel chair, 244–5
Incisions (*see* Wounds, types of)
Incontinence
causes of, 140
definition of, 139–40
effect of on patient morale, 141
patient care, 139–41
training program, 140–1, 243
Incubator for premature infant, how to improvise, 96
Industrial pollution, 12
Infant Care, 13, 91, 305
Infants and children, care of, 91–114
baby's first year (*see* Baby, first year of life)
child
handicapped (*see* Handicapped child)
hospitalized (*see* Hospitalized child)
one to three years (*see* Toddler)
sick (*see* Sick child)
newborn baby (*see* Baby, newborn)
premature baby (*see* Baby, premature)
Infection, 54–75
blood stream, 55
prevention of, 2, 109, 182–4, 291, 293
transmission of, 55–7, 60
treatment of, 54
Influenza, 43, 64–5
Inhalations, steam (*see* Steam inhalations)
Inhalator, steam, how to make, 264–7
funnel for, how to make, 327
Inheritance, genetic, 115
Injuries, disaster-caused, 1, 167–8
chart of, 174–7
recommended action, 174–7

Insect
bites and stings, 160
carrier (*see* Communicable diseases, carrier, insect)
Insurance (*see* Illness, cost of)
International health agencies, 18–20
Intravenous fluids
administration of to disaster patients, 170–1
definition of, 170
instructions to home nurse, 171
reaction to, 177
Iodine
deficiency, 25
essential mineral, 25
trace element, 25
Iron
deficiency, 25
essential mineral, 25
foods rich in, 83
Irrigations, throat (*see* Throat, irrigations of)
Itch (*see* Scabies)

Joints
deformities, prevention of, 200, 236
range of motion, normal, 138, 203
strain on, 5, 122, 200
Journal of the American Medical Association, 124n

Knives, safety in using, 320

Labor
definition of, 86
duration of, 86–7
onset, symptoms of, 86
placenta, expulsion of, 88
stages of, 86–8
Lacerations (*see* Wounds, types of)
Lactation, food guide, recommended during, 84
Lamps
heat, 260
mercury arc, 260
Later years, 115–28
Laxative, indications against, 50, 160
Layette, 85–6
League of Red Cross Societies, 19
Light diet (*see* Diet, light)
Linens (*see* Bedding)
Liquid diet (*see* Diet, liquid)
Local health departments, 14–17
Lockjaw (*see* Tetanus)
Long-term illness, 129–43
behavior patterns during, 132, 140
effect of
on aged persons, 132–3
on children, 132

Pillowcase
  how to put on, 229
  how to remove, 226
Pillows (see Bedding, pillows)
Placenta
  care of in emergency delivery, 88
  description of, 88
  expulsion of after birth, 88
Plague, 19, 55
Plastic bags, danger from, 103
Playpen, 99, 103
Pneumonia, 43
Poison control centers, 163
Poisoning
  accidental, 103–4, 162–3, 291
  food, 161
  by mouth, 103–4, 162–3
  protection against, 103
Poliomyelitis
  disease, communicable, 11, 43, 60, 68–9
  vaccine
    Sabin, 60
    Salk, 60, 68
Poliomyelitis Control, Surgeon General's Committee on, 60
Population, shift in, 17
Positioning the patient (see Posture, positioning the patient)
Posture
  body alignment, 200–1, 211, 249, 275, 316
  body mechanics, 5, 122–3, 182, 200–1
    points to remember, 200–1
  definition of, 200
  emotions, effect on, 122
  of home nurse, 5, 122–3, 182, 200, 211, 223
  moving the patient in bed (see Moving the patient in bed)
  of patient, 5, 122–3, 200, 211, 249
    points to remember, 201–3
  positioning the patient, 137, 173, 201–11, 315
  in preventing disability, 122–3, 137, 200–3, 211
  supports for the bed patient, 137, 173, 201, 203–5, 209, 211 312–16
    lying on his back, 203
    lying on his side, 203–4
    sitting up in bed, 205
Pregnancy
  adjustments to in daily living, 76
  attitudes toward, 76
  blood tests made during
    for anemia, 80
    for blood type, 80
    for clotting time, 80

Pregnancy (continued)
  blood tests made during (continued)
    for Rh factor, 80
    for syphilis, 80
  danger signals during, 82
  dental care during, 76, 80
  diet during, 83–5
  differences in, 76
  fears during, 79
  food during, 83–5
  food guide, recommended, 84
  importance of to both parents, 76
  medical care, 77–9
    during, 76–9
    frequency of visits, 77-8
    objectives of, 76
  nutritional status during, 81
  obstetric physical examination, 79–82
  physical activity during, 78
  physiology of, 79
  protein requirement during, 83–4
  public health nursing services, 77
  sleep and rest during, 78
  toxemia of, 81
  trimesters of, 78
  tuberculosis during, 81–2
  weight during, 81
Premature
  baby (see Baby, premature)
  birth
    adequacy of diet as a factor in, 85
    weight restriction as cause of, 83
Prenatal Care, 79
Pressure
  dressings, 149–50
  sores (see Decubiti)
Professional nurse, 3, 169
Progressive patient care, 130
Protective food (see Food, protective)
Protein
  as an essential nutrient, 21–2
  colostrum, concentration in, 83
  destruction of during illness, 37
  foods containing, 24, 37–8, 84
  requirement
    daily, 24
    during pregnancy, 83–4
Psychiatrist, 52
Psychological age (see Aging, psychological)
Public health, 10–20
  administration, principles of, 11
  administrator, 14–15
  definition of, 10
  funds, 10
  grants-in-aid, 12, 14, 19
  health centers, 14

363

SELECTED TELEPHONE NUMBERS

NAME	NUMBER
Private Physician	
Pharmacy	
Dentist	
Rescue Squad	
Poison Control Center	
Hospital	
Health Department	
Other	